Paediatrics and Neonatology

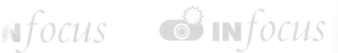 in focus

For Elsevier

Commissioning Editor: *Ellen Green*
Project Development Manager: *Clive Hewat*
Project Controller: *Frances Affleck*
Design Direction: *George Ajayi*

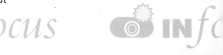

Paediatrics and Neonatology

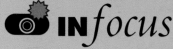 IN *focus*

Roslyn Thomas FRCP FRCPCH

Consultant Paediatrician,
Northwick Park Hospital and Honorary Senior Lecturer,
Imperial College Medical School,
Hammersmith Hospital,
London, UK

David Harvey FRCP FRCPCH

Emeritus Professor of Paediatrics and Neonatal Medicine
Imperial College Medical School,
Hammersmith Hospital,
London, UK

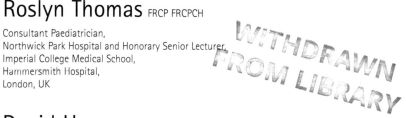

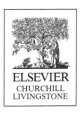

ELSEVIER
CHURCHILL
LIVINGSTONE

EDINBURGH   LONDON   NEW YORK   OXFORD   PHILADELPHIA   ST LOUIS   SYDNEY   TORONTO 2005

ELSEVIER
CHURCHILL
LIVINGSTONE

First published 2005
Some of this material was previously published in
Colour Guide Paediatricsby by R. Thomas and D. Harvey (© 1998 Churchill Livingstone),
Colour Guide Neonatology by R. Thomas and D. Harvey (© 1998 Churchill Livingstone), and
Picture Tests in Neonatology and Paediatrics by R. Thomas, D. Harvey and W. Hyer (© 1998 Churchill Livingstone).

ISBN 0443074364

British Library Cataloguing in Publication Data
A catalogue record for this book is available from the British Library

Library of Congress Cataloging in Publication Data
A catalog record for this book is available from the Library of Congress

Notice
Medical knowledge is constantly changing. Standard safety precautions must be followed, but as new research and clinical experience broaden our knowledge, changes in treatment and drug therapy may become necessary or appropriate. Readers are advised to check the most current product information provided by the manufacturer of each drug to be administered to verify the recommended dose, the method and duration of administration, and contraindications. It is the responsibility of the practitioner, relying on experience and knowledge of the patient, to determine dosages and the best treatment for each individual patient. Neither the Publisher nor the authors assumes any liability for any injury and/or damage to persons or property arising from this publication.

The Publisher

ELSEVIER your source for books, journals and multimedia in the health sciences

www.elsevierhealth.com

The publisher's policy is to use paper manufactured from sustainable forests

Printed in China

Preface

We hope this illustrated introduction to Paediatrics and Neonatology will inspire undergraduate medical students, nurses and midwives to delve further into this exciting specialty. For those already committed to a postgraduate training pathway in paediatrics and child health, the questions will serve as a test of knowledge and preparation for the next hurdle of examinations.

The concise format with a single topic per page is designed to enable the reader to dip into the book while waiting for the next lecture, tutorial, outpatient clinic or bleep summons. The book is not intended to be a comprehensive textbook of the subject. We have focused on conditions which can be displayed in clinical photographs and radiographs, as we believe these provide a useful and stimulating adjunct to learning.

Roslyn Thomas
David Harvey

Contents

Mongolian blue spot

Incidence

Almost universal in non-Caucasian neonates. Particularly obvious in Asian infants and occasionally also occurs in Caucasian infants with dark hair.

Clinical features

Slate grey or bluish pigmentation, usually in the lumbosacral region (Fig. 1), but may occur anywhere on the trunk or limbs (Fig. 2). May be mistaken for bruising by the inexperienced.

Prognosis

Becomes less obvious as the infant grows older.

Erythema toxicum (urticaria of newborn, eosinophil rash)

Incidence

Extremely common, except in preterm infants. Majority of term infants are affected in the first week of life.

Aetiology

Vesicles are full of eosinophils.

Clinical features

Widespread, fluctuating erythematous maculopapular rash (Fig. 3), usually beginning after birth at any time in the first week. Individual lesions consist of a white central papule surrounded by an erythematous flare.

Significance

None, except may occasionally be mistaken for septic spots. Aetiology unknown.

Management

None required, as rash disappears spontaneously.

Milia (milk spots)

Incidence

Very common, seen in 40–50% newborn infants.

Pathology

Milia are hypertrophic sebaceous glands.

Clinical features

Milia are fine white spots seen on the nose and cheeks (Fig. 4).

Management

Disappear spontaneously, but occasionally mistaken for infection. No treatment required.

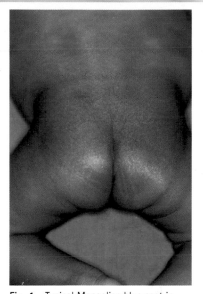

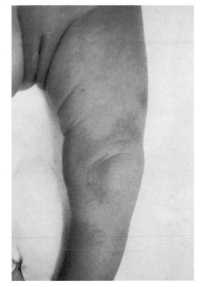

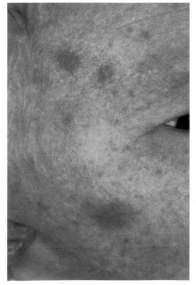

Fig. 1 Typical Mongolian blue spot in lumbosacral region.

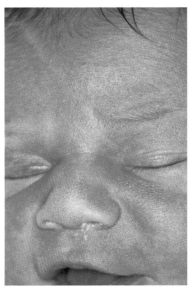

Fig. 2 Mongolian blue spot around the knee.

Fig. 3 Erythema toxicum on the face.

Fig. 4 Milia on nose.

Epithelial pearls

Clinical features

Often occur in clusters as white spots in the mouth (Fig. 5) in midline at junction of hard and soft palate (Epstein's pearls). May also occur on alveolar margin or prepuce.

Pathology

Epithelial pearls are epidermal cysts.

Course and prognosis

They disappear spontaneously. No treatment is required.

Natal teeth

Incidence

Uncommon, but there is often a family history of natal teeth.

Clinical features

Commonly occur in the central lower incisor region (Fig. 6). Usually only loosely attached.

Management

Best removed early in order to prevent aspiration, or ulceration of the tongue. Extraction will not deplete permanent dentition.

Ranula

Clinical features

Mucous retention cyst under the tongue (Fig. 7). Deeper cysts may occur in relation to submandibular or sublingual ducts.

Management

Often disappear spontaneously. Large cysts may occasionally interfere with feeding, and surgery may then be indicated (marsupialization).

Sacral pits and dimples

Clinical features

Common over the sacrum (Fig. 8). Usually blind-ending. Fistulae can usually be excluded by inspection, ultrasound may be helpful. A prominent coccyx can often be palpated in the base.

Associations

Other midline abnormalities (e.g. lipomas, hairy naevi or haemangiomata) may occur higher on the back and may be associated with tethering of cauda equina (diastatomyelia).

Management

None required, providing a fistula has been excluded.

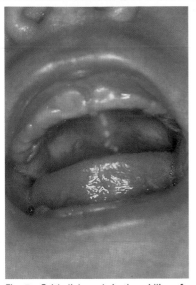

Fig. 5 Epithelial pearls in the midline of the palate.

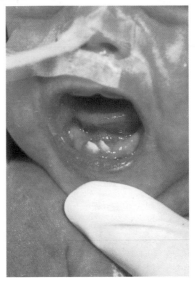

Fig. 6 Natal teeth.

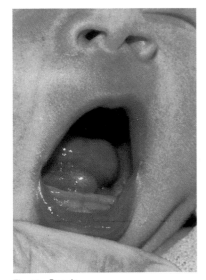

Fig. 7 Ranula.

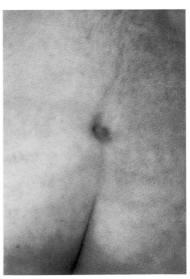

Fig. 8 A dimple over the sacrum.

Hormonal manifestations

Clinical features

Some 30–40% of newborn infants, including male infants, have palpable breast nodules (gynaecomastia) due to placental transfer of maternal oestrogen, progesterone and prolactin. Breast enlargement, often with lactation (witch's milk) is present during the first weeks of life. A tag of mucous membrane is often present in the posterior vulval region of newborn female infants. Discharge of mucus or vaginal bleeding (Fig. 9), occurs in some infants a few days after birth.

Management

No treatment is required. Vulval tags shrivel up within a few weeks. Gradual involution of breast tissue occurs over a few months. Parents can be reassured about the physiological nature of these events and advised not to squeeze the breasts. Antibiotics are only necessary if the breast becomes infected (mastitis), which is rare.

Vernix caseosum

Clinical features

Slimy, ointment-like white substance on skin of some term infants at birth. It is usually found on the face, ears and in folds of neck or groin (Fig. 10), but is occasionally liberally caked all over the body. Vernix is sometimes stained by meconium if there was fetal distress before birth.

Vascular phenomena

Incidence

Very common.

Aetiology

Innocent manifestation of vasomotor instability.

Clinical features

Peripheral cyanosis is very common in the first few days after birth. It occurs in the extremities and around the mouth. There is no central cyanosis. Harlequin colour change is a very rare, but dramatic colour change with vivid midline demarcation of colour (Fig. 11).

Management

None required.

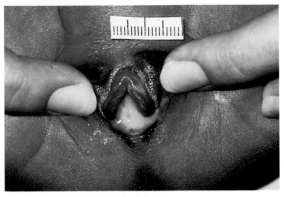

Fig. 9   Normal mucoid vaginal discharge.

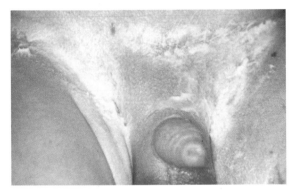

Fig. 10   Vernix caseosum in the groin.

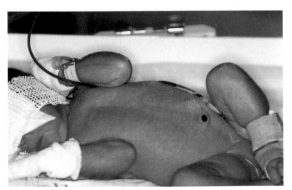

Fig. 11   Harlequin vascular phenomenon.

Umbilical cord

Clinical features

Fleshy translucent cord containing two arteries and one vein (Fig. 12). A single umbilical artery may be associated with other congenital abnormalities. The cord separates within 7–10 days by dry gangrene or with a residual moist base. Frank discharge or cellulitis with a red flare around the umbilicus indicates infection and requires systemic antibiotics. Serosanguineous discharge or a fleshy protuberance from the base may be an umbilical granuloma or rarely a vitello-intestinal remnant or persistent urachus.

Management

Granulomas usually resolve spontaneously or with local application of silver nitrate. Topical antibiotics may actually delay separation. Adherence of umbilical cord beyond 3 weeks may be associated with chronic granulomatous disease.

Sucking pad (sucking callous)

Clinical features

Thickened epithelium of mucous membranes of lips (Fig. 13) in first few weeks of life.

Management

The cause is unknown, but they are not related to pressure or trauma as they occur before suckling and are often present at birth. Sucking pads disappear spontaneously.

Stools

Clinical features

Meconium is sticky, tarry, greenish–black stool (Fig. 14) passed by newborn infants. It is odourless, and contains mucus, epithelial debris and bile from the gastrointestinal tract. Meconium may be passed by the fetus before birth if there is fetal distress. Inhalation of meconium causes pneumonitis with severe respiratory distress. If meconium is present at birth, vigorous suction and resuscitation are indicated before the first spontaneous breath. Failure to pass meconium within 48 h of birth may indicate intestinal obstruction. After feeding, stools gradually change in colour and consistency, becoming softer, greenish in colour and mixed with mucus for a few days. Breast-fed stools are usually soft or semi-formed, but are sometimes liquid and mustard yellow in colour with a faint sweet odour. Frequency varies, but often passed after or during each feed. Formula fed babies usually pass firmer, browner and less frequent stools than breast-fed infants.

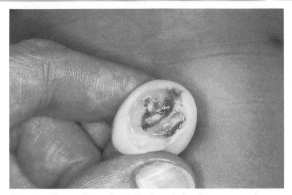

Fig. 12 Cut surface of umbilical cord showing two arteries and one vein.

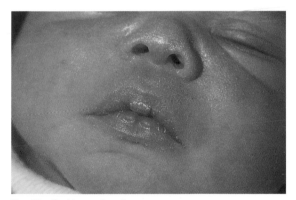

Fig. 13 Sucking pad on lip.

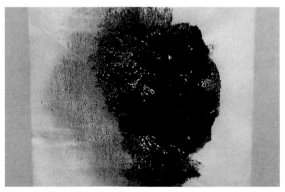

Fig. 14 Meconium.

Jaundice

Incidence

Very common. About 50% of full-term infants and 80% of preterm infants are visibly jaundiced by 3–5 days of age.

Pathology

- Early jaundice occurring within 24–48 h of birth is usually due to abnormal haemolysis, infection, or bruising.
- Physiological jaundice appears after 48 h of age and usually subsides within 7–10 days. It is mainly unconjugated bilirubin due to increased red cell destruction and immaturity of hepatic enzymes.
- Prolonged jaundice lasting beyond 14 days is sometimes seen in normal preterm or breast-fed infants, but other conditions should be excluded, especially hypothyroidism, galactosaemia, liver disease, red cell enzyme defects and biliary atresia.

Clinical features

Yellow staining of the skin (Fig. 15) and conjunctivae. Hepatosplenomegaly indicates the presence of abnormal haemolysis, infection or a metabolic disorder, and is not found in physiological jaundice.

Significance

Very severe unconjugated hyperbilirubinaemia may cause permanent brain damage (kernicterus) with athetoid cerebral palsy and sensorineural deafness.

Management

Observe jaundice clinically and monitor plasma bilirubin level. Investigation may be required if jaundice appears earlier than 48 h, is prolonged beyond 14 days or is unusually high at any stage. Dehydration and drugs such as sulphonamides, which compete with bilirubin for albumin-binding, should be avoided. There is no evidence that extra fluids are needed or hasten the resolution of jaundice in normal infants. Phototherapy (Fig. 16) or exchange transfusion may be required in some infants with high levels of plasma bilirubin. Some jaundiced babies, particularly those with severe rhesus haemolytic disease develop a curious bronze colour under phototherapy (Fig. 17).

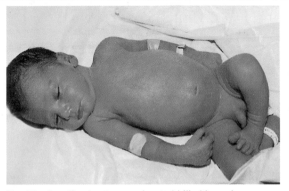

Fig. 15 Jaundice due to unconjugated bilirubinaemia.

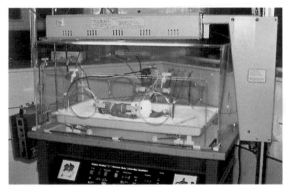

Fig. 16 Phototherapy.

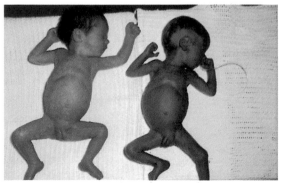

Fig. 17 Bronze baby syndrome with a normal baby.

Neonatal reflexes

There is a large number of primitive neonatal neurological reflexes which disappear spontaneously during early infancy. Presence or absence may be useful in assessment of gestational age and neurological function. Delayed disappearance of certain primitive reflexes may be an early sign of cerebral palsy.

Clinical features

- Moro or startle reflex: the infant is held supine, with trunk and head being supported from below. When the head and shoulders are suddenly allowed to fall back, a startle response with rapid abduction and extension of the upper limbs followed by slower abduction and flexion is elicited. Often accompanied by a cry and may be demonstrated unintentionally when briskly placing an infant in the supine position (Fig. 18). The most common cause of an asymmetric Moro response is a fracture of the humerus or clavicle, or a brachial plexus palsy (Erb's palsy).
- Grasp reflexes: flexion of the digits is a positive response to a finger being placed on the palmar surface of the base of the fingers (Fig. 19) or the plantar surface of the toes.
- Sucking and rooting reflexes: stroking the face near the mouth or cheek causes a sucking and searching response.
- Glabellar tap: a blink of the eyelids is produced in response to tapping the base of the nose.
- Traction reflex: pulling the infant up from the supine position by the wrists results in flexion of the arms and neck.
- Placing reflex: if a foot is brought up under the edge of a surface, the leg is flexed and the baby places the foot on the surface.
- Walking reflex: when the sole of the foot is brought into contact with a surface, there is automatic walking (Fig. 20).
- Galant reflex: if the posterior loin is stroked, the baby swings the buttock towards that side.
- Asymmetric tonic neck reflex: if the head is turned laterally, there is extension of the arm and leg on the same side and flexion of the opposite arm and leg.

Significance

Only very general conclusions can be drawn from examination for primitive reflexes. None of the reflexes is associated with a particular anatomical or pathological lesion. Presence or absence must be considered in association with history, gestational age and other aspects of the neurological examination.

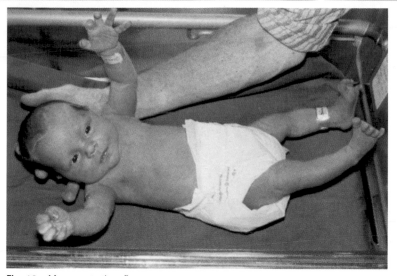

Fig. 18 Moro or startle reflex.

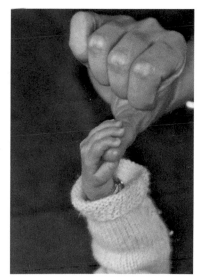

Fig. 19 Grasp reflex.

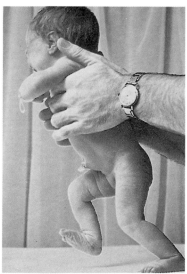

Fig. 20 Automatic walking.

2 Birth trauma

Caput succedaneum

Clinical features

Subcutaneous oedema and bruising of the presenting part (Fig. 21), usually the parietal or occipital region of the head. Swelling is maximal soon after birth, and disappears spontaneously within a few days.

Cephalhaematoma

Clinical features

Soft swelling or lump, often the size and shape of a table tennis ball, with a very discrete edge which never crosses suture lines (Fig. 22) which results from rupture of small vessels in the periosteum. Occurs over the presenting part, usually the parietal bone, is sometimes bilateral and associated with caput. Not apparent at birth, but with ongoing bleeding the maximal size occurs within a few days of birth.

Course and prognosis

Cephalhaematomas disappear spontaneously, sometimes accompanied by calcification, but may take several weeks or months to completely resolve. Jaundice is a common complication.

Obstetric manipulations

Clinical features

Forceps often result in pressure indentation or minor bruising (Fig. 23) and may cause facial palsy or subcutaneous fat necrosis. Both of these complications can also occur after a spontaneous vaginal delivery, particularly after a long labour with slow descent of the presenting part. Subcutaneous fat necrosis can occur over any bony prominence, but is most common on the cheek. It usually appears as an indurated, red area, sometimes followed by calcification. Artificial rupture of membranes, fetal scalp sampling and scalp electrodes may all cause incised wounds. Particular care should be taken when removing scalp clips, as incorrect detachment may result in a core of scalp being removed. Ventouse extraction, by applying suction to the scalp to assist delivery when there is delay in the second stage of labour, frequently causes bruising and a chignon-shaped caput. Sometimes it causes more serious blistering, abrasions or laceration of the presenting part (Fig. 24), and occasionally more serious subaponeurotic haemorrhage.

Prognosis

The lesions are usually trivial, but may become the site of infection. Most resolve spontaneously without significant scarring or more permanent sequelae.

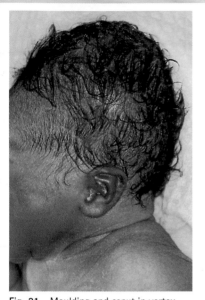

Fig. 21 Moulding and caput in vertex presentation.

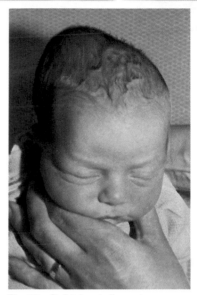

Fig. 22 Parietal cephalhaematoma.

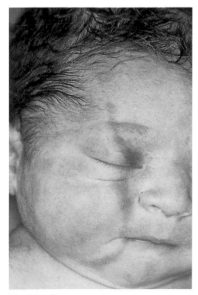

Fig. 23 Forceps mark.

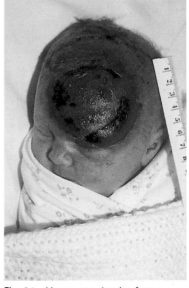

Fig. 24 Very severe abrasion from a prolonged application of ventouse.

3 Deformations

Facial palsy

Aetiology

Facial palsy is due to compression of the facial nerve as it exits from the parotid gland. Often occurs after normal vaginal delivery, but is sometimes caused by pressure from forceps blades.

Clinical features

Weakness, usually unilateral, of facial muscles which may cause drooping of the mouth (Fig. 25) and sometimes dribbling. There is often feeding difficulty and inability to close the eye on the affected side.

Prognosis

Most resolve spontaneously within a few days or weeks after birth.

Erb's palsy

Aetiology

Stretching or tearing of the upper part of the brachial plexus, usually caused by neck traction during breech delivery or with shoulder dystocia. Occasionally may be due to hypoplasia of the brachial plexus, but this is difficult to distinguish in the neonatal period.

Clinical features

The affected arm and hand assume the waiter's tip position (Fig. 26), weakness or paralysis of abduction of shoulder, with flexion at elbow and extension and supination of wrist.

Prognosis

Weakness or paralysis usually responds spontaneously over a period of weeks or months, but paralysis is occasionally permanent. If resolution takes a long time, passive physiotherapy and night splints will prevent contractures. Occasionally surgery may be helpful if paralysis has not resolved by 6–9 months of age.

Postural deformities

Incidence

Postural and compressional effects are common but the majority are mild, transient and do not require treatment.

Clinical features

After a face or brow presentation, the infant may lie with head and neck extended in an opisthotonic posture for several days. After breech delivery, the head is not moulded and legs are often maintained in hip flexion for days (Fig. 27). In many normal infants, feet are often moulded into postural talipes (Fig. 28) which can be fully reduced by passive manipulation, and there is a full range of foot and ankle movement.

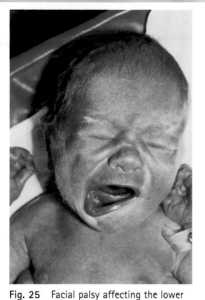

Fig. 25 Facial palsy affecting the lower lip.

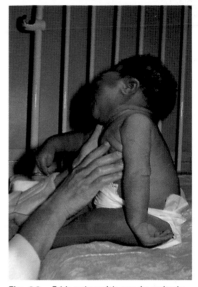

Fig. 26 Erb's palsy with arm in waiter's tip position.

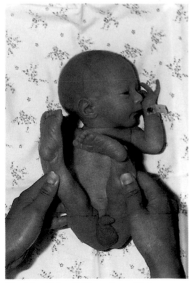

Fig. 27 Extended breech position.

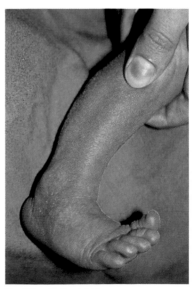

Fig. 28 Postural talipes.

4 Developmental milestones

Gross motor

Birth to 6 weeks

At birth, there is marked head lag when the infant is pulled from the supine position. In ventral suspension with the examiner's hand supporting the chest (Fig. 29), the back is rounded and there is some flexion of the hips and knees. By 6 weeks of age, the infant can lift the head when placed in the prone position and there is some head control when pulled from supine to sitting.

Fine motor and vision

A baby can see at birth, but by 6 weeks can fix his vision on objects and will follow horizontally across to 90 degrees.

Hearing and speech

Response to noise will be indicated by startle or quietening to a soothing voice.

Social behaviour

The infant will stop crying when picked up to be nursed. Infants also begin to smile in response to familiar noises and faces by 5 weeks.

3–6 months

Gross motor

By 6 months, the infant in the prone position kicks well, pushes up from the forearms, lifting the head and chest (Fig. 30), and begins to roll from front to back. They can sit with support or leaning forward into the tripod position. The age of first sitting unsupported ranges from 4–8 months. They begin to weight-bear and to rise to the standing position when supported by the arms or chest.

Fine motor and vision

The infant will reach out for objects with a coarse palmar approach and will clasp and retain small objects placed in the hand. They place objects into the mouth and also begin to release objects.

Hearing and speech

The infant can laugh, gurgle and coo. Around 6 months, they usually begin to babble. They will turn when their name is called.

Social behaviour

The infant holds on to a bottle or feeding cup when fed and frolics when played with. They examine and play with their own hands and feet and place their feet into their mouths (Fig. 31).

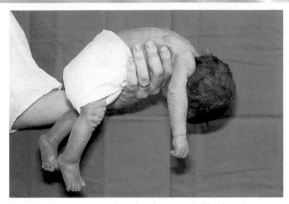

Fig. 29 Ventral suspension showing rounded back.

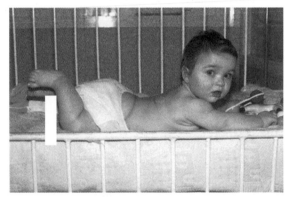

Fig. 30 A press-up at 6 months.

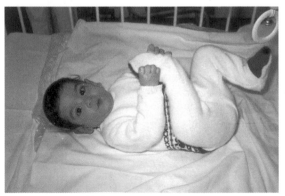

Fig. 31 Playing with feet.

6–9 months

Gross motor

By 6 months, the infant can roll from front to back. They sit unsupported with a straight back. They begin to pivot around on their arms and legs into the crawling position (Fig. 32). They may also begin to crawl on hands and knees.

Fine motor and vision

Small objects are picked up between index finger and thumb in a pincer grasp. Objects are transferred from one hand to the other (Fig. 33).

Hearing and speech

By 9 months they shout to gain attention and vocalize non-specific syllables such as 'dada' and 'mama'.

Social behaviour

The baby turns when being talked to and resists when objects are taken from them. They try to reach objects out of their reach. They like to feed themselves with their fingers.

9–12 months

Gross motor

Most infants are crawling by 9–10 months of age. About 10% of normal infants never crawl, but move around by rolling, paddling or bottom shuffling (Fig. 34). Such children are often late walkers, and other family members may have also exhibited this normal variant of motor development. These children may not walk alone until 2 years of age. Children of 9–12 months begin to pull themselves to standing and to cruise around the room holding on to furniture.

Fine motor and vision

The infant will bang two cubes together. They also look for fallen objects.

Hearing and speech

By 9–12 months, they usually have one or two recognizable single words in addition to 'mama' and 'dada'.

Social behaviour

They enjoy imitative games such as clapping hands and waving goodbye, but are shy with strangers until the end of the first year.

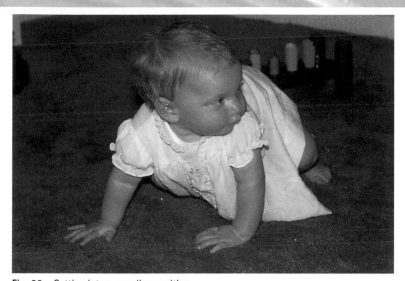

Fig. 32 Getting into a crawling position.

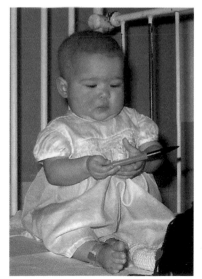

Fig. 33 Transferring objects.

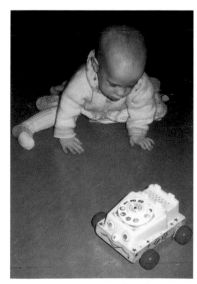

Fig. 34 Normal variant of getting around.

12–18 months

Gross motor

By 12 months, a child can usually walk with hands held (Fig. 35), and begins to stand alone.

Fine motor and vision

The pincer grip becomes more refined and tiny objects can be picked up delicately (Fig. 36). The child also points at objects with the index finger (Fig. 37). They cast objects down repeatedly and can be persuaded to give objects to another person on request. They build a tower with 2–3 bricks.

Hearing and speech

There is a vocabulary of several words and the child usually also repeats their own name. Comprehension is more advanced than speech at this age. They enjoy looking at pictures in a book and often point and babble while doing this.

Social behaviour

By 12 months, children indicate their wants, usually by pointing. They drink from a cup and help to feed themselves. They also begin to help with dressing. The child learns to throw and enjoys simple games such as peek-a-boo (Fig. 38).

18–24 months

Gross motor

Walks confidently and independently. Only 3% have not begun to walk by 18 months of age. The child will be able to climb onto chairs and up stairs, and will also hold onto toys while walking.

Fine motor and vision

Scribbles with a pencil or crayon. Builds a tower of 3–4 bricks.

Speech and language

There will be a vocabulary of at least ten to twelve words and, by 24 months, the child will link several words together in a short 2–3 word sentence.

Social behaviour

The child will spoon and finger feed. They will begin to assert more independence in feeding, dressing and play and will resist the intervention of others who try to assist.

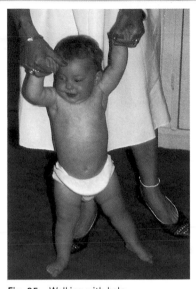

Fig. 35 Walking with help.

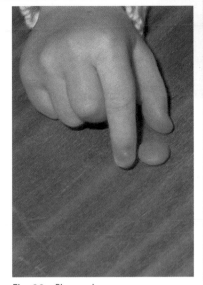

Fig. 36 Pincer grip.

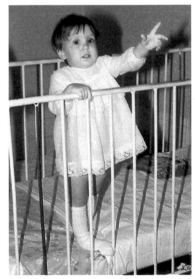

Fig. 37 Pointing.

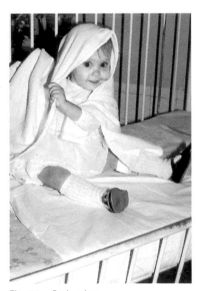

Fig. 38 Peek-a-boo.

Vision

Myelination of the optic pathways is incomplete at term. Early correction of congenital cataracts or severe congenital ptosis is important for normal visual development. At birth, the child will fix on the mother's face, and by 6–8 weeks, follows objects in the direct line of vision. From 9 months, small graded white balls (Stycar test balls) can be used to test visual acuity. After 3 years of age, the child can usually match letters with graded letter cards (Fig. 39).

Hearing

The newborn infant will quieten with soothing noises and within a few weeks of birth reacts to loud noises by startling, or crying. In the UK, routine audiological screening of all newborn infants is now recommended. One commonly used neonatal screening test involves the detection of oto-acoustic emissions (OAEs) from the middle ear. By 7–9 months of age, infants will turn their heads or move their eyes towards a sound stimulus such as a high pitched rattle or bell at ear level (distraction test). Comprehension and imitation of normal speech indicates that severe hearing loss is unlikely.

Speech and language

Most children will be linking 2–3 words into short sentences by 24 months of age, and will have developed full sentences by 3 years of age. By 3 years, the child will talk incessantly and ask many repetitive questions. Referral to a speech and language therapist is indicated if there is not this progression or if the child's speech is not clearly articulated by around 3 years of age.

Drawings

The pictures a child is asked to draw can provide useful clinical information. A child can be asked to 'draw a man' and the parts of the body included in the picture are a good indication of the stage of development. Some pictures may indicate emotional problems that cannot otherwise be communicated to the clinician (Figs 40 and 41). Sometimes the drawing may reveal an undiscovered clinical feature such as hemianopia in a child who only draws on one side of the paper.

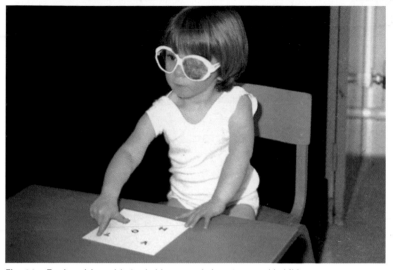

Fig. 39 Testing vision with graded letter cards in a 3-year-old child.

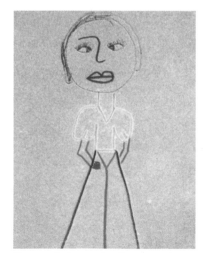

Fig. 40 A picture of a slim woman by a very obese girl.

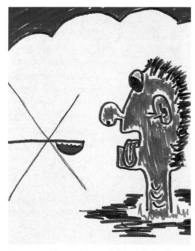

Fig. 41 'A man' by a child with food intolerance.

Breast-feeding has definite advantages (Fig. 42) and should begin in the delivery suite. Formula milk should be discouraged, especially if there is a family history of allergy. The major advantages of breast milk over formula milk are the anti-infective properties, and improved tolerance especially by preterm infants. Breast-feeding is also psychologically important to the maternal–infant relationship. Many preterm infants are unable to suck because of immaturity or respiratory distress, but they can be fed by intermittent gavage feeding through a nasogastric tube. Low birth weight infants require high protein and water intake, and supplements of sodium, iron, vitamins, calcium, phosphate and folic acid are usually necessary. Most children grow similar to their birth centile. Those who are small at birth because of intra-uterine undernutrition are more likely to achieve catch up growth in the early years after birth. Those who are large for gestational age at birth, (e.g. infants of diabetic mothers), are more likely to cross centiles to a lower centile.

Malnutrition

Clinical features

Severe generalized undernutrition (marasmus) (Fig. 43) is usually due to failure to breast-feed and/or inadequate dietary intake. It sometimes occurs in chronic illness. Extreme emaciation and increased susceptibility to gastroenteritis and infection are common. Protein energy malnutrition (kwashiorkor) results from inadequate dietary protein intake and results in oedema, cheilosis, depigmented and scaly skin, and sparse friable reddish hair (Fig. 44). The infant usually has a poor appetite and is listless and irritable. Fatty infiltration of the liver causes hepatomegaly.

Prevention

Community health education should aim to prevent nutritional deficiency states. Breast-feeding should be encouraged, particularly in developing countries where formula milks are often expensive. Cheap nutritious local foods should be introduced into the infant's diet from 4–6 months of age. Early recognition of deficiency states and gradual re-introduction of an adequate local diet. Associated infections may require treatment, and vitamin supplementation is usually necessary.

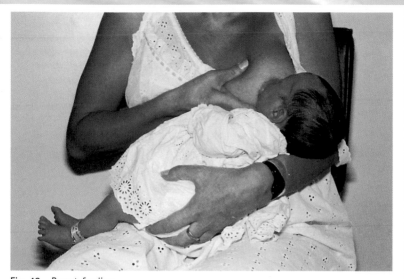

Fig. 42 Breast-feeding.

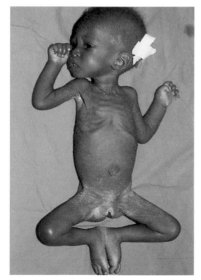

Fig. 43 Marasmus.

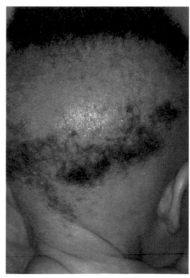

Fig. 44 Sparse friable hair in protein malnutrition (PEM).

Failure to thrive

Aetiology

The most common cause of failure to thrive is inadequate dietary intake. Congenital malformations, chromosomal disorders and specific syndromes can usually be suspected on routine physical examination. The most common causes of malabsorption in childhood are cystic fibrosis and coeliac disease.

Clinical features

Failure to gain weight at normal rate in early childhood. Weight chart will show progressive deviation from birth centile. Buttocks are thin and wasted (Fig. 45). There is loss of subcutaneous fat with poor muscle bulk. If failure to thrive is caused by malabsorption, abdominal distension (Fig. 46) is common and rickets may occur.

Investigation

Dietary intake must be assessed. Anaemia and steatorrhoea suggest malabsorption. Sweat test and jejunal biopsy will confirm cystic fibrosis and coeliac disease respectively.

Rickets

Aetiology

Vitamin D deficiency is usually due to inadequate dietary intake. Rickets is also caused by malabsorption, liver disease, renal failure, renal tubular dysfunction and long-term anticonvulsants.

Clinical features

Swelling of long bone metaphyses, particularly wrist (Fig. 47), bowing of legs, chest deformity, and rachitic rosary. Craniotabes and delayed closure of fontanelle may occur in young infants. The child is often irritable and fretful, and has bone tenderness and muscle weakness.

Diagnosis

Classic biochemical disturbances are hypocalcaemia, hypophosphataemia, vitamin D deficiency, and raised alkaline phosphatase. Radiological signs include splaying of metaphyses of long bones with delayed ossification of epiphyses. Pathological fractures and deformity of weight-bearing long bones may occur.

Management

Vitamin D supplementation and improved dietary intake. High dosage may be necessary in renal rickets or hereditary hypophosphataemic rickets.

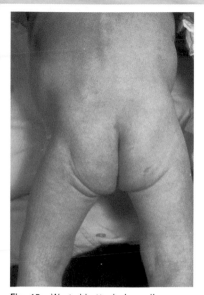

Fig. 45 Wasted buttocks in coeliac disease.

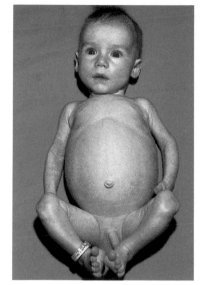

Fig. 46 Failure to thrive with distended abdomen and wasted limbs.

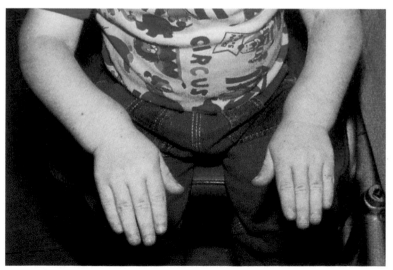

Fig. 47 Swelling of metaphyses at wrists.

Normal growth

Growth is influenced by genetic, nutritional and emotional factors as well as by disease and hormonal deficiencies. Growth in infancy is rapid. There is then slow steady growth in childhood until the adolescent growth spurt, after which final height is reached and epiphyseal fusion takes place. Accurate measurements of height, weight and head circumference should be plotted on centile charts. In most children, growth follows a similar course to centile charts. Height <3rd centile occurs in 3% of normal healthy children. Parental height will help to assess whether short stature is genetic or a disorder of growth. Most preterm infants achieve normal adult size, unless there is severe intrauterine growth restriction. Major postnatal growth in brain and head circumference occurs in the first 3 years of life. Asymmetry of skull (plagiocephaly) and face (Fig. 48) caused by intrauterine posture, or secondary to immaturity (Fig. 49) is common in infancy and improves with age. Premature fusion of skull sutures (craniosynostosis) causing asymmetry is extremely rare.

Short stature

Aetiology

Most short children have short parents. A few have chromosomal abnormalities (e.g. Turner syndrome, hypopituitarism, hypothyroidism, growth hormone deficiency, chondrodysplasia), or iatrogenic causes, including long-term steroid therapy.

Clinical features and investigation

Physical examination usually reveals dysmorphic features in chromosomal abnormalities. In chondrodysplasia, there are usually disproportionately short limbs or trunk (Fig. 50), and abnormal skeletal X-rays. Juvenile hypothyroidism results in progressive growth failure (Fig. 51), severe retardation of bone age, coarse facies and intellectual retardation. In isolated growth hormone deficiency, the child is usually overweight for height. Serial height measurements show reduced growth velocity and pituitary stimulation tests demonstrate lack of growth hormone. Multiple pituitary hormone failure is usually secondary to neoplasia (e.g. craniopharyngioma), radiotherapy or trauma.

Management

Hormonal deficiency requires specific replacement therapy. Catch-up growth and ultimate height depend on age at diagnosis, duration and severity of underlying disorder.

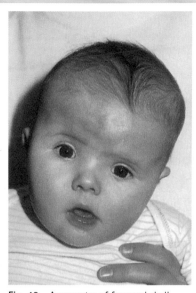

Fig. 48 Asymmetry of face and skull.

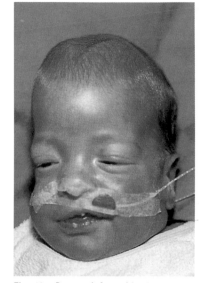

Fig. 49 Preterm infant with narrow, elongated head.

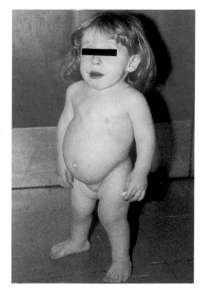

Fig. 50 Short-limbed chondrodysplasia (courtesy of Dr G. Supramanian).

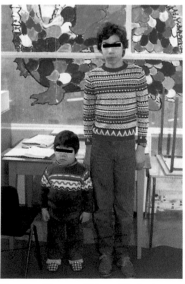

Fig. 51 16-year-old boy with short stature due to hypothyroidism with a normal 16-year-old boy.

Infant of diabetic mother

Incidence

Good control of maternal diabetes throughout pregnancy reduces signs and symptoms in infants of diabetic mothers, but not the increased risk of congenital abnormalities. The frequency of congenital abnormalities (5%) is higher than the general population risk (3%). It is not yet known whether meticulous diabetic control before conception will reduce this high risk.

Clinical features

Large obese infants (Figs 52 and 53) who often develop respiratory distress syndrome due to delayed surfactant production. After birth, there is a risk of hypoglycaemia due to islet cell hyperplasia, and polycythaemia. Infants of diabetic mothers require careful observation in the first few hours after birth, with regular monitoring of blood sugar. Hypoglycaemia usually responds to frequent milk feeds or an intravenous infusion of dextrose.

Course and prognosis

Hypoglycaemia settles within a few days and, provided it has been recognized and treated adequately, will not give rise to sequelae.

Beckwith syndrome

Aetiology

Unknown and usually sporadic occurrence.

Clinical features

Large birth weight infants with glossoptosis (Fig. 54) and omphalocele. Hypoglycaemia due to pancreatic hyperplasia and polycythaemia often occur.

Prognosis

High mortality in the neonatal period.

Obesity

Aetiology

Obesity is a common health problem in Western society, but is rarely due to endocrine disturbance. A genetic component is common.

Clinical features

Weight is greater than expected for height centile, even though the child is often quite tall. Skin fold thickness is excessive.

Management

Established obesity is very difficult to treat, so prevention in early childhood is important.

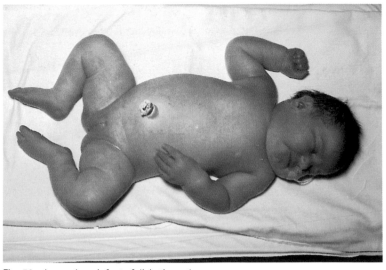

Fig. 52 Large obese infant of diabetic mother.

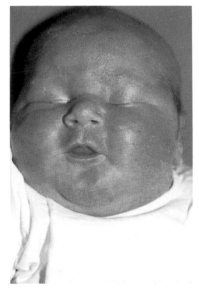

Fig. 53 Cherubic facies of infant of diabetic mother.

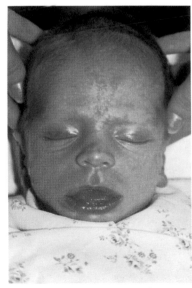

Fig. 54 Beckwith syndrome with glossoptosis.

Hypothyroidism

Incidence

Relatively common, occurs in 1 in 4000 live births.

Aetiology

Congenital hypothyroidism is usually due to thyroid agenesis. Occasionally due to inherited dysgenesis of hormone synthesis.

Clinical features

Coarse facies (Fig. 55), dry skin, hoarse voice and cry, and paucity of spontaneous activity. Hypothermia, hypotonia and poor weight gain are common. Umbilical hernia (Fig. 56), constipation and prolonged jaundice sometimes occur in neonates. Intellectual retardation is the major long-term effect of delayed diagnosis in infancy. Some have cerebellar ataxia, myopia and squints. In juvenile hypothyroidism occurring in later childhood, there is growth failure, but very little intellectual impairment if thyroid function has been normal during the early critical period of brain growth.

Management

Lifelong replacement therapy with L-thyroxine. Dosage is adjusted to achieve normal growth and bone age as well as suppression of thyroid stimulating hormone.

Hyperthyroidism

Incidence

Uncommon. Neonatal thyrotoxicosis may occur in infants of mothers with a history of thyrotoxicosis and thyroid-stimulating immunoglobulins.

Clinical features

Young infants have tachycardia, vomiting, sweating, poor weight gain and irritability. Older children may also have rapid growth, tremor, and proptosis and goitre (Fig. 57).

Management

Antithyroid drugs such as carbimazole until spontaneous remission, usually within a few years. Some require thyroidectomy. Neonatal thyrotoxicosis resolves within a few weeks and sometimes no treatment is needed.

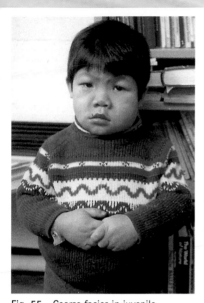

Fig. 55 Coarse facies in juvenile hypothyroidism.

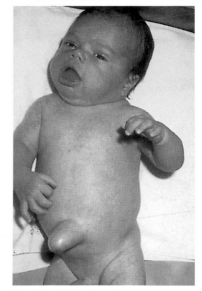

Fig. 56 Umbilical hernia and large tongue.

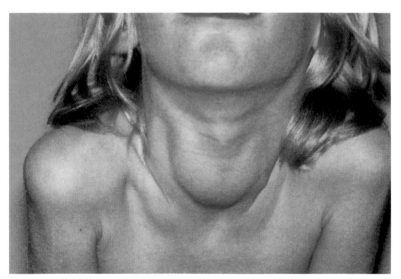

Fig. 57 Goitre in hyperthyroidism.

Congenital adrenal hyperplasia

Aetiology

Autosomal recessive disorder most commonly due to 21-hydroxylase enzyme deficiency resulting in reduced cortisol and aldosterone, and excessive testosterone production. Occurs 1 in 5000 live births. Prenatal diagnosis is possible.

Clinical features

Affected females are virilized (Fig. 58) and may be mistaken for males with severe hypospadias and cryptorchidism. If virilization is not recognized early, infants may collapse with a life-threatening adrenal crisis in the second week of life.

Diagnosis and management

Elevated plasma 17-hydroxyprogesterone level, plasma ACTH and urinary steroid excretion. Salt-losing crises require resuscitation with intravenous saline. Long term replacement hydrocortisone and a salt-retaining steroid fludrocortisone are required.

Precocious puberty

Aetiology

Premature activation of hypothalamo-pituitary-gonadal axis. Early puberty is more common in girls than boys. Isolated breast development (premature thelarche) (Fig. 60) is relatively common. Cerebral tumours, e.g. pineal tumours and exogenous steroid administration also cause early development of secondary sex characteristics (Fig. 59).

Clinical features

Careful physical examination may help to distinguish between physiological but early onset of puberty, and pathological development (<8 years of age in girls and <10 years of age in boys). Discrepancies from the usual sequence of puberty , (e.g. pubic hair but no breast development, are unlikely to be physiological). Abdominal palpation and ultrasound scanning are important in the detection of adrenal or gonadal tumours.

Management

Pathological causes (e.g. hypothyroidism or tumours) require specific treatment. Short stature is the major long-term physical disadvantage of early puberty because of the shorter period of prepubertal growth before epiphyseal fusion. Early puberty is also psychologically upsetting to both child and parents. Drug therapy may be used to suppress gonadotrophin release until the child reaches an appropriate age, but final height will not improve.

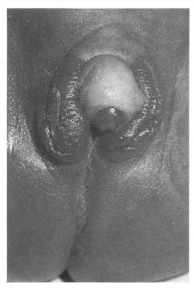

Fig. 58 Enlarged clitoris in congenital adrenal hyperplasia.

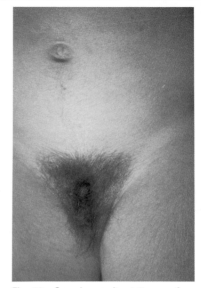

Fig. 59 Sexual precocity at 5 years of age (adrenal tumour).

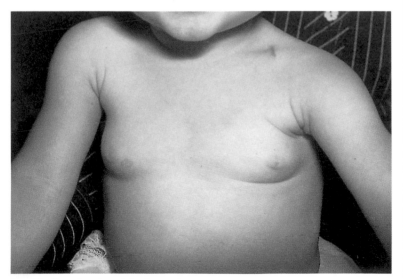

Fig. 60 Premature breast development.

Preterm

Incidence

In the UK, approximately 6–7% of live births are of LBW <2500 g. About two-thirds are preterm <37 weeks' gestation. Infants <1500 g comprise about 1% of births, but nearly 50% of perinatal deaths.

Aetiology

Often unknown. Chorioamnionitis and bacterial vaginosis are associated with preterm labour. Sometimes preterm birth occurs because of maternal complications (e.g. pre-eclampsia, placenta praevia, cervical incompetence, multiple pregnancy, premature rupture of membranes).

Clinical features

Poor muscle tone and tendency to lie in a frog-like position (Fig. 61). Relatively large head and prominent abdomen. Because the skull bones are soft and poorly mineralized, the head of the preterm infant often becomes narrow and elongated, but the shape improves with age. Skin creases are poorly developed, particularly on the soles of the feet (Fig. 62). Lanugo hair is often profuse in babies of 30–36 weeks' gestation, but is less common in very preterm or more mature infants. The pinna is poorly developed with little elastic recoil (Fig. 63). The skin is shiny and transparent with subcutaneous blood vessels readily visible (Fig. 64) and is easily damaged by even minor trauma. Nipples do not appear until 28 weeks' and breast tissue >34 weeks' gestation. The clitoris is relatively large with gaping of the vulva due to prominent labia majora. The scrotum is underdeveloped, and testes may be undescended.

Associations

- Respiratory distress syndrome.
- Periventricular haemorrhage.
- Poor temperature control.
- Increased susceptibility to infection.
- Feeding difficulties and inability to suck.
- Fluid and electrolyte imbalance.

Course and prognosis

Survival is uncommon <24 weeks, but 95% at 30 or >30 weeks' gestation. With optimal care, >90% of preterm infants who survive have no serious neurological handicap. Periventricular leucomalacia, with cysts alongside the ventricles is associated with a high incidence of neurological disability.

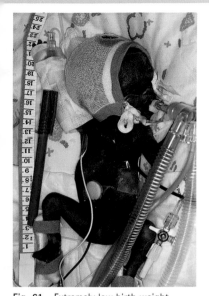

Fig. 61 Extremely low birth weight infant.

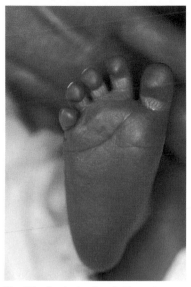

Fig. 62 Poorly developed skin creases on feet.

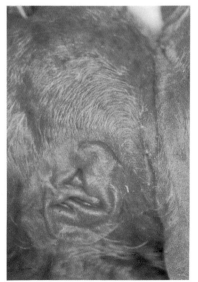

Fig. 63 Profuse lanugo and primitive ear development.

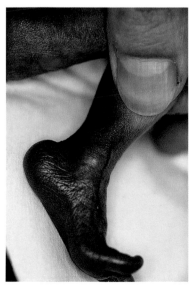

Fig. 64 Thin skin and prominent veins.

Small for gestational age (SGA)

Synonyms

Small for dates; intrauterine growth restriction.

Definition

Birth weight <10th centile for gestational age.

Incidence

Two in 100 live births are SGA and <2500 g.

Aetiology

May be associated with placental insufficiency, maternal pre-eclampsia, hypertension or smoking, and intrauterine viral infection such as rubella , CMV or toxoplasmosis.

Clinical features

The most common SGA infants are usually long and thin, with dry peeling skin (Fig. 65) and long nails. Their physical appearance and behaviour are appropriate for gestational age, not birth weight. Some SGA infants are uniformly small; they are at risk of perinatal asphyxia and often have meconium staining of the skin (Fig. 66), nails and umbilical cord. Unless they are ill or preterm, SGA infants feed very well and require increased caloric intake. Their physiological weight loss is usually insignificant and they gain weight rapidly with adequate postnatal nutrition. They are at risk of hypoglycaemia in the first few days after birth. Hypothermia may also occur. Twins may have a marked difference in prenatal growth (Fig. 67), particularly when there has been chronic feto-fetal transfusion.

Course and prognosis

In the absence of intrauterine infection or neonatal hypoglycaemia, SGA infants are usually of normal intelligence and development. Infants of LBW but appropriate head circumference and length for gestation (asymmetric growth restriction) demonstrate good weight gain providing they receive adequate postnatal nutrition, particularly in the first year of life, and usually achieve normal centiles for all aspects of growth later. If the head circumference, weight and length are all low at birth indicating long-standing intrauterine growth restriction or a genetic influence on growth (symmetric growth restriction), postnatal growth may always remain below the normal centiles. The prognosis for twins with growth discrepancy due to feto-fetal transfusion is much more uncertain and there is a higher risk of poor neurodevelopmental outcome in these infants.

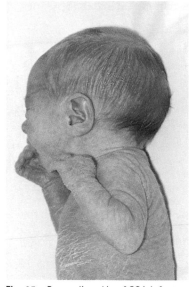

Fig. 65 Dry peeling skin of SGA infant.

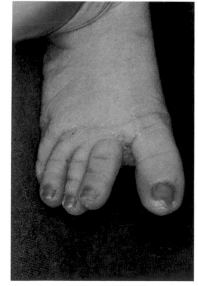

Fig. 66 Meconium staining of skin and nails.

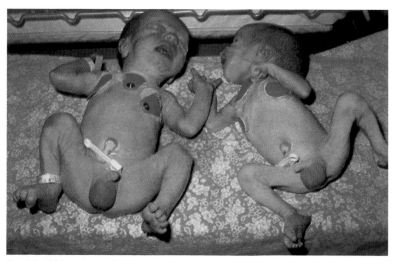

Fig. 67 SGA and normal twins.

Respiratory distress syndrome (hyaline membrane disease, HMD)

Incidence

HMD is the most common respiratory disorder in preterm infants. It is due to surfactant deficiency and structural immaturity of the lungs. It is more common in infants with perinatal asphyxia and infants of diabetic mothers. Gestational age is the main determinant of HMD, but the risk can be reduced by antenatal steroids.

Clinical features

Tachypnoea >60/min, expiratory grunt, cyanosis, intercostal and subcostal recession (Fig. 68) within 4 h of birth. HMD can usually be distinguished from transient tachypnoea due to delayed lung liquid resorption by a characteristic diffuse reticulo-granular pattern due to atelectasis, and an air-bronchogram on chest X-ray (Fig. 69) after 4 h of age. HMD gradually worsens as the infant tires and if uncomplicated, steadily improves from 48 h as natural surfactant is produced. The clinical course is ameliorated by early administration of exogenous surfactant and mechanical ventilation.

Complications

Pneumothoraces develop in approximately 10% of infants with HMD, particularly if ventilation is required. Occasionally, pulmonary interstitial emphysema, pneumomediastinum (Fig. 70), or pneumopericardium occur. About 20–30% extremely LBW infants need prolonged oxygen therapy (chronic lung disease), some even at home after discharge from hospital. Periventricular haemorrhage (PVH), bleeding from the extremely vascular germinal layer of the lateral ventricles is the major cause of morbidity. Germinal layer haemorrhage or intraventricular haemorrhge is common and of no serious significance. Haemorrhage which extends into brain tissue or causes hydrocephalus may be fatal or cause long-term neurological sequelae.

Management

Exogenous surfactant, given into the trachea soon after birth, reduces mortality and severity of HMD. Mechanical ventilation is often required and maintainence of cardiovascular stability is important, particularly in the first few days when PVH may occur.

Prognosis

Survival and long-term prognosis depend on gestation and the occurrence of complications. With improvement in ventilatory techniques in the past decade, PVH is now the main determinant of survival and neurological handicap. With optimal care, <10% of preterm infants suffer major neurodevelopmental disability.

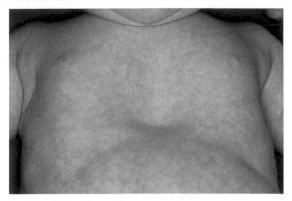

Fig. 68 Subcostal recession.

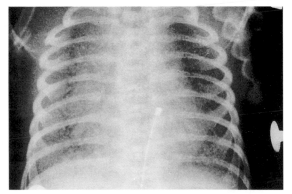

Fig. 69 X-ray appearance of hyaline membrane disease.

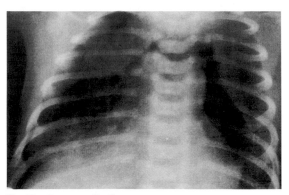

Fig. 70 Pneumonediastinum.

Accessory skin tags and polydactyly

Incidence and inheritance

Common, particularly in Afro-Caribbean infants. Usually autosomal dominant.

Clinical features

Accessory skin tags (accessory auricles) often occur on the face, anterior to the ear (Fig. 71). Accessory nipples are often mistaken for pigmented naevi and may be single or multiple and usually occur in a direct line below the normally situated nipple (Fig. 72). Extra digits (polydactyly) vary from loosely attached skin tags to fully-formed fingers or toes. Occasionally there may be an associated bifid metacarpal or metatarsal bone. Usually only a cosmetic deformity, but extra toes may cause broadening of the forefoot with difficulty in fitting shoes later.

Management

Small pedunculated tags can be ligated if the pedicle and base is very narrow and does not contain cartilage. The tag will become ischaemic, but it is not painful and will usually separate within a few days leaving a small dry scar. If the base is broad, or if the tag has a cartilaginous attachment, plastic surgery will be required.

Amniotic bands, amputations and limb reduction deformities

Aetiology

The most widely accepted hypothesis for amniotic bands is that the developing embryo may lie in a false cavity between the amnion and chorion after traumatic rupture of the amnion in the first trimester. The membranes may then form encircling bands around the limbs. An alternative hypothesis is vascular occlusion secondary to embolization from thrombosed placental vessels. Amniotic bands may be associated with fetal malformations, particularly limb (Fig. 73) or craniofacial defects. An epidemic of limb reduction deformities (Fig. 74) in the early 1960s was due to the effects of a teratogen—thalidomide. Many cases occur without any known cause.

Management

If the deformity is severe and particularly if it will interfere with limb function, early referral to a multi-disciplinary limb-fitting centre will be helpful.

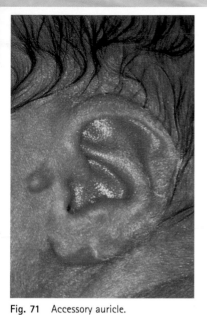

Fig. 71 Accessory auricle.

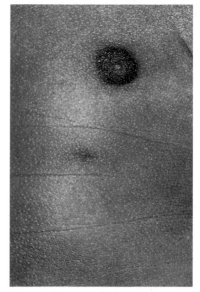

Fig. 72 Accessory nipple.

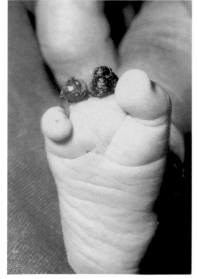

Fig. 73 Gangrene of toes secondary to amniotic bands.

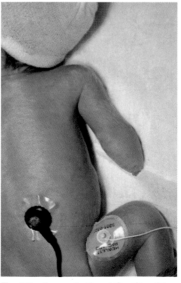

Fig. 74 Arm reduction deformity with vestigial fingers.

Talipes equinovarus (club foot)

Incidence

Occurs in 1 in 1000 live births. The condition is twice as common in males as in females.

Aetiology

Uncertain, probably polygenic inheritance and intrauterine pressure play a part.

Clinical features

The affected foot is held in a fixed flexion (equinus) and inturned (varus) position (Fig. 75). It can be differentiated from positional talipes because the deformity in true talipes cannot be passively corrected. Usually occurs as an isolated deformity but may occur in association with meningomyelocele, oligohydramnios and congenital dislocation of the hip.

Management

Correction of the deformity is usually initially attempted by splinting, but if correction is difficult, surgical release of the contracted structures in the calf and ankle may be necessary.

Foot and toe deformities

Incidence

Common—particularly syndactyly.

Inheritance

Mostly autosomal dominant.

Clinical features

Syndactyly usually occurs as webbing of the second and third toes (Fig. 76). Overlapping of the little toe over the fourth toe is usually bilateral. Hammer toe (Fig. 77) usually occurs in the big toe and results from a congenital contracture of the flexor tendons. In-toeing occurs when the feet tend to curve medially because of adduction of the forefoot (metatarsus varus).

Management

Syndactyly of toes does not require surgery. The position of the toes in hammer toe or overlapping little toe is usually uncomfortable and surgical correction may be needed. Metatarsus varus improves with age and growth of the foot, although surgery is occasionally required.

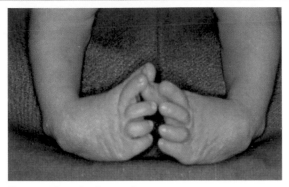

Fig. 75 Bilateral talipes equinovarus.

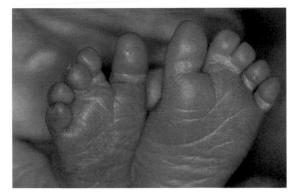

Fig. 76 Syndactyly of second and third toes.

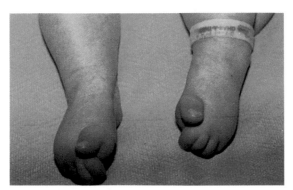

Fig. 77 Bilateral hammer toes.

Developmental dysplasia of the hip

Synonym

Congenital dislocation of the hip.

Incidence

Dislocated or dislocatible hip at birth may be as common as 1 in 100 live births. With early detection and treatment, the prevalence of dislocated hip after the first year of life has been reduced from 1:1000 to 1:10 000. It is more common in girls and after breech presentation.

Inheritance

Familial. There is no simple Mendelian pattern of inheritance.

Clinical features

The majority should be detected by routine screening tests in the neonatal period. Fixed dislocation can be diagnosed by finding restricted abduction of the hip and sometimes shortening of the affected leg. To examine for a reducible dislocation, the infant should be placed on its back on a firm surface. Holding the thighs between finger and thumb with the hips and knees both flexed (Fig. 78), each hip should be slowly abducted through 90 degrees starting from the midline (Figs 79 and 80). A palpable 'clunk' will be felt as a posteriorly dislocated hip slips back into the acetabulum. A gentle attempt should then be made to diagnose a dislocatible hip. With the leg adducted, pressure is applied with the thumb on the upper part of the femur; the leg is then abducted, as above. Ultrasound is useful in diagnosis, but is labour-intensive, has a high false-positive rate and in the UK is therefore used mainly as an adjunct in screening high risk babies or where a clinical abnormality has been detected. The role of ultrasound as a primary screening test is unproven.

Management

Abduction splinting is required for at least 6 weeks. Even a dislocatible hip which resolves spontaneously should be observed until the child is walking. X-ray all hips at 4–6 months of age when neonatal examinations have aroused suspicion. Delay in diagnosis may involve more prolonged splinting or surgery. With early diagnosis and treatment, the majority of infants with developmental dysplasia of the hip should have no delay in crawling or walking.

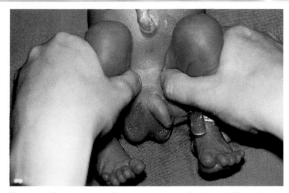

Fig. 78 Examination of the hips starting in the midline with hips and knees flexed.

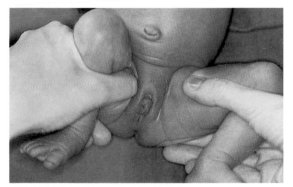

Fig. 79 Abduction of the hip holding the thigh between fingers and thumb.

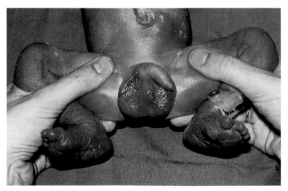

Fig. 80 Full abduction of both hips through 90°.

Cleft lip and palate

Incidence

Common; approximately 1 in 600 live births.

Inheritance

Familial; probably polygenic, there is no simple Mendelian pattern.

Clinical features

Isolated clefts of the palate always occur in the midline. The least obvious type is the submucous cleft which is often associated with a bifid uvula. Cleft lip and palate may be unilateral or bilateral (Fig. 81).

Associations

Feeding difficulties and orthodontic deformities are common. Speech problems may occur with cleft palate, particularly after late closure. Deafness may arise secondary to regurgitation and sepsis in the nasopharynx.

Management

Some infants can breast-feed; most infants feed well through a large teat. Tube or spoon feeding may occasionally be needed. Surgery is performed in several stages. Timing of repair of cleft lip to correct the cosmetic deformity requires consideration of short- and long-term benefits of early closure. Palatal repair is done later, but always within the first year of life when an excellent cosmetic result is usually achieved and speech difficulties of late closure are minimized. If initial deformity is severe, secondary repair of the lip or nose, or pharyngoplasty may be required later (Fig. 82).

Cystic hygroma

Aetiology

Uncommon hamartoma of jugular lymphatic vessels.

Clinical features

Soft, multicystic and ill-defined fluctuant lymphatic swelling in the lateral part of the neck (Fig. 83). Cystic hygromas transilluminate and enlarge slowly during the first few months or years of life. The effect on the child depends on size and site of the abnormality, but can occasionally cause dysphagia or respiratory obstruction, particularly if it enlarges rapidly. Occasionally enlargement may be due to infection or haemorrhage.

Management

Surgical excision is difficult because of the invasive, ill-defined nature of the lymphatic channels, but it is usually necessary.

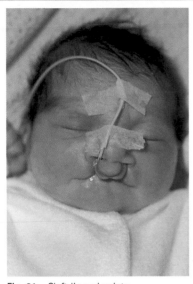

Fig. 81 Cleft lip and palate.

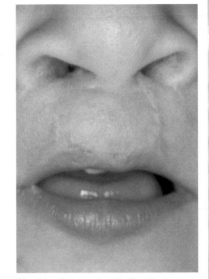

Fig. 82 Same patient in Fig. 81 at 4 years of age, after surgery.

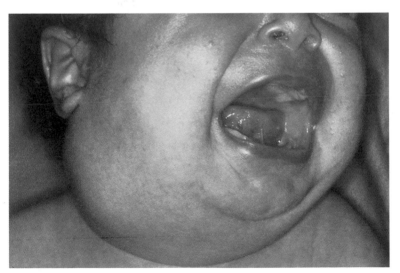

Fig. 83 Cystic hygroma in the neck.

Neural tube defects

Incidence

Prevalence is falling due to antenatal screening and improved maternal nutrition. Spina bifida occulta occurs in approximately 1% of people.

Aetiology

Unknown, but peri-conceptual maternal folic acid supplementation reduces the risk of neural tube defect in high risk families.

Inheritance

Polygenic. After one affected child, 1 in 20 risk of recurrence of neural tube defect in subsequent pregnancies.

Antenatal diagnosis

Elevated alpha fetoprotein concentrations in amniotic fluid and maternal plasma occur in second trimester of pregnancy. Defects are usually apparent on ultrasound examination.

Clinical features

Meningomyelocele and meningocele
Sac containing fluid and/or neural tissue (meningomyelocele), with underlying defect of spinal arch in lumbosacral region in 94% cases (Fig. 84). The degree of handicap depends on the level and severity of the defect. Flaccid paralysis of lower limbs, sensory loss, neurogenic bladder, urinary incontinence, and patulous anus (Fig. 85) with faecal incontinence may occur. Meningoceles often occur in thoracic (Fig. 86) or cervical spine.

Encephalocele
Herniation of meninges and brain through skull.

Anencephaly
Absence of forebrain and skull vault, with distortion of face and ears; incompatible with life although a few may survive for several hours or occasionally days. Other abnormalities are common, particularly cleft palate and abnormal cervical vertebrae.

Associations

Hydrocephaly occurs in 70% of meningomyeloceles. Developmental dysplasia of hip, and talipes equinovarus are common. Urinary tract infections often occur.

Management

Surgery may be indicated in some infants after careful assessment of congenital abnormalities and neurological state of infant in first few days of life. Skin closure initially (Fig. 87), but may require management of hydrocephaly, orthopaedic and urinary problems. Meningoceles in thoracic or cervical regions usually have excellent prognosis and fewer neurological sequelae.

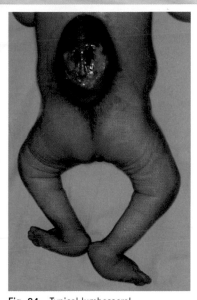

Fig. 84 Typical lumbosacral meningomyelocele.

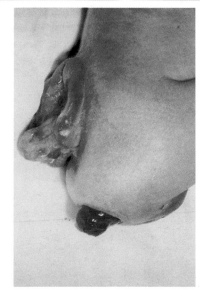

Fig. 85 Meningomyelocele with paralysed anus. There is a rectal prolapse.

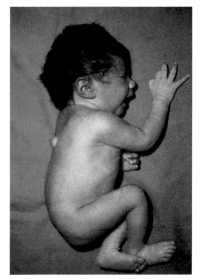

Fig. 86 Thoracic meningocele.

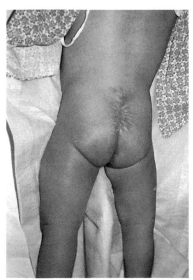

Fig. 87 Repaired meningomyelocele.

Hydrocephaly

Aetiology

May occur as an isolated congenital abnormality. The condition is most commonly due to congenital aqueduct stenosis, or is secondary to peri-ventricular haemorrhage or neonatal meningitis. It is a common association of neural tube defects.

Clinical features

Accelerated rate of growth of the skull gives rise to a disproportinate increase in head circumference (Fig. 88), and widening of the fontanelles and sutures. Increasing ventricular index will be seen on routine cranial ultrasonography in preterm infants with post-haemorrhagic hydrocephaly. Associated symptoms of raised intra-cranial pressure (e.g. lethargy, apnoea, and vomiting) may occur but may be subtle in the early stages. When severe and untreated, hydrocephaly may give rise to a setting-sun appearance of the eyes, upper motor neurone signs particularly in the legs, and neurodevelopmental problems.

Management

Depends on aetiology and severity. Cranial ultrasonography and computed tomography scan will confirm the diagnosis. If there is evidence of continuing deviation from the normal rate of growth of the ventricles or skull circumference, a ventriculoperitoneal (Fig. 89) or ventriculoatrial shunt may be required.

Course and prognosis

Not all infants with hydrocephaly require neurosurgery. Particularly after peri-ventricular haemorrhage, hydrocephaly may be transient and symptoms may be conrolled by serial lumbar punctures until arrest or resolution of ventriculomegaly occurs. When shunt surgery is required, prognosis depends on the underlying aetiology, extent of preceding brain damage and occurrence of shunt complications.

Microcephaly

Clinical features

Head circumference <3rd centile for age and gestation, and which is inappropriately small for the length and weight of the infant (Fig. 90).

Aetiology

Usually unknown; often associated with intellectual retardation. Sometimes a clear prenatal cause is known (e.g. congenital rubella or cytomegalovirus infection).

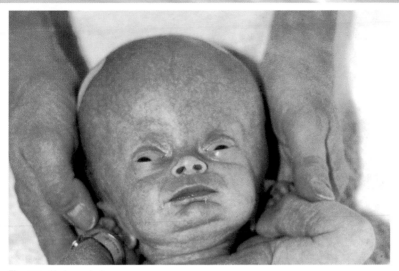

Fig. 88   Hydrocephalus.

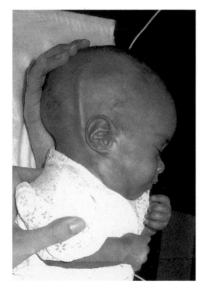

Fig. 89   Ventriculoperitoneal shunt.

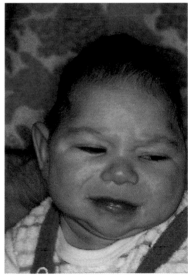

Fig. 90   Microcephaly at 11 months of age.

Syndromes

Down syndrome

Synonyms	Trisomy 21; used to be called mongolism.
Incidence	Occurs in 1 in 600 live births. It is the most common chromosomal abnormality.
Inheritance	Increased incidence of trisomy 21 with older maternal age (1 in 100 live births after maternal age of 40 years and 1 in 50, over 45 years), but most infants with Down syndrome are born to young mothers. General risk of recurrence is 1%, but may be higher if there is translocation.
Aetiology	Trisomy 21 occurs in 94% infants, translocation in 3% and mosaicism in 3%.
Clinical features	Low birth weight and growth restriction are common. Flat moon-shaped facies with upward slanting eyes (Fig. 91), prominent epicanthic folds, generalized hypotonia, brachycephaly with a flattened occiput, a third fontanelle and single transverse palmar creases (simian crease (Fig. 92) are usually present. There may also be incurving of short fifth finger (clinodactyly), a wide gap between second and third toe (sandal gap), marked plantar crease, and Brushfield spots (Fig. 93). Congenital heart disease, most commonly atrio-ventriculo-septal defects, occur in 30% children with Down syndrome and routine echocardiogram should be performed.
Associations	Respiratory infection, acute myeloid leukaemia, hypothyroidism, duodenal atresia, Hirschsprung's disease and alopecia.
Course and prognosis	Short stature and intellectual retardation are always present. Average IQ is <50, although social performance is often beyond that expected for mental age. Many of these children are now educated in normal schools. Males are invariably infertile, but females are not necessarily so. Average life span is 30–40 years.
Antenatal diagnosis	Women at high risk can be identified by a combination of maternal biochemical tests (triple test) antenatally. Amniocentesis or chorionic villus sampling will provide cells for chromosomal analysis or fluorescence *in situ* hybridization.

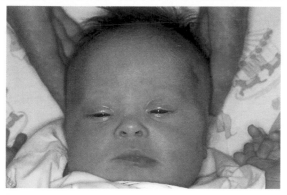

Fig. 91　Typical facies of Down syndrome.

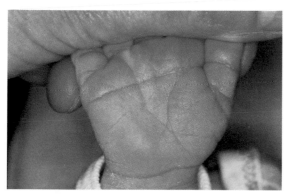

Fig. 92　Single transverse palmar crease (Simian crease).

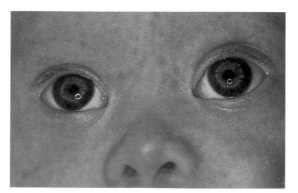

Fig. 93　Prominent epicanthic folds in Down syndrome. Note Brushfield spots on the iris.

Edward syndrome (trisomy 18; E-trisomy)

Incidence

Occurs in 1 in 3000 live births; second most common chromosomal abnormality.

Clinical features

Small for gestational age, microcephaly, severe mental retardation, hypoplastic lungs, congenital heart disease, abnormal posture with flexion deformities of hips and limbs (Fig. 94), clenched hands with overlapping of index finger over third, and fifth finger over fourth finger (Fig. 95), rocker-bottom feet, renal abnormalities, cryptorchidism, craniofacial abnormalities with prominent occiput, micrognathia, hirsutism, short palpebral fissures, microstomia, facial palsy and low-set ears.

Course and prognosis

Most die within first few weeks. Fewer than 10% survive >1 year.

Patau syndrome (trisomy 13; D-trisomy)

Clinical features

Midline defects of face, eyes and forebrain, cleft lip and palate, microcephaly, severe mental retardation, deafness, rocker-bottom feet ,cryptorchidism, congenital heart defects.

Course and prognosis

Fewer than 20% survive the first year of life.

Turner syndrome

Incidence

Appoximately 1 in 5000 live births; usually sporadic occurrence.

Aetiology

Premature ovarian failure. Single X chromosome (XO).

Clinical features

Low birth weight, transient congenital lymphoedema of hands and feet (Fig. 96), webbing of the neck, broad chest with widely-spaced nipples, low hairline and short neck and a wide carrying angle (cubitus valgus). Coarctation of the aorta, deafness and mild mental deficiency occur in about 10%. Short stature and failure of secondary sexual development become apparent in later childhood.

Management

Cyclical oestrogen replacement therapy given from adolescence will induce secondary sexual development. Infertility is invariable. Recombinant growth hormone will improve final height.

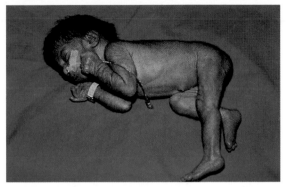

Fig. 94 Edward syndrome with typical flexion deformities of hips and limbs.

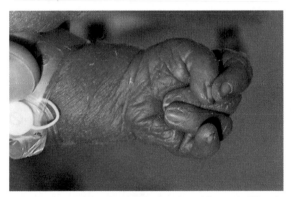

Fig. 95 Clenched hands with overlapping of fingers in Edward syndrome.

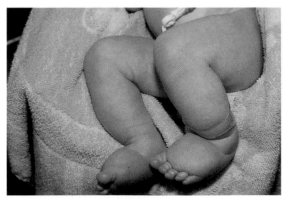

Fig. 96 Congenital lymphoedema of feet.

Short-limbed dwarfism

Incidence

Achondroplasia, the most common chondrodysplasia, occurs in 1 in 10 000 live births.

Inheritance

Autosomal dominant inheritance but approximately 90% occur as a fresh mutation. The lethal forms of chondrodysplasia (asphyxiating thoracic dystrophy or thanatophoric dwarfism) are usually autosomal recessive (Fig. 97).

Clinical features

Short limbs (Fig. 98), large head (macrocephaly) and prominent forehead with broad nasal bridge.

Course and prognosis

Intelligence is usually normal in achondroplastic dwarfs, but early motor development may be slow.

Osteogenesis imperfecta (brittle bone disease)

Inheritance

The severe congenital broad-boned type of osteogenesis imperfecta is usually autosomal recessive. Other less severe forms may be autosomal dominant.

Aetiology

Abnormality of collagen formation of uncertain cause.

Clinical features

Poorly mineralized skull and long bones with multiple fractures and callus formation. In the severe form, they often have short, deformed limbs at birth due to intrauterine fractures (Fig. 99). Crepitus may be felt in bones with recent fractures. Blue sclerae are sometimes present, but may be difficult to diagnose in the neonatal period.

Prognosis

Wide variability in the natural history of this disorder, with stillbirth or early mortality among severely affected infants. Beyond infancy, the outlook for survival is good, but the child is often handicapped by orthopaedic deformity (Fig. 100) and deafness secondary to otosclerosis.

Management

Careful nursing is mandatory. Orthopaedic treatment of fractures is the only form of treatment that can be offered, but optimal management will limit deformity.

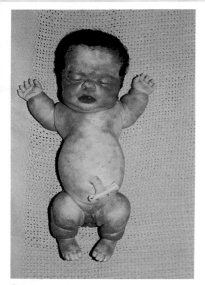

Fig. 97   Asphyxiating thoracic dystrophy.

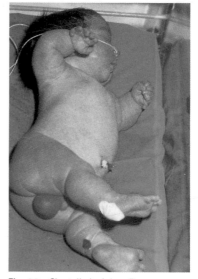

Fig. 98   Short-limbed dwarfism.

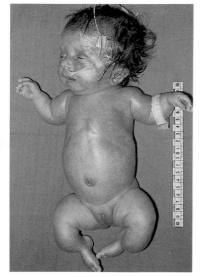

Fig. 99   Osteogenesis imperfecta.

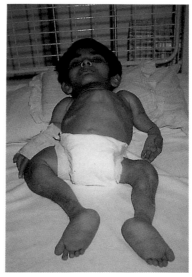

Fig. 100   Osteogenesis imperfecta with bony deformity.

Pierre–Robin syndrome

Incidence Relatively common.

Inheritance Usually sporadic occurrence.

Aetiology Early developmental anomaly with mandibular hypoplasia, posterior location of the tongue and impaired closure of the posterior palate.

Clinical features Severe micrognathia and wide posterior midline cleft palate (Figs 101 and 102).

Complications Acute respiratory obstruction because of a tendency of the tongue to fall back into the cleft palate; feeding difficulties.

Management Expert nursing is required, often with the infant in the face-down posture to prevent respiratory obstruction. Surgical closure of the cleft palate should be performed after 3 months of age.

Course and prognosis High mortality in early infancy due to acute respiratory obstruction. Micrognathia and glossoptosis improve during infancy.

Branchial arch syndrome

Synonym Facio-auriculovertebral syndrome.

Incidence Relatively common. Often associated with ocular or vertebral anomalies or epibulbar dermoids (Goldenhar syndrome).

Clinical features Hypoplastic pinna with absent external auditory meatus (Fig. 103). Usually unilateral. Accessory pre-auricular tags are common. Unilateral hearing loss is common, but speech is usually normal if hearing is normal on the other side. Facial hypoplasia, and branchial cleft remnants in the anterolateral neck are common.

Management Early assessment of hearing is important. Cosmetic surgery is usually desirable, but not always satisfactory.

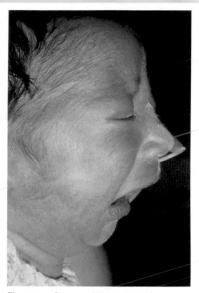

Fig. 101 Severe micrognathia of Pierre–Robin syndrome.

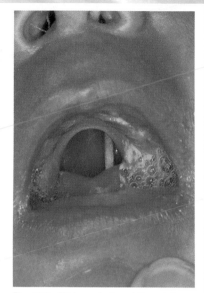

Fig. 102 Wide posterior midline cleft palate.

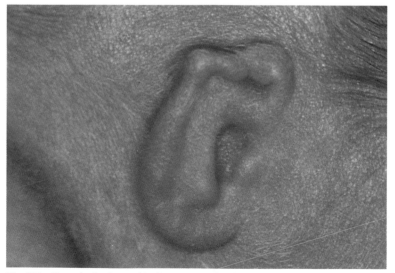

Fig. 103 Hypoplastic pinna with absent external auditory meatus.

Potter syndrome

Synonym	Renal agenesis.
Incidence	Occurs in 1 in 3000 live births. Routine antenatal ultrasonography will show severe oligohydramnios.
Aetiology	The classic syndrome described by Potter was due to renal agenesis of unknown aetiology. Other renal defects (infantile polycystic kidneys or chronic urinary tract obstruction) or chronic leakage of amniotic fluid, may also give rise to oligohydramnios and similar clinical manifestations (e.g. contractures of limbs and hypoplastic lungs).
Inheritance	Sporadic occurrence.
Clinical features	Low birth weight, low set ears (Fig. 104), compression abnormalities with flexion contractures of limbs, hypoplastic lungs, and renal failure.
Course and prognosis	Renal failure and progressive biochemical derangement occur. Death is normally due to respiratory failure soon after birth.

Prune-belly syndrome

Incidence	Uncommon.
Inheritance	Sporadic occurrence.
Clinical features	Deficient abdominal wall musculature giving a rugose, prune-belly appearance (Fig. 105), undescended testis and multiple renal anomalies, usually obstructive uropathopathies (Fig. 106).
Management	Surgical management of renal abnormalities if appropriate. Reconstitution of abdominal wall at a later stage.
Prognosis	Depends on the severity of the renal abnormalities and the effect on renal function. Chronic renal failure is common.

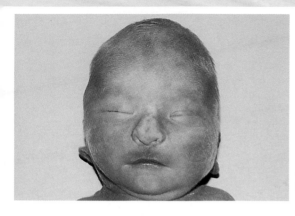

Fig. 104 Potter syndrome (courtesy of Dr G. Gau).

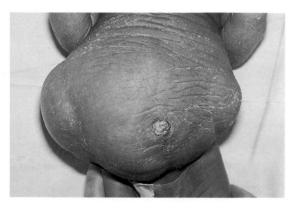

Fig. 105 Prune-belly syndrome with lax abdominal wall musculature.

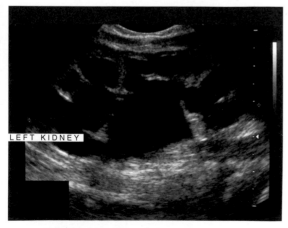

Fig. 106 Gross hydronephrosis in obstructive uropathy.

LEFT KIDNEY

Ectodermal dysplasia

Incidence and inheritance

Rare; X-linked and autosomal dominant inheritance described.

Clinical features

Hypoplastic or absent nails and teeth. Hair is usually fine and sparse. Abnormalities of sweat and sebaceous glands also occur in some varieties.

Nail–patella syndrome

Clinical features

Hypoplastic or absent nails (Fig. 107) and absent patellae. Osteoarthritis of the knees develops in adult life.

Menkes syndrome (Menkes kinky hair syndrome)

Inheritance

Rare, X-linked recessive.

Aetiology

Probably a defect of copper-binding metalloprotein.

Clinical features

Characteristic sparse, twisted kinky hair (Figs 108 and 109) which has partial breakages and twists on microscopic examination. There is profound progressive neurological deterioration and failure to thrive from early infancy. Death is usual within the first few years.

Antenatal diagnosis

Excessive copper uptake in cultured amniotic cells has been demonstrated.

de Lange syndrome

Inheritance

Sporadic condition of unknown aetiology.

Clinical features

Short stature, failure to thrive, and hirsutism are invariable. Bushy eyebrows, long curling eyelashes, micrognathia, small nose with anteverted nostrils, and down-turned mouth give a characteristic facial appearance (Fig. 110).

Course and prognosis

All are severely mentally retarded and death usually occurs in early childhood.

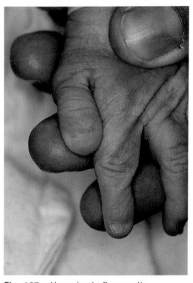

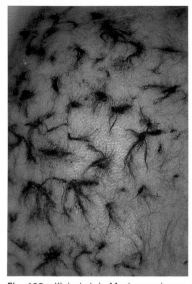

Fig. 107 Hypoplastic fingernails.

Fig. 108 Kinky hair in Menkes syndrome.

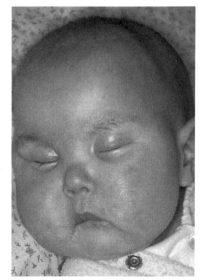

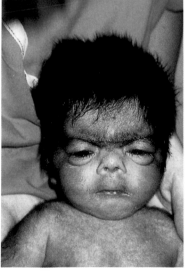

Fig. 109 Facies of Menkes syndrome showing puffy cheeks and kinky eyebrows.

Fig. 110 Characteristic hirsuite facial appearance of de Lange syndrome.

Tuberous sclerosis

Incidence Uncommon, but mild forms may be underdiagnosed.

Inheritance Autosomal dominant, but at least 80% are due to a new mutation.

Clinical features Severity and expression of the syndrome varies enormously, even within families. Usually epilepsy, mental deficiency and some skin manifestations occur. All have granulomatous, lesions (tubers) in the brain which become visible on CT scan by 7–8 years of age. Skin manifestations include the typical adenoma sebaceum (Fig. 111), fibromas, shagreen patch, café-au-lait spots, and depigmented patches (Fig. 112). Visceral hamartomas and retinal lesions are common.

Waardenburg syndrome

Incidence Uncommon.

Inheritance Autosomal dominant.

Clinical features White forelock (Fig. 113) or partial albinism and congenital deafness are usual. Sometimes there is heterochromia of the iris and vitiligo of the skin.

Prognosis Deafness is the most serious feature; usually bilateral and severe sensorineural deafness.

Lesch–Nyhan syndrome

Incidence Rare.

Inheritance X-linked.

Aetiology Enzyme deficiency resulting in excess production of uric acid. Antenatal diagnosis is now available for high-risk families.

Clinical features Mental retardation, athetoid or choreiform movements, dysarthria, muscle weakness, brisk tendon reflexes and extensor plantar responses. Characteristic self-mutilation (Fig. 114) due to uncontrollable aggressive impulses which appear to be unrelated to impaired sensation or hyperuricaemia.

Management Hyperuricaemia can be controlled with allopurinol, but clinical course remains unchanged.

Prognosis Poor. Most die in childhood.

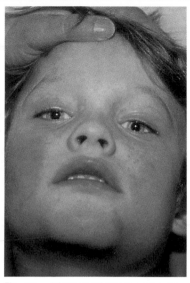

Fig. 111 Adenoma sebaceum on the chin.

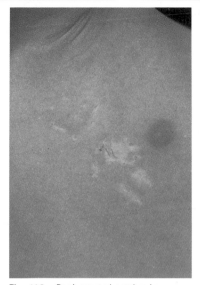

Fig. 112 Depigmented patches in tuberous sclerosis.

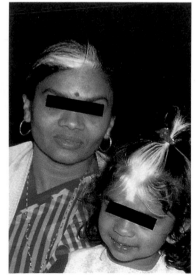

Fig. 113 White forelock of Waardenburg syndrome.

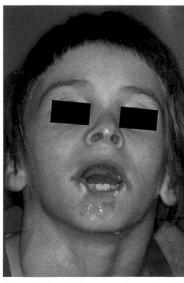

Fig. 114 Lesch-Nyhan syndrome showing effects of self-mutilation.

Mucopolysaccharidoses

Inheritance and incidence

Autosomal recessive; uncommon.

Aetiology

Various specific enzyme deficiencies which result in accumulation of cytoplasmic mucopolysaccharides. Most common types are Hurler (type I) (Fig. 115), Hunter (type II), Morquio (type IV) and Sanfilippo (type VII) syndromes.

Clinical features

The infant appears normal at birth. Coarse facies, growth retardation, mental retardation, skeletal abnormalities and hepatosplenomegaly develop within the first 2 years of life (Fig. 116). Cloudy cornea is found in Hurler syndrome. In Morquio syndrome, there is severe skeletal deformity and growth retardation, but normal intelligence.

Management

There is no cure, but bone marrow transplantation may be a useful form of treatment to halt the progression of the condition, and may cause it to regress.

Russell–Silver syndrome

Inheritance and incidence

Usually sporadic; uncommon.

Clinical features

A syndrome of extreme growth retardation of prenatal onset (Fig. 117), asymmetry of the limbs and shortened incurved fifth finger. There is craniofacial dysostosis with small triangular facies and a small down-turned mouth.

Course and prognosis

Gradual improvement in growth rate may occur in later childhood, but final adult height remains small.

Cockayne syndrome

Inheritance and incidence

Rare autosomal recessive; antenatal diagnosis possible.

Clinical features

Short stature with loss of subcutaneous fat from infancy. Dorsal kyphosis (Fig. 118), limitation of joint movement, grey sparse hair and mental retardation are present. Retinal pigmentation and photosensitive skin are common.

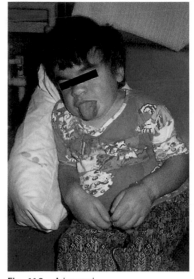

Fig. 115   Hurler syndrome.

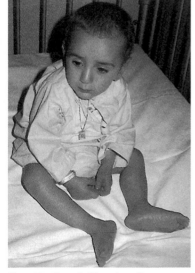

Fig. 116   Advanced
mucopolysaccharidosis.

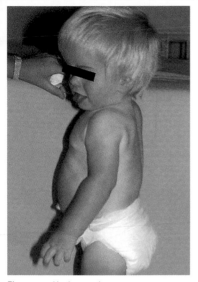

Fig. 117   Russell–Silver dwarfism.

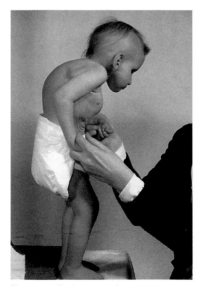

Fig. 118   Cockayne syndrome.

Crouzon syndrome

Incidence

Uncommon.

Inheritance

Autosomal dominant with variable expression.

Clinical features

Cranial facial dysostosis with craniosynostosis of coronal, lambdoid and sagittal sutures. Ocular proptosis because of shallow orbits and hypertelorism give a characteristic facial appearance (Fig. 119).

Management

Surgery to allow normal brain growth when craniosynostosis is severe, or for cosmetic reasons.

Prognosis

Good if surgery is performed early.

Progeria

Incidence and inheritance

Extremely rare syndrome of unknown aetiology. Most cases are sporadic.

Clinical features

Premature and rapid ageing (Fig. 120) with onset in infancy. Severe growth retardation, loss of subcutaneous fat and generalized atherosclerosis. Alopecia, hypoplastic nails and flexion deformities sometimes occur.

Course and prognosis

There is normal brain development and intelligence. Life expectancy is severely shortened (average 15 years) and death is usually due to myocardial infarction.

Lowe syndrome

Synonym

Oculo-cerebro-renal syndrome

Inheritance and incidence

X-linked; rare.

Clinical features

Mental retardation, hypotonia, joint hypermobility, hyperactivity and growth retardation are common. Cataracts and blindness (Fig. 121) usually occur. Renal tubular dysfunction and cryptorchidism are also found.

Prognosis

Poor.

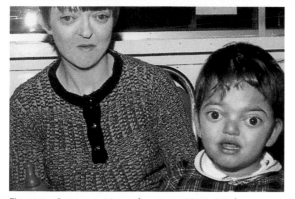

Fig. 119 Crouzon syndrome (courtesy of Dr A. Kilby).

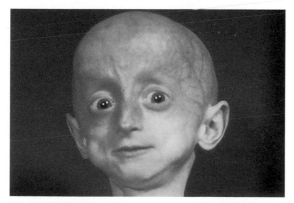

Fig. 120 Progeria.

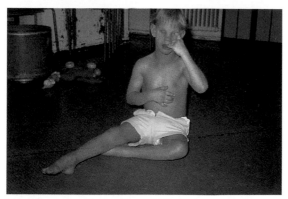

Fig. 121 A mentally handicapped blind child with Lowe syndrome.

Hydrops fetalis

Incidence

Less common since prevention of rhesus haemolytic disease has been possible with antenatal anti-D administration.

Aetiology

• Haemolytic disease, particularly rhesus isoimmunization.
• Alpha-thalassaemia major.
• Intrauterine viral infections, particularly cytomegalovirus.
• Congenital syphilis.
• Supraventricular tachycardia with congestive cardiac failure.
• Congenital nephrotic syndrome.
• Congenital parvovirus infection.
• Placental angioma.

Clinical features

Pallor, gross generalized oedema (Figs 122 and 123), ascites, pleural effusions, congestive heart failure, and severe respiratory distress due to pulmonary oedema or pulmonary hypoplasia.

Management

Depends on the cause of hydrops. If hydrops is secondary to haemolytic disease, exchange transfusions and ventilatory support are the mainstay of treatment. In the presence of cardiac failure secondary to a tachyarrhythmia, treatment is directed towards correcting the arrhythmia with drugs or defibrillation, and supportive treatment of cardiac failure.

Prognosis

Depends on underlying cause; usually good if infant survives neonatal period.

Klippel–Feil syndrome

Inheritance and incidence

Sporadic occurrence of unknown aetiology; occurs in 1 in 40 000 live births; female predominance.

Clinical features

Short immobile neck, secondary webbing of neck, low hairline (Fig. 124) and fusion of cervical vertebrae. Hemivertebrae, rib defects, scoliosis and Sprengel's shoulder sometimes occur.

Associations

Deafness in approximately 30% of cases. May occur as part of a more serious defect of neural tube development.

Prognosis

Variable and dependant on the underlying skeletal abnormality.

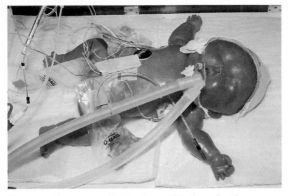

Fig. 122   Gross generalized oedema of hydrops fetalis.

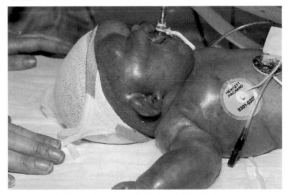

Fig. 123   Pallor and oedema in hydrops fetalis due to rhesus haemolytic disease.

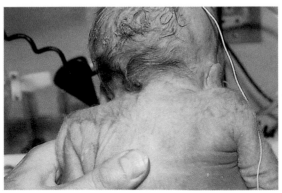

Fig. 124   Short neck and low hairline in Klippel–Feil syndrome.

Strawberry naevi

Incidence

Common, particularly in preterm infants.

Pathology

Dilated capillaries +/– endothelial proliferation.

Clinical features

Raised, soft, pitted, bright red haemangiomata with a discrete edge. Not usually present at birth, but appear within the first few weeks of life. Often preceded by a small and slightly raised, bright red spot, which evolves into a strawberry naevus. May be single or multiple and occur anywhere on the body. Majority increase rapidly in size during the first year of life. Ulceration and subsequent infection may occur in the centre of the lesion. All strawberry naevi regress slowly over a few years. Involution has started when pale grey areas of fibrosis appear in the centre of the naevus (Fig. 125). They eventually disappear completely and leave only a flat, pale depigmented area.

Course and prognosis

No treatment is required, unless there is haemorrhage, infection or severe cosmetic deformity interfering with function of affected part. All forms of treatment except steroids will leave some scarring of skin; natural resolution is the optimal management in majority of strawberry naevi. When there is pressure on a vital organ or severe bleeding, steroids may sometimes be helpful.

Simple naevus (stork bite naevus)

Incidence

Very common; seen in 30–50% of infants.

Pathology

Capillary haemangioma.

Clinical features

Bright pink 'macular' capillary haemangiomata seen on eyelids, bridge of nose (Fig. 126), upper lip and nape of neck (Fig. 127). On the forehead, there is sometimes a V-shaped lesion said in folklore to be the mark of the stork's beak. Simple naevi do not blanch on pressure.

Course and prognosis

All simple naevi on the face disappear spontaneously in the first year. Those on the nape of the neck are usually permanent, but never require treatment.

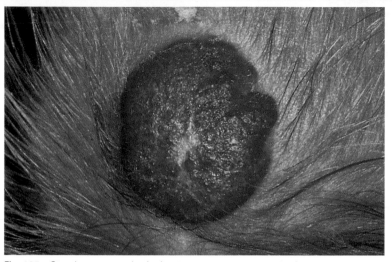

Fig. 125 Strawberry naevus beginning to regress.

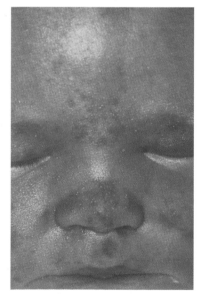

Fig. 126 Simple naevus on eyelids, nose and upper lip.

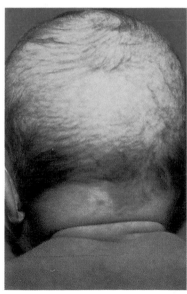

Fig. 127 Simple naevus on nape of the neck.

Cavernous haemangiomata

Clinical features

Soft, subcutaneous bluish-red mass (Fig. 128) with a less distinct edge than a strawberry naevus; dilated blood-filled cavities with venous anastamoses and often a surface capillary element.

Course and prognosis

The majority do not regress and may actually increase in size. Haemorrhage and infection sometimes occur, and occasionally sequestration of platelets within the naevus may cause thrombocytopenia.

Management

Surgical excision is often difficult. Injection of sclerosing agents under anaesthetic may promote fibrosis.

Port wine stains (naevus flammeus)

Clinical features

Sharply demarcated 'flat' capillary haemangiomata which may vary in colour from pale pink to deep purple. They are present at birth and do not increase in size after birth. May occur anywhere on the body (Fig. 129), but are most common on the face.

Course and prognosis

The majority remain as permanent discoloration of the skin.

Associations

Most port wine stains occur as an isolated defect but sometimes are partly cavernous, involve other organs or form part of a recognizable vascular syndrome, (e.g. Sturge–Weber syndrome).

Management

Surgery is cosmetically unsatisfactory. Cosmetic cover-up cream may be helpful in older children. Laser treatment is helpful for some and early referral to a specialist is recommended.

Sturge–Weber syndrome

Inheritance

Majority sporadic; occasionally autosomal dominant.

Clinical features

Facial port-wine stain (Fig. 130), characteristically in trigeminal distribution, seizures and sometimes mental retardation. Meningeal haemangioma often present on same side and may cause contralateral hemiplegia, cerebral atrophy, cerebral calcification and macrocephaly.

BMA Library

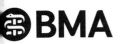 **BMA**

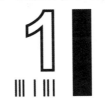 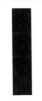

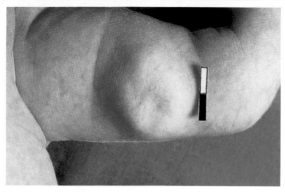

Fig. 128   Cavernous haemangioma.

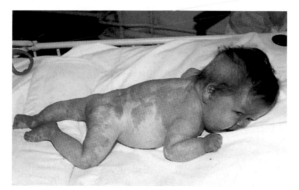

Fig. 129   Extensive port wine stain.

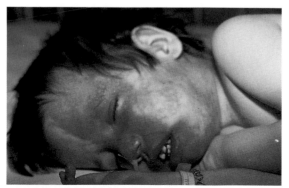

Fig. 130   Facial naevus of Sturge–Weber syndrome.

Pigmented naevus

Incidence

Uncommon in neonatal period except for Mongolian blue spots which are very common, particularly in infants with dark skin.

Clinical features

Small localized brown or black pigmented naevi (Fig. 131) are of no clinical significance and are usually not elevated during childhood, but may become palpable during adult life. Some congenital pigmented naevi contain hair follicles. Severe cosmetic deformity may occur with the rare giant bathing trunk naevus. Incontinentia pigmenti, a rare sex-linked hereditary disorder, initially consists of inflammatory bullae in the neonatal period which progress to pigmented streaks (Fig. 132).

Associations

Majority are harmless. Multiple pigmented naevi are seen in certain syndromes such as neurofibromatosis. Junctional naevi occasionally develop into malignant melanoma in adults, but this is rare.

Management

Depends on the cosmetic deformity and co-existence of associated disorders. Giant bathing trunk naevi are often grossly disfiguring and may be improved by dermabrasion in the first few months.

Depigmented naevus

Incidence

Uncommon and may occur as an isolated finding.

Clinical features

Occasionally, areas of skin or hair depigmentation may be the only manifestation of tuberous sclerosis in the neonatal period.

Sebaceous naevus

Clinical features

Waxy, yellow, pitted but hairless plaque usually found around the hairline or scalp (Fig. 133) in newborn infants.

Course and prognosis

Malignant transformation may occur in lesions which persist, hence excision is advised in adolescence.

Associations

Rarely, may be associated with convulsions and neurodevelopmental problems.

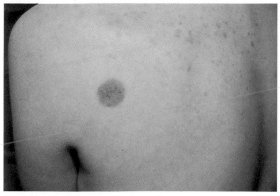

Fig. 131 Multiple pigmented naevi.

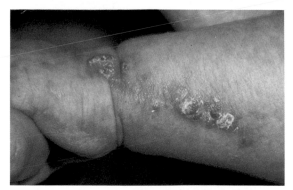

Fig. 132 Lesions of incontinentia pigmenti in a linear distribution.

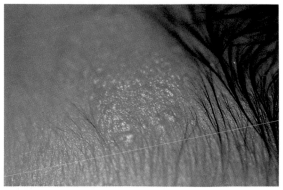

Fig. 133 Sebaceous naevus near the hairline.

Alopecia areata

Incidence

Uncommon; alopecia areata totalis is very rare. There is an increased incidence in Down syndrome.

Aetiology

Unknown; sometimes occurs during periods of stress.

Clinical features

Alopecia areata commonly causes localized hair loss on the scalp (Fig. 134). It can usually be distinguished from tinea capitis by the characteristic margin of exclamation mark hair shafts, and the absence of erythema and scaling.

Course and prognosis

Usually self-limiting; but occasionally may progress to alopecia totalis which results in total body hair loss. No effective treatment.

Partial thickness skin defects

Incidence

Rare.

Aetiology

Unknown.

Clinical features

The lesion is usually a superficial area of ulceration, most commonly found on the scalp (Fig. 135). Partial thickness skin defects of the scalp sometimes occur in trisomy 13 (Patau syndrome), but most occur as an isolated congenital anomaly. Small scalp defects are sometimes mistakenly attributed to obstetric trauma (e.g. fetal scalp sampling or scalp electrodes). Obstetric manipulations usually only cause minor skin trauma (Fig. 136) which heal without scarring or hair loss providing care is taken when removing scalp clips.

Course and prognosis

The defect heals by granulation. If it is not superficial, or if secondary infection occurs, healing may result in scar formation and contraction. A permanent bald patch may be left on the scalp.

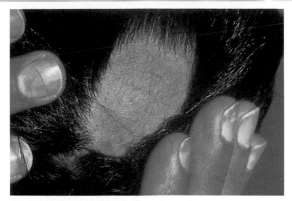

Fig. 134 Scalp hair loss in alopecia areata.

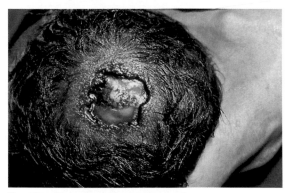

Fig. 135 Scalp skin defect in trisomy 13.

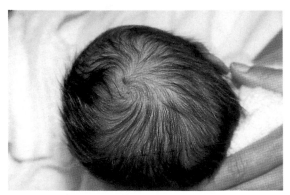

Fig. 136 Wound from a scalp clip used for fetal heart monitoring.

Napkin or diaper rash

Aetiology

Usually due to irritation from prolonged wearing of wet napkins; sometimes called 'ammonical dermatitis'. Monilial infection and seborrhoeic dermatitis are the other main rashes in the napkin area.

Clinical features

Erythema, umbilicated pustules, and ulceration of the perineum and sometimes the genitalia, but usually sparing the groin flexures (Fig. 137). The presence of discrete satellite lesions or involvement of the flexures is suggestive of monilial infection (Fig. 138). In babies with loose stools, there is often perianal erythema.

Management

Napkins should be changed frequently. In simple napkin rash, exposure of the perineum and a protective barrier cream is all that is required. Monilial infection responds to topical nystatin or miconazole cream. Monilia should always be considered when a rash does not respond to simple treatment. Seborrhoeic dermatitis often requires the application of a weak steroid cream.

Seborrhoeic dermatitis

Aetiology

Very common in young infants; aetiology unknown.

Clinical features

Distinctive greasy, scaly, erythematous rash or plaques, which usually appear within the first few months of life. The eyebrows (Fig. 139), skin behind the ears, and perineum are commonly affected. Thick greasy scales are often found on the scalp where the condition is commonly called 'cradle cap'. Occasionally, there may be discoid lesions on the trunk spreading up from a napkin rash (napkin psoriasis). In mild forms, seborrhoeic dermatitis may be mistakenly diagnosed as atopic eczema, particularly when the rash affects the flexures. There is never any systemic illness, even with widespread seborrhoeic dermatitis (Leiner syndrome), but secondary infection sometimes occurs.

Management

Mild corticosteroid cream such as 1% hydrocortisone. Cradle cap usually responds to a keratolytic shampoo or cream, but often recurs.

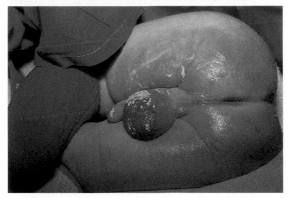

Fig. 137 Simple napkin rash.

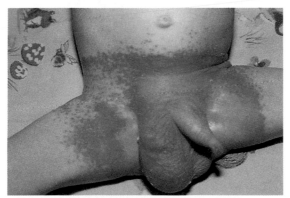

Fig. 138 Monilial infection with discrete satellite lesions.

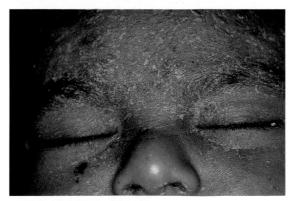

Fig. 139 Seborrhoeic dermatitis.

Epidermolysis bullosa

Incidence and inheritance

Very rare; usually autosomal recessive.

Pathology

Subepidermal bullae with blisters between basement membrane of epidermis and connective tissue of dermis.

Clinical features

Bullae, often resulting from minor trauma, occur at or soon after birth and cover large areas of the body (Fig. 140). High mortality in the neonatal form. Later onset in infancy, is usually autosomal dominant and often dystrophic, resulting in scar formation.

Differential diagnosis

Epidermolysis bullosa may be similar in appearance to widespread staphylococcal skin infection (pemphigus neonatorum or toxic epidermal necrolysis).

Management

Good nursing care is required, with particular emphasis on minimal handling because of the dramatic effect of minor trauma on the skin. Antibiotics may be required if there is secondary bacterial infection.

Antenatal diagnosis

Possible when there is DNA from a previously affected infant.

Collodion baby and harlequin fetus

Incidence

Very rare; unknown aetiology.

Clinical features

At birth, the infant is encased in a shiny, brownish–yellow, cellophane-like membrane which may distort facial features and extremities (Fig. 141). Respiratory embarrassment may occur because of restriction of chest expansion. Harlequin fetus is a more serious condition which is usually fatal, with a similar appearance of the skin, but also deep fissures between scale-like areas of skin, and sometimes ectropion and everted lips (fish-mouth).

Course and prognosis

Desquamation of the membranous skin occurs after birth. No particular treatment apart from copious lubrication of skin with creams (Fig. 142). Secondary infection should be treated promptly. Most collodion babies have normal skin in later childhood, a few develop ichthyotic skin changes later.

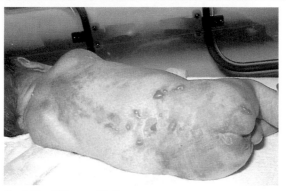

Fig. 140 Widespread bullae.

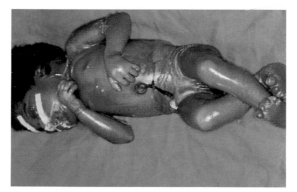

Fig. 141 Collodion baby.

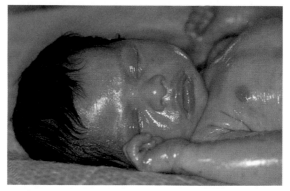

Fig. 142 Improvement is seen after 20 days. Note the oiled skin.

Eczema

Incidence	Common; affects 3% of children. Onset usually within first few years of life.
Inheritance	Often family history of other atopic disorders (e.g. asthma, hay-fever, allergy).
Clinical features	Itchy plaques with excoriation and lichenification, characteristically occurring on the face, behind the knees, antecubital fossae and wrists (Fig. 143), but can occur anywhere. The skin is often dry, and itching is a prominent symptom. Secondary infection is common because of scratching.
Investigation	Eosinophilia, raised serum IgE or positive skin tests are sometimes helpful in the general diagnosis of atopy, but are rarely useful in clinical management, as multiple factors are usually involved.
Management	Soap should be avoided, and emollient oil or emulsifying ointment used instead. Aqueous cream can be used liberally on the dry skin. Weak corticosteroid cream may be applied sparingly to bad patches during acute flare-ups. Systemic antihistamines are sometimes useful to control itching and scratching, which occur particularly during sleep. When there is a clear history of aggravation by certain foods, an exclusion diet may help.
Course and prognosis	Fluctuating course; usually improves in later childhood.

Psoriasis

Incidence	Uncommon in childhood; when it occurs there is usually a strong family history. Aetiology unknown.
Clinical features	Erythematous, scaly lesions which form plaques (Fig. 144), typically on the elbows, knees, around the hairline and scalp (Fig. 145).
Management and course	The tendency to psoriasis is usually life-long. Treatment depends on severity of the lesions. Corticosteroids, coal-tar and salicylic acid ointments are the mainstay of treatment.

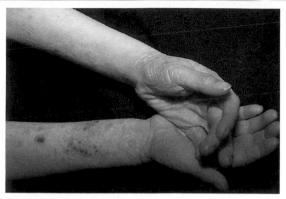

Fig. 143 Typical eczematous rash on arms.

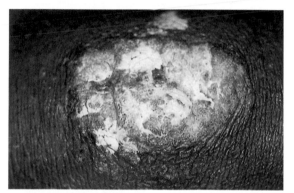

Fig. 144 Severe psoriasis.

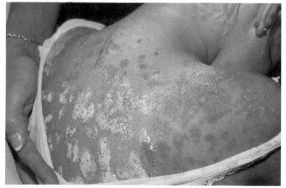

Fig. 145 Multiple plaques of psoriasis.

Urticaria

Aetiology

Common allergic manifestation, but the offending allergen is often not identified. Some recurrent cases are caused by sensitivity to food colouring agents.

Clinical features

Intensely itchy, erythematous rash with wheals. The pattern of the rash is constantly changing and may leave areas of bruising when the wheals subside. There is often marked oedema, particularly around the eyes and mouth, where it is called 'angioneurotic oedema' (Fig. 146).

Management

Acute respiratory obstruction caused by severe swelling of the mouth and tongue may be life-threatening; it responds to subcutaneous adrenaline. Systemic antihistamines may be helpful in urticaria. Food exclusion diets may help some children with recurrent urticaria. Some cases of chronic or recurrent urticaria are due to familial acetylcholinesterase deficiency.

Erythema multiforme and Stevens–Johnson syndrome

Aetiology

Idiosyncratic reactions, often to drugs (e.g. penicillin or sulphonamides).

Clinical features

Erythema multiforme shows widespread target lesions (Fig. 147). Stevens–Johnson is a more severe illness; it begins as a bullous eruption which rapidly progresses to widespread skin loss (Fig. 148). There is always involvement of the mucous membranes of the mouth, rectum, vagina or conjunctiva.

Management

Discontinue the offending drug. Barrier nursing, strict fluid and electrolyte balance and prevention of infection are important. In severe Stevens–Johnson syndrome mortality is high, particularly if septicaemia occurs.

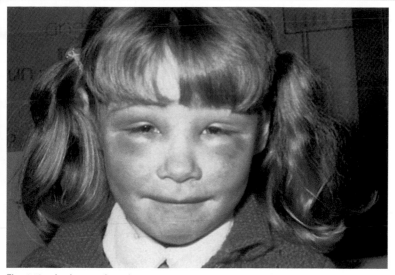

Fig. 146 Angioneurotic oedema.

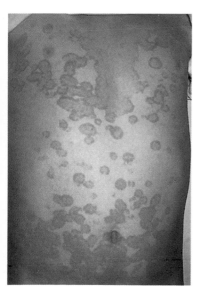

Fig. 147 Target lesions of erythema multiforme.

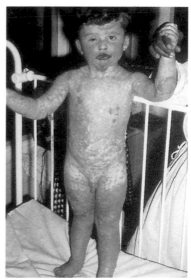

Fig. 148 Stevens–Johnson syndrome.

Henoch–Schönlein purpura (anaphylactoid purpura)

Incidence

Common; often occurs in small epidemics.

Aetiology

Diffuse vasculitis of unknown aetiology; there is often a history of a recent viral upper respiratory tract infection.

Clinical features

Pathognomonic feature is a purpuric rash on buttocks, extensor surfaces of legs (Figs 149, 150 and 151), arms, and sometimes face. Lesions are often papular and bullae sometimes occur. Localized oedema of face, hands, feet and scrotum often accompany the typical rash, and flitting arthritis affecting peripheral joints is common. Colicky abdominal pain is a troublesome symptom. Haematemesis, melaena or intussusception occur in a minority of cases. Haematuria occurs in approximately 70% but progressive renal disease occurs <1%.

Management

Other causes of purpura should always be excluded. Treatment is symptomatic. Corticosteroids may be indicated if there are severe gastrointestinal symptoms or progressive renal involvement.

Course and prognosis

Majority resolve rapidly, although further episodes or recurrences are common in the first few weeks. Prognosis is more serious if acute nephritis or nephrotic syndrome occurs.

Erythema nodosum

Incidence

Common, particularly in black children.

Aetiology

May be associated with streptococcal infection, tuberculosis, sarcoidosis, mycoplasma infection, drug sensitivity (particularly to sulphonamides), or inflammatory bowel disease. In the majority of cases, no underlying condition will be found.

Clinical features

Exquisitely tender, raised, erythematous nodules most frequently occurring over the pretibial region (Fig. 152), but may also occur around the elbows and on the forearms. Often occur in crops over several weeks or occasionally months; may be associated with fever and arthralgia, particularly when nodules occur over joints. Skin lesions resolve with the same colour changes as a bruise.

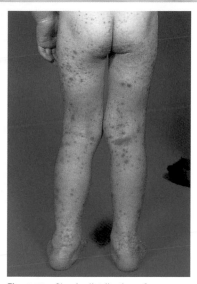

Fig. 149 Classic distribution of Henoch–Schönlein purpura.

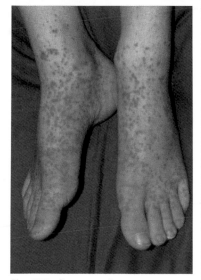

Fig. 150 Purpura on feet.

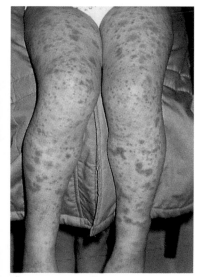

Fig. 151 Widespread Henoch–Schönlein purpura.

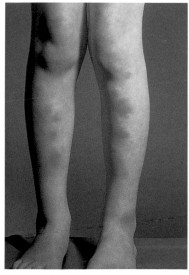

Fig. 152 Erythema nodosum.

Kawasaki disease

Incidence

Most common in Japan, but reported worldwide.

Clinical features

Prolonged febrile illness with fleeting erythematous rash, sore tongue, cracked lips and lymphadenopathy. During the second week after the fever has subsided, there is typical peeling of the hands and feet (Fig. 153).

Management

Coronary artery aneurysms associated with thrombocytosis occur in a minority of infants. Salicylates and intravenous gamma globulin prevent this serious complication.

Fungal infections and infestations

Scabies

Intensely itchy, excoriated, erythematous papular rash (Fig. 154), sometimes with burrows visible to the naked eye. Scabies may occur anywhere on the body, but is most common between the fingers and around the wrists. It is spread by close human contact, so the whole family should be treated with topical lindane. Clothes and bed-linen should be thoroughly washed if recurrence is to be avoided.

Tinea (ringworm)

Causes circular erythematous patches with a scaly centre. When tinea affects the scalp, there may be hair loss with circular patches of baldness. Tinea corporis usually responds to topical antifungals such as miconazole. Systemic griseofulvin may be necessary when there is extensive hair or nail involvement.

Monilia

Oral thrush (Fig. 155) is common in young infants. Candida also gives rise to a characteristic napkin rash with erythematous ulcerated satellite lesions. In later childhood, oral thrush may occur when the child is taking corticosteroids or when there is an immunodeficiency syndrome.

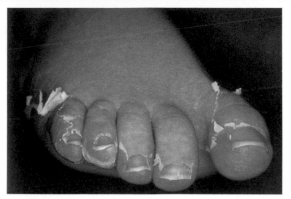

Fig. 153 Peeling toes in Kawasaki disease (courtesy of Dr R. Briggs).

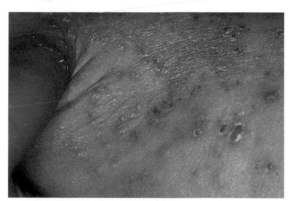

Fig. 154 Scabies infestation with excoriation.

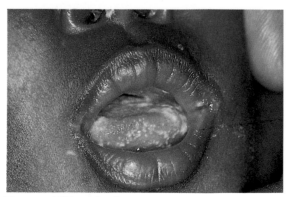

Fig. 155 Mild oral thrush.

Iatrogenic skin lesions

Incidence

Iatrogenic skin lesions associated with neonatal intensive care are becoming more common with increasing survival of low birth weight infants.

Clinical features

Abrasions are often associated with the use of adhesive tape (Fig. 156), name bands or starched sheets. Radiant heaters increase insensitive water loss through the skin of low birth weight infants and may cause drying of fragile skin. Transcutaneous skin monitors for monitoring O_2 and CO_2 leave a transient, superficial, pink burn which does not usually cause scarring unless the electrode has been left *in situ* for a prolonged period, but depigmented circular areas are often seen later in dark-skinned infants. Peripheral artery puncture and repeated heel pricking may leave scars. Intercostal catheters for draining pneumothoraces should be sited carefully, avoiding the area around the nipple in order to prevent damage to the breast (Fig. 157). Catheters in major vessels may occasionally cause obstruction and ischaemic necrosis of distal extremities, thrombosis or embolism. Transient cyanosis of the leg is sometimes seen after insertion of an umbilical arterial catheter, but if it does not resolve rapidly or if there is associated pallor or absence of arterial pulses, the catheter should be removed immediately. With prolonged catheterization, the risk of infection and necrotizing enterocolitis increases. Peripheral intravenous infusion sites may be associated with oedema or extravasation of infusion fluid. Infusions containing irritants such as calcium or sodium bicarbonate may cause serious tissue necrosis and lead to ulceration and later scar formation.

Management and prevention

Avoid excessive use of adhesive plasters whenever possible. Protective covering may limit insensible water loss by evaporation soon after birth. Within a few days of birth, the skin becomes thicker and less prone to traumatic damage, even in very immature infants. Care should be taken in siting peripheral infusions to avoid veins near joints because contractures may occur later if there is scarring (Fig. 158). Central catheters should always be removed if there is persistent cyanosis of extremities, or if there are signs of catheter occlusion or impaired circulation to the limbs, kidneys or gut. Arterial catheters should be removed as soon as the infant's clinical condition improves, and when sampling for blood gas analysis is required less often.

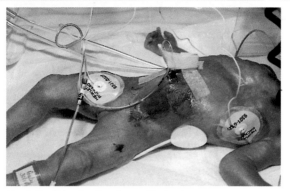

Fig. 156   Skin abrasions from adhesive tape.

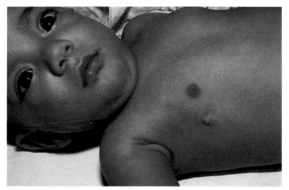

Fig. 157   Scar from a drain for pneumothorax.

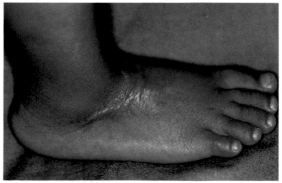

Fig. 158   A scar after an ulcer had healed.

Neonatal ophthalmia

Incidence

Minor sticky eye is extremely common.

Aetiology

Conjunctivitis may be due to a variety of organisms, most commonly Gram-negative organisms (e.g. *Escherichia coli*) acquired from the maternal genital tract during birth. The most serious causes of neonatal conjunctivitis are the sexually transmitted organisms, *Neisseria gonorrhoeae and Chlamydia trachomatis*.

Clinical features

Manifestations vary from a mild sticky eye (Fig. 159), to severe conjunctival inflammation with a purulent discharge and periorbital oedema. Gonococcal ophthalmia (Fig. 160) causes severe signs within 48 h of birth. Chlamydia infection (Fig. 161) often does not become apparent until the second week of life and may coexist with gonorrhoea.

Diagnosis

Appropriate swabs should be taken and an urgent Gram stain should be done. Treatment with high dose penicillin or cefotaxime should be commenced immediately if gonorrhoea is suspected.

Mangement

Minor sticky eyes are usually non-infective and respond to saline eye washes. Gonococcal ophthalmia should be treated with high-dose penicillin or cefotaxime, given both topically and systemically. *Chlamydia trachomatis* infection will be eradicated with chlortetracycline eye ointment and systemic erythromycin. Most other minor infections will respond to neomycin or chloramphenicol eye drops or ointment. When gonorrhoea or chlamydia are diagnosed, both parents will require genital swabs and treatment.

Complications

Inadequate treatment of gonococcal ophthalmia may lead to corneal scarring and blindness. In developing countries, chlamydia frequently causes blindness from trachoma, but this is uncommon in developed countries. The reason for this different outcome from the same organism is unclear.

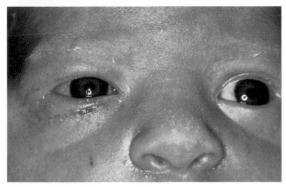

Fig. 159 Minor sticky eye with conjunctival inflammation.

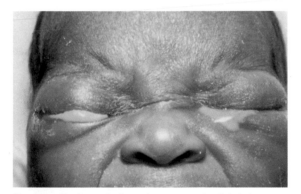

Fig. 160 Frank pus discharge in gonococcal ophthalmia.

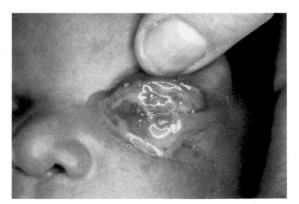

Fig. 161 Chlamydia ophthalmia.

Staphylococcal infection

Incidence

Serious staphylococcal infection is now uncommon, but not minor superficial infections.

Aetiology

Bacterial infection caused by Gram-positive cocci, *Staphylococcus aureus*. Some strains of this bacterium produce a toxin called exfoliatin.

Clinical features

Superficial staphylococcal infections result in small pustules anywhere on the skin (Figs 162 and 163). Umbilical sepsis is common, and if there is a frank discharge or periumbilical cellulitis, systemic antibiotics will be required. Paronychiae of the fingers and toes, although apparently minor infections, may cause more serious sepsis if not promptly treated. Occasionally, toxic epidermal necrolysis (scalded skin syndrome or Ritter disease) with extensive epidermal separation may develop (Fig. 164).

Complications

Septicaemia, meningitis and osteomyelitis.

Management

All superficial infections in young infants should be promptly treated with broad-spectrum systemic antibiotics after appropriate swabs and cultures.

Osteomyelitis

Clinical features

About 90% of cases are caused by *Staphylococcus aureus*. The metaphyses of the long bones are usually affected. There are local signs of acute inflammation and exquisite bony tenderness. Fever and toxaemia often occur.

Diagnosis and management

Blood cultures usually identify the organism. Magnetic resonance imaging and radioisotope bone scans will reveal the site of infection earlier than X-rays which rarely show any abnormality before the second week. Surgical aspiration is helpful for identifying the organism especially when blood cultures are negative. Surgical drainage is sometimes necessary. Systemic antibiotics are given for at least 6 weeks. With adequate treatment, chronic osteomyelitis (Fig. 165) is now rare.

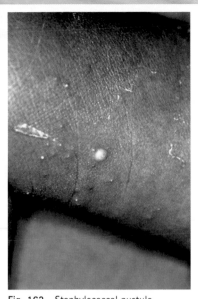

Fig. 162 Staphylococcal pustule.

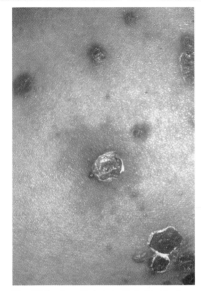

Fig. 163 Impetiginous staphylococcal lesions.

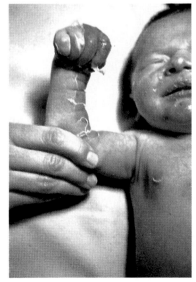

Fig. 164 Toxic epidermal necrolysis.

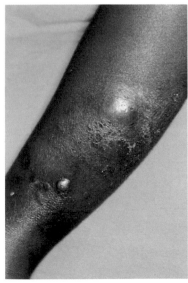

Fig. 165 Chronic osteomyelitis.

Erysipelas

Aetiology

Streptococcal skin infection.

Clinical features

Spreading cellulitis with a well-defined edge (Fig. 166). A red flare is sometimes seen spreading along the draining lymphatics.

Management

High dose intravenous penicillin.

Meningococcaemia

Clinical features

Acute fulminating septicaemia with shock and a purpuric rash (Fig. 167). Meningococcal septicaemia has a high mortality.

Diagnosis

Blood cultures should always be taken. Antigen testing is very useful, particularly when antibiotics have already been given. Lumbar puncture should be considered, but may be contraindicated in a very ill child.

Management

High dose intramuscular or intravenous penicillin or cefotaxime should be given immediately to any child with a suspicious rash. Early support of circulatory failure is critical to survival.

Meningitis

Aetiology

Common organisms causing bacterial meningitis in children <age of 5 years are *Haemophilus influenzae*, meningococci and pneumococci. The incidence of *Haemophilus influenzae* B and meningococcal C infection can be reduced by immunization.

Clinical features

Specific signs such as headache and neck stiffness occur in older children but are often absent in young infants. Infants often present with non-specific signs of irritability, drowsiness, vomiting, anorexia, convulsions or fever. Bulging fontanelle, high pitched cry and arching of the back (opisthotonos; Fig. 168) are late signs.

Diagnosis

High index of suspicion in any ill child with unexplained fever or convulsions. Cerebrospinal fluid examination and culture will confirm the diagnosis.

Management

Broad-spectrum antibiotics should be given until the organism and sensitivities are known.

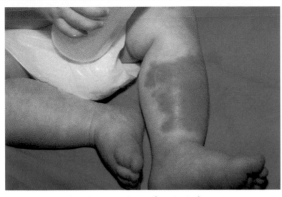

Fig. 166   Well-defined erythema (erysipelas).

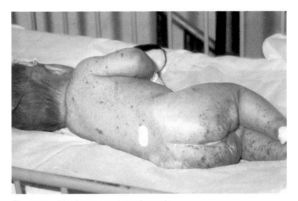

Fig. 167   Meningococcal septicaemia.

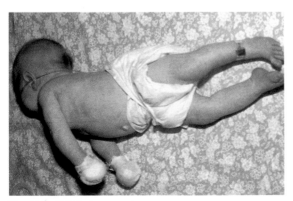

Fig. 168   Opisthotonos.

Measles

Clinical features

Incubation period 10–14 days. Prodromal illness with fever, coryza, conjunctivitis and cough. The child is extremely miserable as the rash begins to appear. Tiny white spots on a bright red background (Koplik's spots) may be seen on the buccal mucosa. After 3–4 days, a florid, maculopapular rash appears initially on the face and behind the ears. (Fig. 169). The rash becomes more confluent as it spreads down the trunk; bronzing and desquamation occur after about 7 days.

Complications

Bronchopneumonia and otitis media are common; encephalitis occurs in 1 in 1000 children. Mortality is high in children with malnutrition or immunodeficiency. Rarely, a slowly progressive neurodegenerative disorder (subacute sclerosing panencephalitis) occurs some years after acute measles.

Immunization

A triple vaccine with mumps and rubella (MMR) is very effective and usually given around 12–15 months of age.

German measles (rubella)

Clinical features

Incubation period 14–21 days. Mild illness with transient, non-specific macular rash lasting only a few days. Generalized lymphadenopathy, particularly of suboccipital nodes, is common.

Complications

Thrombocytopenia occasionally occurs. Arthritis is more common in adolescent females. Congenital rubella syndrome affecting the developing fetus in the first trimester of pregnancy is the most devastating complication.

Immunization

In the UK, MMR vaccine is given routinely at 12–15 months of age. All girls should be vaccinated before pregnancy.

Molluscum contagiosum

Clinical features

Pearly papules with a central punctum (Fig. 170) caused by pox virus.

Treatment

Usually asymptomatic and no treatment required. Cryotherapy or needling reduces the duration and is useful if the lesions are widespread, or cosmetically unacceptable.

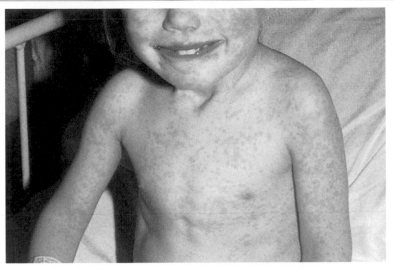

Fig. 169 Measles rash.

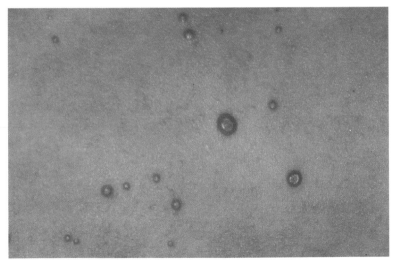

Fig. 170 Typical punctate lesions of molloscum contagiosum.

Mumps

Clinical features

Fever and enlargement of one or both parotid glands (Fig. 171) occur 14–21 days after contact by a susceptible individual. Subclinical infection is common. The brawny, swollen glands are painful, tender and often accompanied by earache or trismus. Submandibular salivary glands may also be affected.

Complications

Mild meningitis is common and may precede or occur in the absence of parotid swelling. Pancreatitis and epididymo-orchitis occur more often in adults.

Immunization

Part of routine MMR at 12–15 months of age.

Haemophilus cellulitis

Clinical features

Haemophilus influenzae may cause severe cellulitis affecting the face, particularly the cheek, periorbital region and neck (Fig. 172). Now uncommon as a result of haemophilus B immunization.

Management

Responds to an appropriate antibiotic (e.g. systemic ampicillin, or a cephalosporin).

Infectious mononucleosis (glandular fever)

Clinical features

Sporadic infection caused by the Epstein–Barr virus after an incubation period of 4–14 days. Anorexia, malaise, fever and generalized lymphadenopathy are prominent symptoms. Petechiae on the palate, and severe exudative tonsillitis often occur. A macular rash occurs in approximately 20% of cases, and in 90% if ampicillin is given (Fig. 173).

Diagnosis

Atypical mononuclear cells appear in the blood film, and agglutination tests (e.g. Paul-Bunnell test) may be positive in early weeks.

Complications

Hepatitis is common. Non-specific symptoms of fever and malaise may persist for several weeks or occasionally months.

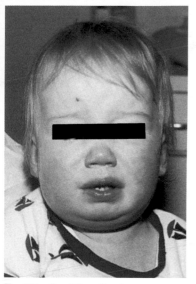

Fig. 171 Parotid swelling in mumps.

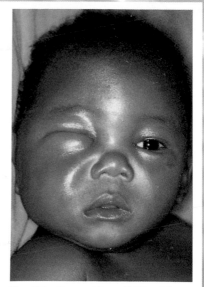

Fig. 172 Haemophilus cellulitis of the face.

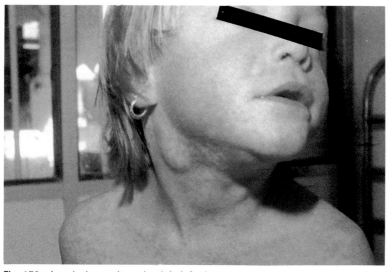

Fig. 173 Lymphadenopathy and rash in infectious mononucleosis.

Herpes simplex

Clinical features

Primary infection with type 1 virus may cause severe gingivostomatitis. Multiple painful blisters or ulcers occur around the mouth, on the lips (Fig. 174) and buccal mucous membranes. The child is usually extremely miserable with excessive dribbling and salivation, fever, irritability and difficulty in swallowing. Recurrent herpes simplex causes the simple common cold sore. Neonatal herpes infection with a generalized vesicular eruption, usually type II virus, is acquired by the infant during delivery through a genital tract with active herpes infection.

Complications

Dehydration may occur when there is inadequate fluid intake because of the painful mouth and difficulty in swallowing. Herpes encephalitis is a rare but serious complication with high mortality and high risk of neurodevelopmental disability in survivors.

Management

Sympathetic nursing, analgesia and adequate fluid intake. Primary infection is usually self-limiting within 2 weeks. Early infection within 48 h of onset may respond to topical acyclovir. Intravenous acyclovir is also used for systemic complications. Elective Caesarean section should be considered if active maternal genital herpes has been present in late pregnancy.

Herpes zoster: chicken pox (varicella)

Clinical features

Incubation period 14–21 days. The spots occur in crops which rapidly progress from macules to papules to vesicles (Figs 175 and 176). The vesicle becomes crusted and the child remains infectious until the scales separate 10–14 days later, often leaving pitted scars. Usually a mild illness, except when the child is immunodeficient. Encephalitis is rare, but when it occurs, the predominant sign is ataxia with onset several weeks after the acute illness.

Complications

Haemorrhagic chicken pox is a rare, but severe form of the illness.

Shingles (herpes zoster)

Uncommon in children. Vesicles have the typical dermatome distribution (Fig. 177). Itching is a common symptom, but post-herpetic neuralgia is uncommon in children.

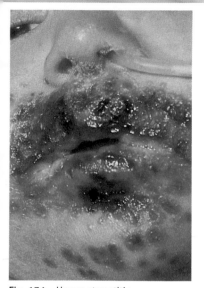

Fig. 174 Herpes stomatitis.

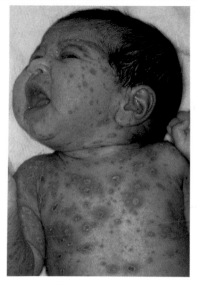

Fig. 175 Chicken pox in a young infant born to a non-immune mother.

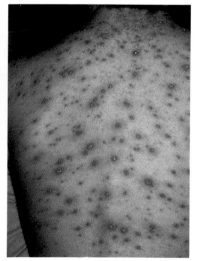

Fig. 176 Typical chicken pox in an older child.

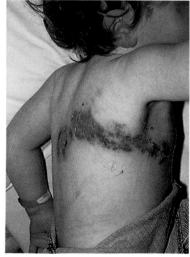

Fig. 177 Shingles involving dermatome.

Human immunodeficiency virus (HIV) infection

Incidence

Becoming more common as a result of the epidemic throughout the world. Most children are infected by vertical transmission during vaginal delivery. Breast-feeding increases the risk of infection.

Clinical features

Most babies with HIV infection are healthy at birth. AIDS-defining illness does not usually develop until the baby is several months old. Recurrent candida infection, recurrent parotitis, failure to thrive, pneumocystis pneumonia, generalized lymphadenopathy (Fig. 178), and chronic diarrhoea are common.

Prevention

If maternal viral load is reduced by anti-retroviral therapy during pregnancy, the risk of perinatal transmission can be reduced to <2%. Avoidance of breast-feeding and elective Caesarean section, also reduce the risk of infection, but may not be appropriate in developing countries.

Tuberculosis

Aetiology

Mycobacterium tuberculosis (Fig. 179). Primary infection may present in the lung or as enlarged lymph nodes. It is contracted by droplet spread, usually from asymptomatic adults.

Clinical features

Primary tuberculosis is usually asymptomatic. Haematogenous spread and meningitis are most common in the very young, and in children with malnutrition or intercurrent infection. Pulmonary tuberculosis with chronic cough occurs in later life.

Diagnosis

Sensitivity to tuberculin as shown by a positive Mantoux reaction (Fig. 180) develops within 4–8 weeks after infection. Chest X-ray may show hilar lymphadenopathy or a segmental lesion.

Management

Combination chemotherapy with isoniazid and rifampicin for 6–12 months, and occasionally other drugs, particularly if there is miliary spread or tuberculous meningitis.

Prevention

Bacille Calmette-Guérin vaccination provides up to 80% protection.

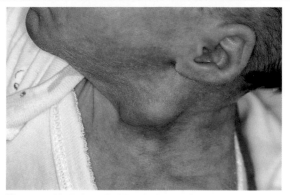

Fig. 178 Marked cervical lymphadenopathy.

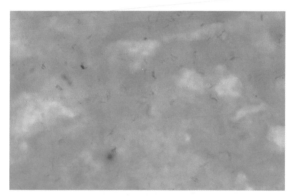

Fig. 179 Acid fast bacilli of *Mycobacterium tuberculosis*.

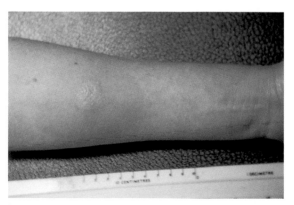

Fig. 180 Positive Mantoux reaction.

Cytomegalovirus (CMV)

Clinical features

Microcephaly, anaemia, hepatosplenomegaly, purpura (Fig. 181), jaundice, lymphadenopathy, intra-cranial calcification, and pneumonia. Deafness, mental handicap, cerebral palsy and epilepsy may occur later.

Prognosis

Some 1% of asymptomatic neonates excrete CMV in urine, majority have no sequelae. Approximately 5% develop deafness, and 1% more serious neurological manifestations.

Toxoplasmosis

Incidence

Less common in the UK than in continental Europe. Infection is acquired from eating raw infected meat or from cat faeces.

Clinical features

Hepatosplenomegaly, purpura, jaundice, growth retardation, intra-cranial lesions (Fig. 182) and calcification, chorioretinitis and hydrocephalus. Rarely, neurological damage may be severe.

Diagnosis

Toxoplasma-specific IgM confirms infection, but IgM-negative babies may still be infected and need follow-up for many months.

Management

Spiramycin is used in pregnancy after proven infection and continued after birth. Pyrimethamine and sulphadiazine are used for infants after the neonatal period. Treatment is particularly important in chorioretinitis.

Prognosis

Variable. Many children only have eye lesions, and rarely, neurological damage may be severe.

Listeriosis

Incidence

More common in France than in the UK. The bacterium is present in many foods, such as soft unpasteurized cheeses or in salads.

Clinical features

Intra-uterine infection resulting in abortion or premature delivery is common. Neonatal pneumonia and meningitis and discrete ulceration of the skin (Fig. 183).

Management and prognosis

Early treatment with ampicillin may provide intact survival.

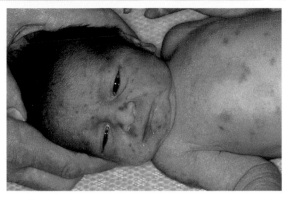

Fig. 181 Infant with purpura and an intra-uterine viral infection.

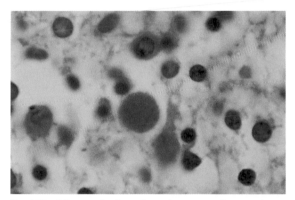

Fig. 182 Microscopic view of toxoplasma cysts in a new born brain.

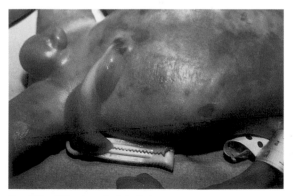

Fig. 183 Skin ulcers in listeriosis.

Haematological disorders

Leukaemia

Incidence

The most common childhood malignancy; 85% have acute lymphoblastic leukaemia (ALL).

Clinical features

Pallor, lethargy, recurrent infections, fever and spontaneous bruising are common. Hepatosplenomegaly, lymphadenopathy and bone tenderness sometimes occur. Neonatal leukaemia, though rare, may present with characteristic subcutaneous deposits (Fig. 184). Anaemia, thrombocytopenia and blast cells in peripheral blood. Excessive blast cells (Fig. 185) in bone marrow confirm the diagnosis.

Management

Full discussion of treatment and prognosis with the family is very important. Transfusions of blood, platelets or granulocytes are often necessary. Maintenance chemotherapy with several cytotoxic drugs will continue for several years. Bone marrow transplantation is becoming an important method of treatment.

Prognosis

At least 70% 5-year survival now occurs in ALL.

Langerhan cell histiocytosis

Pathology

Abnormal proliferation of histiocytes; variable disease spectrum which sometimes runs a malignant course.

Clinical features

Clearly defined lytic bone lesions, often involving the skull, are usually benign (eosinophilic granuloma). Systemic disease with fever, hepatosplenomegaly, lymphadenopathy, seborrhoeic rash (Fig. 186) or skin deposits is more serious.

Management

Systemic disease may respond to cytotoxic chemotherapy similar to treatment for acute leukaemia.

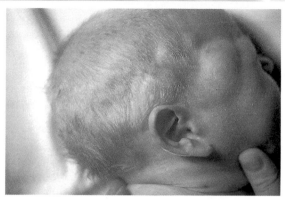

Fig. 184   Subcutaneous lesions of neonatal leukaemia.

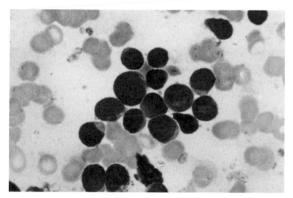

Fig. 185   Bone marrow showing many blast cells.

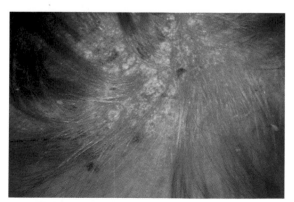

Fig. 186   Seborrhoeic scalp lesions of histiocytosis.

Sickle cell disease

Aetiology

Common. Haemoglobinopathy with sickle cell trait is found in 15% of black people. Inheritance is autosomal recessive.

Clinical features

Chronic anaemia, recurrent bone pains with tenderness and swelling, fever and jaundice (Fig. 187). Chronic leg ulcers, haematuria, chest and abdominal pain are common.

Management

Symptomatic treatment of painful crises. Prompt antibiotic treatment of infection. Prophylactic penicillin and pneumococcal vaccines to prevent serious pneumococcal infections.

Idiopathic thrombocytopenic purpura (ITP)

Aetiology

Often occurs after viral infections, especially rubella. Platelet antibodies are usually detectable.

Clinical features

Spontaneous petechiae and superficial bruising (Fig. 188). Other more serious causes of thrombocytopenia must be excluded.

Prognosis

Majority recover spontaneously within a few months; occasionally chronic, requiring splenectomy.

Management

Platelet transfusions if count falls <30 000. Steroids and intravenous gammaglobulin may also be helpful.

Aplastic anaemia

Clinical features

Pallor, anaemia, hirsutism, and palatal petechiae (Fig. 189).

Diagnosis

Blood tests show anaemia, thrombocytopenia, and neutropenia. Bone marrow confirms absence of precursors.

Management

Matched bone marrow transplant or stem cells from umbilical blood may be curative and are now the preferred treatment. Supportive treatment includes blood and platelet transfusions, immunosuppression with corticosteroids, ciclosporin, and antithymocyte or antilymphocyte globulin, or androgens. Early aggressive management of sepsis with broad spectrum antibiotics.

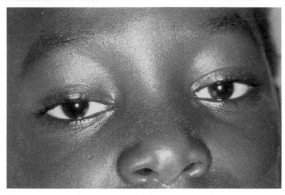

Fig. 187 Jaundiced sclera in sickle cell anaemia.

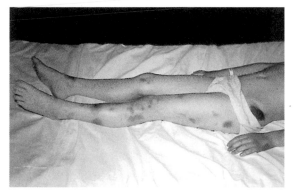

Fig. 188 Bruising in ITP.

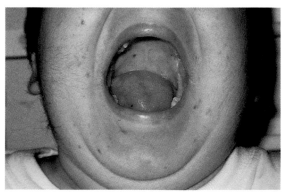

Fig. 189 Pallor, hisutism and petechiae on face and palate.

Thalassaemia

Aetiology and inheritance

Failure of synthesis of alpha or beta globin chains. Autosomal recessive; 1 in 4 risk of homozygous major disease in infants of parents with thalassaemia trait.

Clinical features

Alpha-thalassaemia is more common in Asians. Homozygous α-thalassaemia results in hydrops fetalis (Fig. 190) with intrauterine or early neonatal death. Beta-thalassaemia occurs mainly in Mediterranean populations. When fetal haemoglobin levels decline after the first few months, severe anaemia, hepatosplenomegaly due to extramedullary haemopoiesis, and sometimes cardiac failure occur. Compensatory bone marrow hyperplasia produces characteristic expansion of the skull and facial bones in older children (Fig. 191). Skull X-rays show characteristic hair-on-end appearance.

Management

Lifelong regular blood transfusions. Matched bone marrow transplant is curative, but a suitable donor may be difficult to find.

Complications

Frequent transfusions cause chronic iron overload. Subcutaneous infusions of an iron chelating agent (desferrioxamine) improve survival. Cardiomyopathy occurs in early adult life; growth and puberty failure, diabetes mellitus, skin pigmentation and liver damage are other manifestations of untreated chronic iron overload.

Antenatal diagnosis

Affected fetuses may be detected by analysis of globin chain synthesis of fetal blood or DNA analysis of chorionic villus samples.

Bleeding disorders

Aetiology

Haemophilia A (factor VIII deficiency) is the most common.

Clinical features

Spontaneous bruising or excessive bleeding after minimal trauma cause haemarthrosis (Fig. 192), deep haematomas or mucosal haemorrhage.

Management

Early treatment of trauma and surgical procedures with intravenous factor concentrates may reduce chronic joint damage.

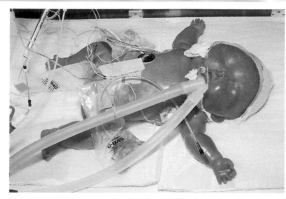

Fig. 190   Gross generalized oedema of hydrops fetalis.

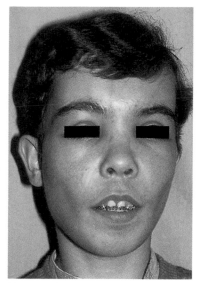

Fig. 191   Bone hyperplasia in β-thalassaemia intermedia.

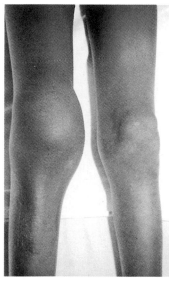

Fig. 192   Haemarthrosis in haemophilia (courtesy of Dr A. Kilby).

Wilms tumour (nephroblastoma) and neuroblastoma

Clinical features

Asymptomatic abdominal mass (Fig. 193). Haematuria and abdominal pain common in Wilms tumour.

Diagnosis

Ultrasound shows distortion of renal pelvicalyceal system in Wilms tumour. Abdominal X-ray may show tumour calcification in neuroblastoma. Adrenal tumours displace the kidney but do not usually distort the pelvicalyceal system. Elevated urinary catecholamine levels (VMA and HVA) confirm diagnosis of neuroblastoma in 90% cases and are a sensitive indicator of recurrence. Bony metastases (Fig. 195) sometimes occur in neuroblastoma.

Management and prognosis

Wilms tumour: chemotherapy reduces tumour mass before surgery. Sometimes postoperative radiotherapy. The 5-year survival is at least 80%. Metastases are common, but frequently respond to therapy. Neuroblastoma: surgical excision followed by radiotherapy. The 5-year survival is 60%; occasional spontaneous recovery reported.

Cerebral tumour

Incidence

Second most common childhood malignancy.

Clinical features

Headache, vomiting, ataxia or visual disturbance are common presenting symptoms. Behavioural disturbance, mood change, convulsions sometimes occur. Cranial nerve palsies (Fig. 194) are often found in brain stem tumours.

Management and prognosis

Surgical resection, but often difficult. Medulloblastomas are often radiosensitive and 5-year survival is now at least 60%. Long-term complications of tumour or treatment, particularly growth and endocrine disturbance, are almost invariable in survivors.

Other malignancies

Solid tumours are uncommon in childhood, but retinoblastoma, rhabdomyosarcoma, osteosarcoma, Hodgkin's disease, and lymphoma may occur. Bilateral retinoblastoma has a strong familial incidence and a good prognosis for survival with early treatment.

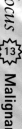

INfocus 13 Malignancy

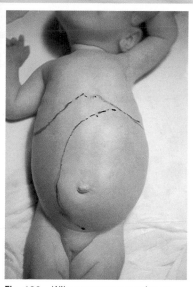

Fig. 193 Wilms tumour presenting as abdominal distension.

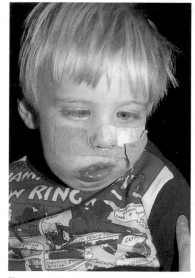

Fig. 194 VI and VII nerve palsies due to brain stem glioma.

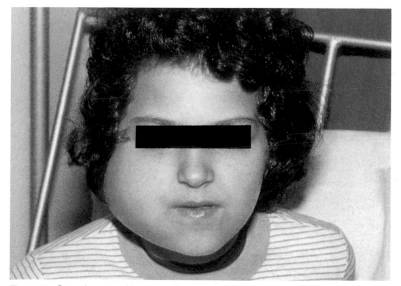

Fig. 195 Secondary neuroblastoma of mandible.

Common clinical forms

Pyogenic arthritis

Usually sudden onset of a single, hot, swollen, tender joint with painful restriction of movement. *Staphylococcus aureus* is the most common infective organism. Surgical drainage is often necessary for diagnosis and treatment.

Rheumatic fever

There has been a dramatic reduction in the incidence of this disease in developed countries. Classically there is an acute migratory polyarthritis associated with fever, rash and sometimes subcutaneous nodules. Carditis is the most serious long-term complication, resulting in permanent valvular damage.

Henoch–Schönlein purpura

A common allergic vasculitis which causes an easily recognizable clinical picture. There is a characteristic purpuric rash (Figs 149, 150, 151, 198), flitting arthritis or arthralgia, abdominal pain and haematuria. The majority resolve rapidly and require only rest and analgesia. Occasionally recurrent over a period of several months.

Juvenile chronic arthritis (JCA)

The peak incidence of systemic disease (Still's disease) is between 1–5 years of age. Fever, weight loss and mild anaemia are associated findings. Recurrent painful swelling and stiffness of both small (Fig. 196) and large joints (Figs 197 and 198) is common in older children. Psoriasis is associated with a small number of children presenting with arthritis, and skin and nail manifestations may be subtle in the early years of the disease. Joint inflammation can be reduced by appropriate choice of anti-inflammatory drugs. Exercise, physiotherapy, hydrotherapy and night splints help to limit deformity. Acute inflammatory episodes often remit spontaneously, but sometimes only after many years.

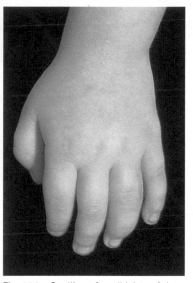

Fig. 196 Swelling of small joints of the hand in JCA (courtesy of Dr B. Ansell).

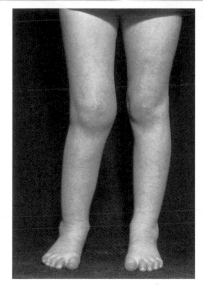

Fig. 197 Monoarthritis of knee (courtesy of Dr B. Ansell).

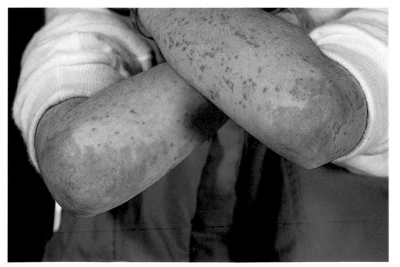

Fig. 198 Henoch–Schönlein purpura on the elbows.

15 Neuromuscular disorders

The floppy baby

Aetiology

Describes the clinical condition of the hypotonic infant in the first year of life. There are many possible underlying causes. Paralytic causes include neuromuscular disorders and cerebral palsy. Non-paralytic causes are hypothyroidism, malnutrition and Down syndrome. A few may have delayed, but eventually normal motor development (benign congenital hypotonia). Benign hypotonia is often familial.

Clinical features

A useful method of assessment is to hold the young infant in ventral suspension and pull the infant from supine to sitting posture (Fig. 199).

Spinal muscular atrophy (Werdnig–Hoffmann disease)

Inheritance and incidence

Autosomal recessive inheritance; occurs in 1 in 20 000 live births.

Clinical features

Infants are often weak and floppy from birth (Fig. 200) Rapidly progressive with death from respiratory failure within 12–18 months.

Antenatal diagnosis

Now available for some affected families.

Arthrogryposis multiplex congenita

Clinical features

Clinical syndrome of flexion contractures and sometimes dislocation of joints (Fig. 201), and gross muscle wasting.

Aetiology

Precise diagnosis may be difficult. Sometimes primary muscle hypoplasia or secondary to oligohydramnios.

Prognosis and management

Depends on severity of muscle hypoplasia. Long-term physiotherapy reduces contractures. Surgery may be helpful later.

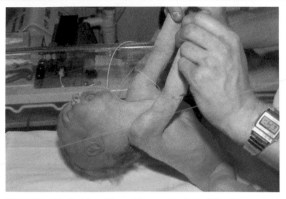

Fig. 199   Marked head lag of floppy newborn infant.

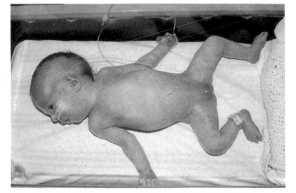

Fig. 200   Frog-like posture of infant with Werdnig–Hoffmann disease.

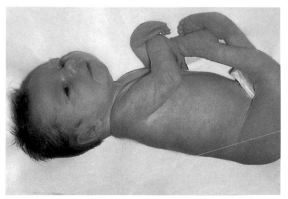

Fig. 201   Arthrogryposis multiplex congenita.

Cerebral palsy

Incidence and aetiology

Approximately 2 per 1000 live births. Cause is often obscure. A few are due to hypoxic brain damage in fetal or early neonatal life. Increasingly, thrombotic tendencies (e.g. protein C, protein S, anti-thrombin 3 and factor V Leiden), are being identified in children with hemipareses secondary to neonatal stroke. Spastic diplegia is more common in preterm infants.

Clinical features

Permanent, but non-progressive disorder of movement and posture. Clinical features often change because the child is continuing to grow and develop. Infants often show poor sucking, feeding difficulties, hypotonia, hypertonia, or irritability. About 70% of children with cerebral palsy have spastic manifestations with scissoring of legs, opisthotonos, hypertonia (Fig. 202), clonus and brisk tendon reflexes. One or several limbs may be involved, giving rise to hemiplegia, diplegia or quadriplegia. Ataxic cerebral palsy with hypotonia and weakness occurs in approximately 10%. Choreoathetosis characterized by irregular involuntary movements accounts for another 10% and is sometimes associated with hyperbilirubinaemia (kernicterus).

Diagnosis

Cerebral palsy is often not apparent for several months, until delayed or abnormal motor development become more obvious. Infants at high risk (e.g. preterm and infants with unexplained neonatal seizures) should have routine ultrasonography in the neonatal period and long-term neurodevelopmental follow-up. Magnetic resonance imaging or computed tomography brain scans are also helpful in establishing a cause, but may not be routinely available.

Complications

Mental retardation, epilepsy and sensory handicap are present in at least 60% of children with cerebral palsy.

Management

A multidisciplinary approach to assessment and long-term management is essential. Physiotherapy may encourage normal motor development and prevent contractures. The 'wind-swept' deformity (Fig. 203) seen after prolonged immobilization should be avoidable.

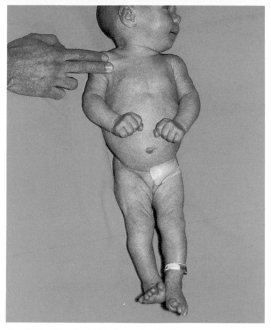

Fig. 202 Clenched fists in cerebral palsy.

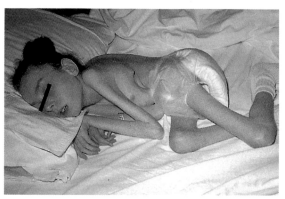

Fig. 203 'Wind-swept' deformity.

Duchenne muscular dystrophy

Incidence

Most common muscular dystrophy; occurs in 1 in 4000 male infants.

Inheritance

Sex-linked recessive, but mutations are frequent. Female carriers are usually asymptomatic but can often be identified. The disorder usually presents within the first 5 years because of difficulty in climbing stairs and frequent falls. The calf muscles are prominent (Fig. 204) though weak. When attempting to rise to standing from sitting or lying position, the boy 'climbs up' his legs using his hands for support (Gower's sign).

Diagnosis

Elevated creatine phosphokinase (CPK); abnormal electromyogram and muscle biopsy.

Course and prognosis

Progressive weakness resulting in most boys being confined to a wheelchair by teenage years. Death, usually from respiratory infections, occurs in early adult life.

Antenatal diagnosis

An affected male fetus can be identified using DNA analysis. Some carrier females have a mildly elevated CPK.

Neurofibromatosis (Von Recklinghausen's disease)

Incidence

1 in 3000 live births.

Inheritance

Autosomal dominant; but at least 50% due to new mutation.

Clinical features

Most have areas of skin hypo- or hyperpigmentation (café-au-lait spots) (Fig. 205). Pigmented spots in the axillae are characteristic. Subcutaneous fibromata, scoliosis (Fig. 206), neurofibromata of peripheral nerves and viscera are common. Many have skeletal abnormalities and pseudoarthroses. Limb hemi-hypertrophy (Fig. 207) occasionally occurs.

Complications

Phaeochromocytoma and glioma are common. At least 50% develop some neurological impairment.

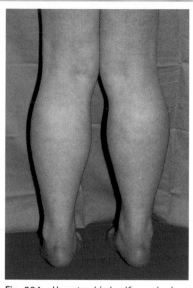

Fig. 204 Hypertrophied calf muscles in Duchenne muscular dystrophy.

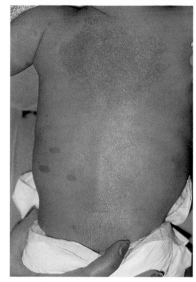

Fig. 205 Café-au-lait spots and shagreen patch in neurofibromatosis.

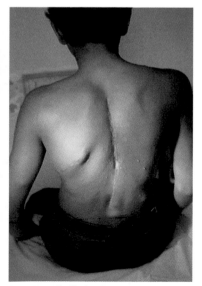

Fig. 206 Scoliosis after surgery.

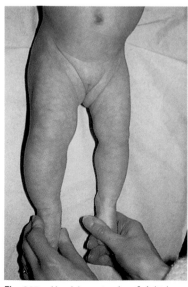

Fig. 207 Hemi-hypertrophy of right leg.

Poliomyelitis

Incidence

Uncommon in countries with a successful immunization policy.

Clinical features

Initially a mild viral illness with fever, sore throat, headache and vomiting, lasting several days. About 1 week later, in approximately 30% of cases, there are more severe symptoms of headache, neck stiffness, leg and back pains, and progressive asymmetrical weakness with muscular paralysis due to anterior horn cell damage.

Course and prognosis

In severe cases, death may occur from respiratory failure and bulbar paralysis in the acute illness. In the majority there is gradual improvement over 12–18 months. Many children have residual muscle wasting and paralysis (Fig. 208).

Myasthenia gravis

Incidence

Uncommon in early childhood. Peak incidence in adolescent girls.

Aetiology

Autoimmune disorder; anticholinesterase antibodies can be demonstrated in the majority.

Clinical features

Gradual onset of muscle weakness, with early fatigue. Loss of facial expression, arm weakness, chewing difficulty and ptosis (Fig. 209) are common. A transient form of myasthenia gravis occurs in newborn infants of mothers with the disease due to transplacental passage of antibodies.

Diagnosis

Clinically confirmed by showing prompt improvement with intravenous edrophonium (Tensilon).

Management

Long-acting anticholinesterase drugs such as pyridostigmine. Thymectomy often helpful.

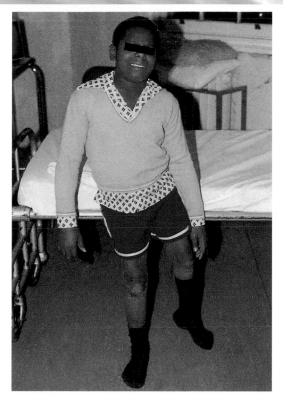

Fig. 208   Old poliomyelitis with shortening of leg.

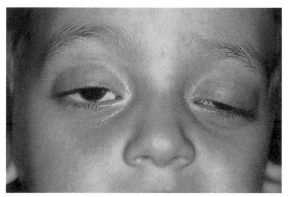

Fig. 209   Ptosis in myasthenia gravis.

Orthopaedic problems

Scoliosis

Aetiology

Usually idiopathic; occurs mainly in adolescent girls.

Clinical features

Spinal curvature is best detected by asking the child to bend forwards. Usually asymptomatic, but is a cosmetic deformity. Severe scoliosis may cause respiratory embarrassment or spinal cord complications. Midline lesions, such as haemangiomas (Fig. 210), hairy naevi, or lipomas, may indicate an underlying vertebral anomaly, particularly when they occur in the lumbosacral region.

Management

Bracing or surgical correction when deformity progresses.

Postural deformities of the leg and foot

Common clinical types

Bow legs

In the first 2 years of life, the tibia of the normal child has an outward curve and internal rotation. This bow-legged appearance (Fig. 211) is often more apparent when walking begins. Spontaneous improvement occurs.

Knock-knees

After 2 years of age, there may be unequal growth of the femoral condyles which gives rise to the knock-knee posture (genu valgum) (Fig. 212). Girls are more commonly affected. Gradual improvement occurs and by 6–7 years of age, the legs are usually straight.

In-toeing

The most common cause is metatarsus varus. The feet tend to curve medially because of adduction of the forefoot. The natural tendency is for improvement with growth, although surgery is occasionally necessary. Excessive internal rotation of the femora is common in girls and this also causes in-toeing. Treatment is unnecessary because spontaneous resolution occurs.

Overlapping toes

Overlapping of the little toe over the fourth toe (Fig. 213) is common and often bilateral. Surgical correction may be required as shoes may be uncomfortable and callous formation is common in later childhood.

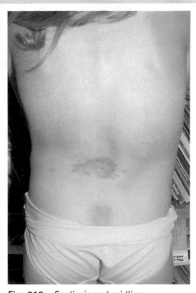

Fig. 210 Scoliosis and midline haemangioma.

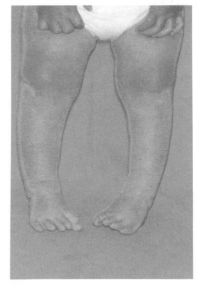

Fig. 211 Normal bow legs in infancy.

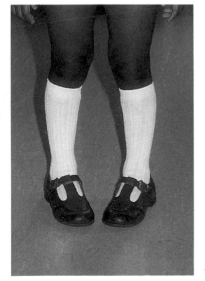

Fig. 212 Knock-knee.

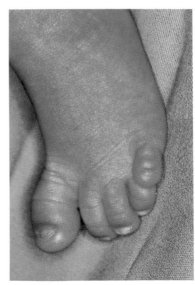

Fig. 213 Overriding little toe.

Developmental limb anomalies

Incidence

Common, particularly anomalies of the hand and arms.

Aetiology

Usually unknown. Absent radius or limb reduction defects may occur after a major vascular catastrophe in fetal life. Phocomelia is known to occur with maternal ingestion of drugs such as thalidomide in early pregnancy.

Clinical features

Polydactyly: extra digits of the hands (Fig. 214) and feet are extremely common and are often of autosomal dominant inheritance.

Management

Extra digits on the hand usually require surgical excision in early life. Polydactyly of the toes may require excision as the provision of comfortable footwear is difficult when the child is older.

Clinical features

Syndactyly: webbing, particularly of the 2nd and 3rd toes is extremely common and is never of any functional significance.

Management

Syndactyly of the fingers is uncommon, but surgery will be necessary as it is of functional as well as cosmetic significance.

Clinical features

Amputation deformities: absent radius and thumb is sometimes found in association with thrombocytopenia or anaemia. Missing digits (Fig. 215) sometimes occur. Complete absence of the hand is the most common limb reduction deformity. Sometimes almost the whole limb is missing—phocomelia (see Fig. 7.4).

Management

When there are upper limb reduction anomalies, prosthetic substitutes should be provided before the age of acquisition of skills requiring hand coordination.

Clinical features

Claw deformities: claw hand (Fig. 216) and foot are uncommon anomalies of major functional significance.

Management

Surgery is usually considered, but is not always necessary.

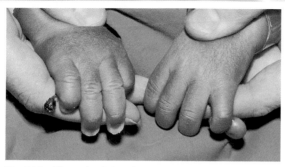

Fig. 214   Bilateral polydactyly.

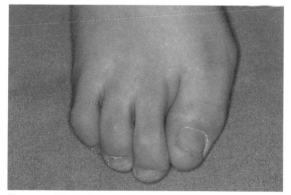

Fig. 215   Missing digit.

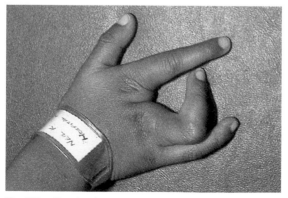

Fig. 216   Claw hand.

Hip disorders

Incidence and aetiology

Transient synovitis (irritable hip), or trauma is most common cause of limp or hip pain. Avascular necrosis of femoral head (Perthes' disease) occurs in boys 5–10 years of age. Obese teenage boys are at risk of slipped upper femoral epiphyses.

Clinical features

Usually sudden onset of limp and hip pain. There is restriction of abduction, extension and internal rotation.

Diagnosis

X-rays are diagnostic in Perthes' disease (Fig. 217) and slipped femoral epiphyses. Irritable hip is diagnosed after exclusion of infection and specific joint and bone disorders.

Management

Irritable hip recovers with a few days or weeks of bed-rest. Limb traction, surgery or internal fixation may be necessary in Perthes' disease and slipped femoral epiphyses.

Fractures

Clinical features

Pain, swelling and loss of function of a limb. A history of trauma is not always obtained, particularly in the very young. Extremely low birth weight infants (ELBW) <1000 g birth weight and <26 weeks' gestation, particularly those requiring prolonged parenteral nutrition, are at high risk of osteopenia of prematurity (neonatal rickets) and pathological fractures.

Management

Exact anatomical repositioning is not always necessary in children, as efficient remodelling ensures a good end result. Fracture of the humerus in young infants (usually due to birth trauma) requires only a collar-and-cuff sling (Fig. 218). Callus formation and healing is more rapid in young children. Even a major fracture of the femur will heal rapidly after a few weeks of immobilization in gallows traction (Fig. 219). ELBW infants should receive at least 400 U vitamin D daily and adequate long term phosphate intake.

Complications

Arterial ischaemia or nerve injury are the major complications of any fracture.

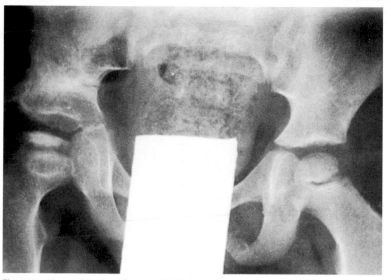

Fig. 217 X-ray of Perthes' disease of right hip.

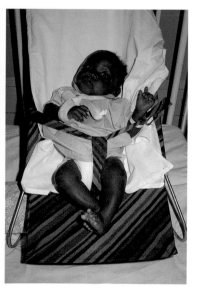

Fig. 218 Collar-and-cuff sling.

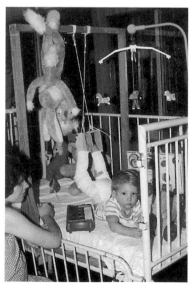

Fig. 219 Gallows traction. Legs in traction, but still partly mobile!

17 Surgical disorders

Inguinal hernia

Incidence
Most common condition requiring surgery during infancy; 1 in 50 live male births, highest incidence in first 3 months of life.

Aetiology
Persistent patency of the processus vaginalis, accompanied by herniation of small bowel.

Clinical features
Intermittent swelling in inguinal region (Fig. 220) or scrotum, often noticed after crying or straining. Herniae are usually easily reducible, but high risk of strangulation if irreducible.

Management
Surgical repair (herniorraphy) as soon as possible after diagnosis of an uncomplicated hernia. Strangulation, with a tense, tender, irreducible swelling sometimes accompanied by signs of gut obstruction (e.g. vomiting, abdominal distension) is a surgical emergency.

Umbilical hernia

Incidence
Approximately 20% of infants and 60% of black infants. High incidence in preterm.

Clinical features
Central defect in abdominal wall at umbilicus, with herniation of bowel into redundant skin (Fig. 221). On crying, straining or coughing, the skin covering the bowel-filled hernia often becomes tense, shiny and bluish but is not painful. Umbilical herniae always reduce easily when the infant is lying quietly or when asleep.

Significance
Cosmetic deformity only. Strangulation is extremely rare in central umbilical herniae, but may occur in para-umbilical herniae (defect in linea alba adjacent to umbilicus).

Management
Most close spontaneously within the first few years of life; occasionally surgical repair around 3 years of age. Strapping does not hasten spontaneous resolution.

Umbilical granuloma

Soft, spongy, pink umbilical mass (Fig. 222) which is often accompanied by sero-sanguinous discharge. Topical application of silver nitrate may hasten resolution but most do not require treatment.

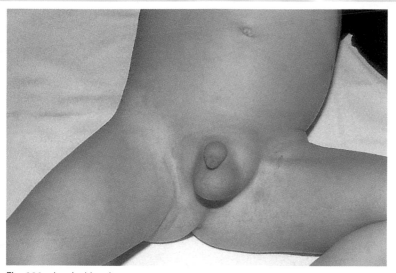

Fig. 220 Inguinal hernia.

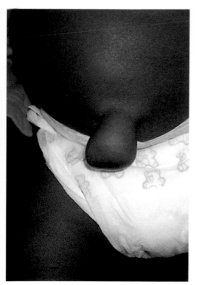

Fig. 221 Umbilical hernia.

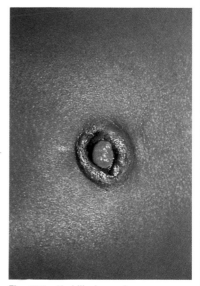

Fig. 222 Umbilical granuloma.

Hydrocele

Incidence and aetiology

Common; patent processus vaginalis.

Clinical features

Painless, fluid-filled cyst anterior to testes which is usually easily palpable within the scrotum. Brightly translucent (Fig. 223) and not emptied by pressure, although it may vary in size. Can be differentiated from a hernia because it does not extend up to the inguinal ring.

Management

Majority resolve spontaneously in the first year of life, but those presenting later often require surgery.

Hypospadias

Incidence

Glandular hypospadias is common; 1 in 350 male infants.

Clinical features

The urethral orifice is situated on the ventral aspect of the penis at a site proximal to the normal opening (Fig. 224), with severity varying from a glandular orifice to a scrotal or perineal site. Usually accompanied by a redundant dorsal hooded prepuce and sometimes associated with ventral curvature called chordee (Fig. 225).

Management

Mild glandular hypospadias without chordee is usually insignificant but minor cosmetic surgery is usually required. Surgical repair is indicated if the urethral orifice is situated proximal to the glans, or if chordee is present. Circumcision should be delayed until corrective surgery is performed, as the prepuce may be required for urethroplasty.

Ectopia vesicae

Incidence

Very rare; more common in males.

Clinical features

Wide separation of pubic symphysis with ventral herniation of bladder, exposure of bladder mucosa (Fig. 226) and a deficiency of pelvic floor leading to rectal prolapse. The condition is often accompanied by epispadias, undescended testis and an inguinal hernia. In the female, the clitoris is frequently septate or duplicated. Abnormalities of the kidneys are common.

Management

Surgical reconstruction is difficult. Continence is rare.

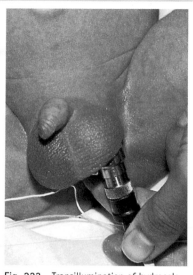

Fig. 223 Transillumination of hydrocele.

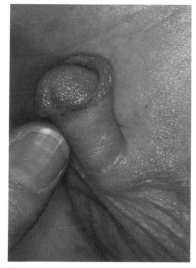

Fig. 224 Hypospadias with dorsal hooded prepuce.

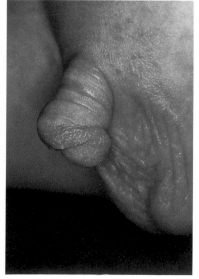

Fig. 225 Ventral curvature of penis (chordee).

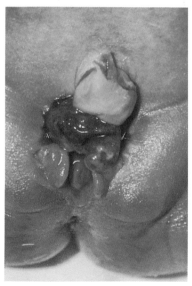

Fig. 226 Ectopia vesicae.

Undescended testes

Incidence

Undescended testes are common in young infants, particularly preterm (Fig. 227).

Clinical features

Retractile testes due to an active cremasteric reflex are extremely common and entirely normal. Bilateral undescended testes (cryptorchidism) are associated with hypoplastic scrotum (Fig. 228).

Investigations

Ultrasound examination of the inguinal region will identify testes in the inguinal canal. Infants with cryptorchidism will require chromosome analysis and exclusion of virilizing syndromes (e.g. congenital adrenal hyperplasia).

Management

Some 98% of testes descend spontaneously. Exploration and orchidopexy is indicated if the testes fail to descend by 1 year of age.

Circumcision

The prepuce is closely adherent to the glans during early childhood and retraction is unnecessary and undesirable. Spontaneous separation occurs after some years. The only medical indications for circumcision are phimosis, paraphimosis, recurrent balanitis and recurrent urinary tract infections associated with vesicoureteric reflux.

Vaginal defects

Incidence

Uncommon.

Clinical features

Imperforate hymen is a rare condition which may present in the neonatal period with an accumulation of mucus beneath the imperforate membrane (mucocolpos) which bulges out between the labia minora. Paravaginal cysts (Fig. 229) may be confused with an imperforate hymen, but it is possible to pass a probe into the vagina alongside the cyst.

Management

Imperforate hymen requires surgical drainage and excision of the membrane. Paravaginal cysts usually rupture spontaneously.

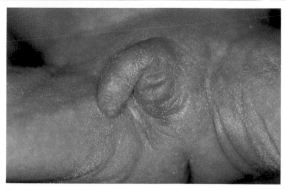

Fig. 227 Immature male genitalia with underdeveloped scrotum and undescended testes.

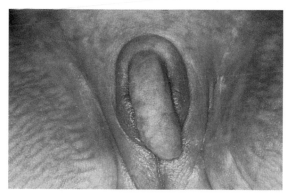

Fig. 228 Cryptorchidism—undescended testes.

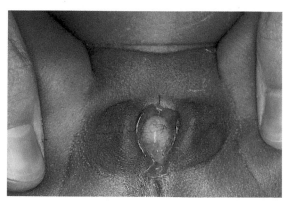

Fig. 229 Paravaginal cyst.

Exomphalos (omphalocele)

Incidence and aetiology

Uncommon anomaly of unknown aetiology.

Pathology

Failure of rotation and re-entry of gut into abdominal cavity during fetal development.

Clinical features

Congenital herniation of abdominal viscera through midline abdominal wall defect with umbilical cord at apex, and sometimes with a covering of peritoneum (Figs 230 and 231). Exomphalos can be differentiated from gastroschisis where there is no sac, and the umbilical cord is inserted at edge of the defect.

Associations

Other congenital anomalies are common, particularly cardiac or bowel defects.

Management

Surgical closure. The bowel should be carefully inspected to exclude stenosis or atresia. With large defects, definitive repair is often delayed until the peritoneal cavity is able to accommodate the contents. The sac and contents are usually enclosed in an artificial membrane, and gradually reduced in size over some weeks as the contents are slowly replaced into the abdominal cavity.

Imperforate anus (anal atresia, covered anus, rectal atresia)

Clinical features

Usually diagnosed during routine examination immediately after birth (Fig. 232), but occasionally presents later as intestinal obstruction or delayed passage of meconium.

Associations

Other congenital abnormalities are found in approximately 60% of cases. Recto–genito–urinary fistulae are common, particularly in high rectal atresia. Urinary tract infections are common, particularly when there is a fistula.

Management

A simple covered anus can be incised. More often, colostomy is performed in the neonatal period. A thorough search should be made for fistulae, particularly in females. Rectoplasty and a pull-through procedure are done later, at 6–12 months of age. Continence is achieved in approximately 70% of cases after final surgery.

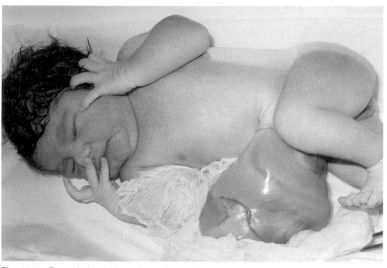

Fig. 230 Exomphalos with peritoneal covering.

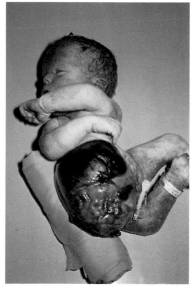

Fig. 231 Massive exomphalos with herniation of entire abdominal contents.

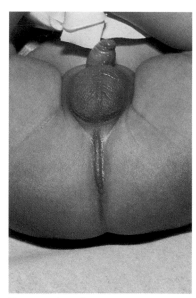

Fig. 232 Imperforate anus.

Necrotizing enterocolitis (NEC)

Incidence

Variable; more common in preterm infants. Associated with severe intrauterine growth restriction, birth asphyxia, umbilical catheterization, early feeding and artificial milk formulae. Clusters of cases may occur.

Aetiology

Unknown. Probably related to gut ischaemia and secondary infection with invasion by gut flora.

Pathology

Histological evidence of impaired gut perfusion, bowel ischaemia and necrosis, usually affecting terminal ileum, caecum and proximal transverse colon.

Clinical signs

Abdominal distension, vomiting and passage of bloody stools. NEC is sometimes accompanied by peritonitis, shiny bluish discoloration and oedema of anterior abdominal wall (Fig. 233), dilated abdominal veins or a palpable mass. Invasion by gas-forming organisms or diffusion of intraluminal gas into the bowel wall gives rise to the pathognomonic sign of pneumatosis intestinalis (intramural bubbles of gas) on plain abdominal X-ray (Fig. 234).

Management

Enteral feeds should be discontinued and parenteral nutrition will be required. Antibiotics, including those for anaerobes, are usually given, but specific pathogens are rarely isolated. Mechanical ventilation, analgesia and continuous nasogastric suction may be indicated. Maintenance of circulation with intravenous fluid and inotropes is essential. Persistent metabolic acidosis, thrombocytopenia or coagulopathy are signs of poor prognosis. If there is no improvement after 48 h conservative treatment, laparotomy may be indicated to assess and excise non-viable gut. Perforation (Fig. 235) is the only indication for laparotomy in the acute stages of NEC when mortality with surgery is high.

Course and prognosis

With conservative management, mortality has improved, but gut obstruction secondary to adhesions or stricture may require surgical intervention at a later stage in approximately 25% of survivors.

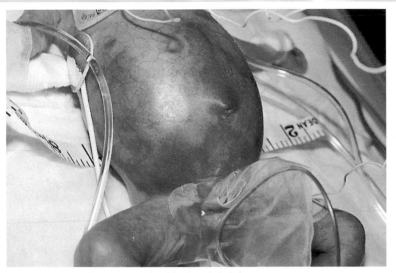

Fig. 233 Necrotizing enterocolitis with distended abdomen.

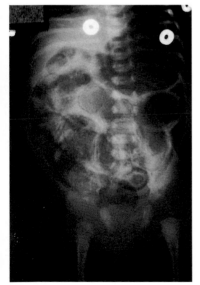

Fig. 234 X-ray showing intramural gas.

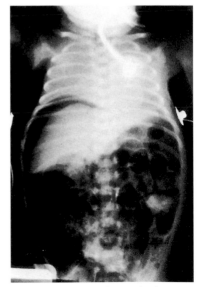

Fig. 235 X-ray showing gas in the peritoneal cavity from perforation.

Diaphragmatic hernia

Incidence

Occurs in 1 in 1500 live births.

Aetiology

Failure of fusion or muscularization of the anterior and posterior leaves of the diaphragm. The condition is most commonly due to persistence of the pleuroperitoneal canal, usually on the left side and resulting in a posterolateral hernia through the foramen of Bochdalek.

Antenatal diagnosis

When herniation occurs early in gestation, absence of the abdominal stomach bubble may be diagnosed on routine antenatal anomaly ultrasonography. Those detected early have a poor prognosis because pulmonary hypoplasia is likely to be severe. Herniation in later gestation may not be diagnosable until after birth.

Clinical features

Most diaphragmatic herniae are large and produce cardio-respiratory symptoms soon after birth. The signs and symptoms depend on the size of the hernia and include respiratory distress, cyanosis, dextrocardia and scaphoid abdomen with reduced or absent abdominal contents (Fig. 236).

Associations

Pulmonary hypoplasia; gut anomalies.

Management

The mother should be delivered in a perinatal centre with a paediatric surgical service. Confirm the diagnosis with a chest X-ray after birth (Fig. 237). Preoperative decompression of the gut with a large nasogastric tube and mechanical ventilation are usually required. Pulmonary hypertension is common and when significant should be treated with pulmonary vasodilators, including nitric oxide, before surgical repair is undertaken. Surgery is usually not technically difficult, but delay in surgical repair of the diaphragmatic defect until the baby's condition is stable, improves the chances of survival.

Prognosis

Mortality is high even after successful surgery. Survival depends on the severity of pulmonary hypoplasia. Better treatment of pulmonary hypertension and delayed surgery has not improved survival in recent years.

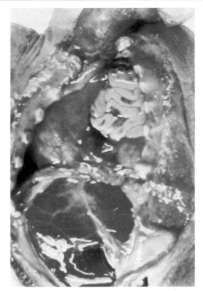

Fig. 236 Post-mortem appearance of diaphragmatic hernia (courtesy of Dr S. Gould).

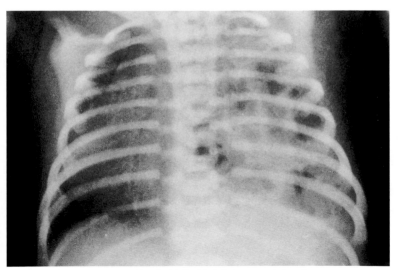

Fig. 237 X-ray appearance of typical left-sided diaphragmatic hernia.

Pyloric stenosis

Aetiology

Hypertrophy of the smooth muscle of pylorus of obscure aetiology. First born male infants often affected.

Clinical features

Onset of vomiting within a few weeks of birth. Classically, there is projectile vomiting with failure to thrive and constipation. During feeding, a pyloric mass (Fig. 238) can usually be palpated and visible peristalsis may be seen in the upper abdomen. Ultrasound examination is helpful for confirmation of the diagnosis.

Management

Surgery (Ramstedt's pyloromyotomy) after rehydration and correction of electrolyte imbalance.

Intussusception

Incidence

Common cause of gut obstruction in infancy.

Clinical features

Sudden onset of colicky abdominal pain, with loose stools often blood-stained (red-currant jelly stools). A sausage-shaped bowel mass may be palpable.

Management

Gentle barium or air enema (Fig. 239) will confirm the diagnosis and may be curative in cases of recent onset. Surgery may be required for intussusception when the diagnosis is delayed.

Hirschsprung's disease

Aetiology

Congenital absence of ganglionic cells in the colon.

Clinical features

May cause acute neonatal intestinal obstruction (Fig. 240) or chronic constipation in older children.

Diagnosis

Barium enema and anorectal manometry assist in the diagnosis; rectal biopsy is always necessary for confirmation.

Management

Colostomy relieves acute obstruction; resection of the aganglionic segment and a pull-through anastomosis are performed later.

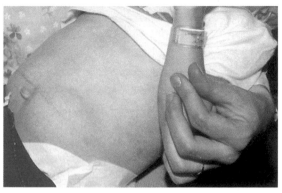

Fig. 238   Visible peristalsis in pyloric stenosis.

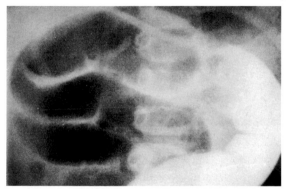

Fig. 239   Intussusception.

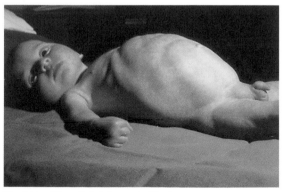

Fig. 240   Distended abdomen in Hirschsprung's disease
(courtesy of Dr T. Lissauer).

Choanal atresia

Incidence

Rare anomaly with absence or narrowing of posterior nares.

Clinical features

Bilateral choanal atresia causes cyanosis and respiratory obstruction in the newborn. In unilateral choanal atresia, the condition causes unilateral rhinorrhoea and diagnosis is often not made until later in childhood.

Management

Urgent provision of an oral airway is needed in bilateral choanal atresia. The membranous posterior nares are then surgically excised and a small tube left in situ (Fig. 241) until the new orifice has epithelialized.

Bat ears

Incidence

Often autosomal dominant.

Clinical features

Large protruding ears, usually bilateral (Fig. 242).

Pathology

Defect in normal folding of the anti-helix. Surgery when protrusion of ears is cosmetically unacceptable.

Torticollis

Aetiology

Usually acute onset of unknown aetiology. Chronic painless torticollis may be secondary to sternomastoid fibrosis, intrauterine posture, cervical hemivertebrae, or ocular imbalance. In acute painful torticollis or the common wry-neck (Fig. 243), there is a sudden onset of limitation of neck rotation with an intensely painful sternomastoid muscle. The head is sometimes tilted towards the affected side.

Management

Spontaneous recovery occurs within days in acute torticollis or months in postural torticollis. Gentle physiotherapy may be helpful.

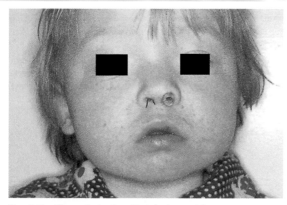

Fig. 241   Choanal atresia with tube in nostril.

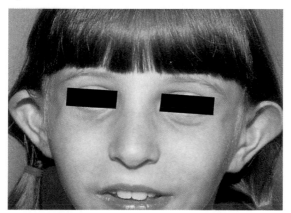

Fig. 242   Bat ears.

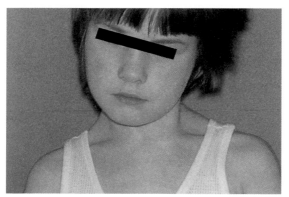

Fig. 243   Acute torticollis.

Burns and scalds

Clinical features

The most common scald happens to the toddler who pulls boiling water onto the face, neck, shoulder and upper arm (Fig. 244). Flame burns tend to happen to older children. When clothes catch fire, burns may involve extensive areas of the body (Fig. 245) and are often deep.

Management

Treatment depends on the extent and severity of the burn. Emergency measures consist of appropriate pain relief (particularly for superficial scalds), ensuring an adequate airway, and resuscitation with plasma volume expanders when there are signs of shock. If burns involve more than 10% of the child's surface area, intravenous fluid therapy will be necessary. Large quantities of fluid, blood and protein are lost from burned areas. Tetanus toxoid should always be given. Infection should be prevented by barrier nursing of exposed burns or by the closed method with topical antibiotics such as silver sulphadiazine under occlusive dressings (Fig. 246). Systemic antibiotics are given if there are specific indications. All but the most minor scalds should be managed by a team of experienced paediatric intensivists, nurses and plastic surgeons. Children involved in house fires may develop severe respiratory distress due to smoke inhalation and should always be admitted to hospital for observation even if there are no signs of burns to the skin.

Course and prognosis

Superficial burns quickly form a protective eschar when left exposed. This eschar gradually lifts off when new epithelium has formed (Fig. 247). Skin grafts may be necessary for deep burns, extensive burns or to relieve tight contractures.

Prevention

Burns and scalds in children should be preventable by education of families and the public, and by safeguards in design of heating appliances and children's clothing.

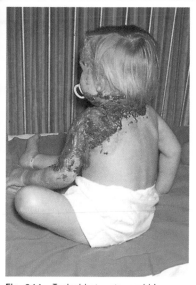

Fig. 244 Typical hot water scald in toddler.

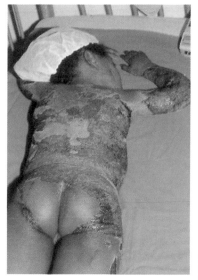

Fig. 245 Extensive flame burns.

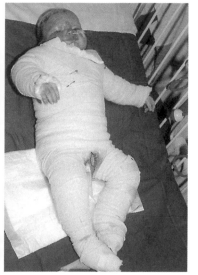

Fig. 246 Extensive burns treated by closed dressings.

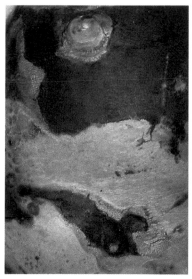

Fig. 247 New epithelium forming after a scald.

18 Renal disorders

Urinary tract infection (UTI)

Incidence

Very common infection; occurs in 1–2% of girls.

Clinical features

Young infants may have non-specific symptoms of poor weight gain, fever, vomiting and irritability. Older children may complain of urinary frequency, dysuria and loin pain.

Diagnosis

High index of suspicion; must obtain adequate urine sample for urinalysis and culture. Suprapubic aspirate is often necessary in young infants because skin contamination may make bag or clean-catch specimens difficult to interpret, particularly in girls. Occasionally catheter specimen, particularly if very unwell and antibiotic treatment is considered urgent.

Management

Acute infection requires antibiotic therapy. Proven UTIs require investigation of the renal tract with ultrasound examination and sometimes, radioisotope scans or micturating cystourethrogram. At least 50% have an underlying abnormality, most commonly vesicoureteric reflux (Fig. 248). Prophylactic antibiotics may protect against renal scarring. New scars rarely develop after the age of 7 years. Surgery (ureteric reimplantation) is occasionally necessary when there is progression of renal scarring or recurrent breakthrough infections, despite prophylaxis.

Renal tract anomalies

Incidence

Relatively common; most are asymptomatic and functionally insignificant. Many are now diagnosed on routine antenatal anomaly ultrasonography.

Clinical features

Ureteric duplication is usually asymptomatic but may predispose to infection, obstruction or reflux. Posterior urethral valves in male infants cause poor urinary stream, and obstruction may cause renal failure. Horseshoe kidneys, pelvic kidneys, unilateral renal dysplasia are often asymptomatic unless there is infection. Severe anomalies of the renal tract such as renal agenesis or prune-belly (see Fig. 105) syndrome are usually diagnosed on routine antenatal anomaly ultrasound scans. Mild antenatally detected renal tract dilatation (Fig. 249) is common and needs investigation after birth, but only occasionally is due to an obstructive uropathy (Fig. 250) requiring surgery.

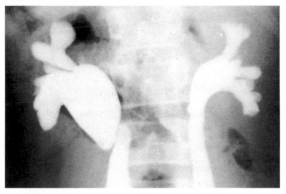

Fig. 248 Vesicoureteric reflux (bilateral grade III).

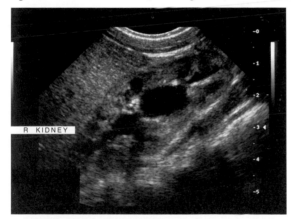

Fig. 249 Minimal renal pelvic dilatation.

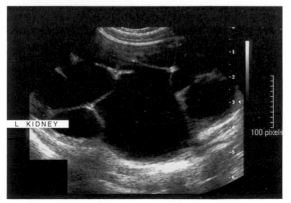

Fig. 250 Grossly dilated renal pelvi-calyceal system.

Nephrotic syndrome

Incidence

1 in 20 000 children. Boys are more commonly affected. The peak age incidence is 1–5 years.

Aetiology

Cause unknown; immunological basis likely.

Clinical features

Periorbital (Fig. 251) and generalized oedema, abdominal pain and ascites. Gross proteinuria may lead to hypovolaemia and acute circulatory collapse. Prone to pneumococcal peritonitis. Renal biopsy is indicated in children with hypertension or haematuria, in whom a more serious underlying diagnosis is likely to be found.

Management

Bedrest and high protein, salt-restricted diet until diuresis occurs, usually within 10–14 days of starting oral corticosteroids. Hypovolaemia responds to infusion of plasma or salt-free albumin. Prophylactic penicillin during relapses and pneumoccal vaccination is recommended.

Course and prognosis

Majority have minimal change lesion and recover completely within 2 years. Relapses are common, but normally respond to steroids. Azothiaprine therapy is occasionally helpful in children who have frequent relapses or unacceptable side effects on steroids.

Acute glomerulonephritis

Incidence and aetiology

Uncommon. May be secondary to recent streptococcal or viral infection. May occur in association with Henoch–Schönlein purpura (Fig. 252).

Clinical features

Pallor, lethargy, smoky urine due to microscopic haematuria, oliguria and hypertension.

Management

Bed-rest, treatment of significant hypertension and careful fluid balance until spontaneous improvement occurs.

Course and prognosis

Most recover within a few weeks, but microscopic haematuria may persist for months.

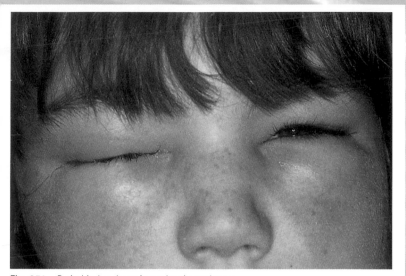

Fig. 251 Periorbital oedema in nephrotic syndrome.

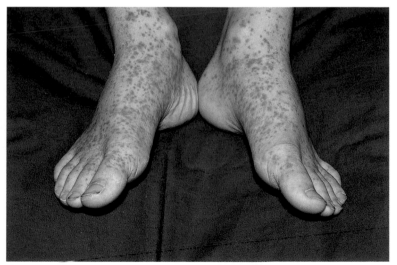

Fig. 252 Henoch–Schönlein purpura on the feet.

Gastroenteritis

Incidence

The most common cause of death in young infants in developing countries where early weaning and malnutrition are common.

Aetiology

Rotavirus infection is a common cause of gastroenteritis in infants in winter months. *Esherichia coli*, Salmonella, Shigella and Campylobacter are the common causes of bacterial gastroenteritis.

Clinical features

Diarrhoea, vomiting and colicky abdominal pain. The most serious complication is dehydration due to excessive water loss or inadequate fluid intake. In mild to moderate dehydration (up to 5%) the child is thirsty, lethargic, has sunken eyes and loss of skin turgor (Figs 253 and 254). In moderate to severe dehydration (5–10%) there may be tachycardia and signs of peripheral circulatory collapse.

Management

Recognition of dehydration and adequate fluid and electrolyte replacement is important. Frequent administration of an oral glucose electrolyte solution is usually possible, except when there is shock. Intravenous therapy will then be necessary.

Intestinal parasites

Incidence

Common cause of malabsorption, anaemia and chronic diarrhoea in developing countries.

Aetiology and clinical features

Giardia lamblia is a protozoal infestation which causes acute diarrhoea and sometimes chronic malabsorption. *Ascaris lumbricoides* (roundworm) (Fig. 255) causes colicky abdominal pain and gut obstruction. Ankylostoma (hookworm) is a common cause of iron deficiency anaemia in tropical countries.

Treatment

Appropriate anti-helminthic drug therapy.

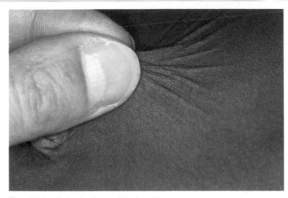

Fig. 253 Dehydration with dry skin.

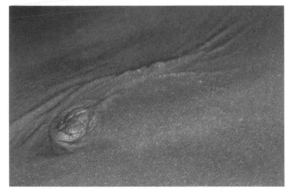

Fig. 254 Dehydration showing poor skin turgor after release.

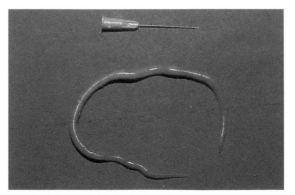

Fig. 255 *Ascaris lumbricoides* (roundworm).

Coeliac disease

Aetiology
Gluten sensitivity; gluten intolerance. Permanent intolerance of dietary wheat, rye and sometimes barley and oats.

Incidence
About 1 in 2000 in the UK.

Clinical features
Most children have signs in infancy (e.g. poor weight gain after introduction of gluten-containing solids), but signs are often insidious. Vomiting, diarrhoea and abdominal distension are common. Anorexia, irritability with miserable facies (Fig. 256), hypotonia and wasted buttocks occur. Sometimes failure to thrive or growth failure is the only sign and may not be diagnosed until adolescence.

Diagnosis
Jejunal biopsy, showing total villus atrophy and inflammatory infiltration of the lamina propria, is the definitive investigation. Anti-gliadin antibodies are often found in blood.

Management
Gluten-free diet. Supplementation with iron and vitamins is often necessary after diagnosis. Lactose or cow's milk protein intolerance sometimes occurs.

Course and prognosis
Gastrointestinal symptoms, mood disturbance and growth failure improve with a gluten-free diet. There is an increased risk of intestinal lymphoma in adult life.

Inflammatory bowel disorders

Clinical features
Abdominal pain, chronic diarrhoea, weight loss, pallor, fever, mouth (Fig. 257) and anal (Fig. 258) ulceration and growth failure.

Diagnosis
Barium meal and follow-through, colonoscopy and biopsy are usually required to differentiate between Crohn's disease and ulcerative colitis.

Management
Crohn's disease may be difficult to treat, but oral steroids, azothiaprine, cyclosporin or an elemental or polymeric diet may induce remission. Hemi-colectomy is ultimately necessary in ulcerative colitis if unresponsive to steroids.

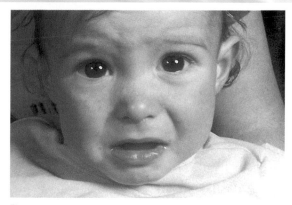

Fig. 256 Miserable facies of coeliac child.

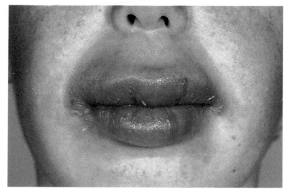

Fig. 257 Swelling of lips and angular cheilitis in Crohn's disease.

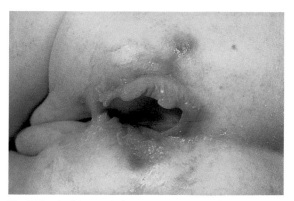

Fig. 258 Anal tags and sinuses.

Bronchiolitis

Incidence

Commonly occurs in infants in winter epidemics; usually due to respiratory syncytial virus.

Clinical features

Coryzal symptoms, then gradual onset of cough, wheeze, tachypnoea and feeding difficulty. The child may develop over-inflation of the lungs, producing a barrel-shaped chest, cyanosis, subcostal recession (Fig. 259) and occasionally heart failure.

Management

Supportive care with added oxygen when necessary. Tube feeding or intravenous fluids are often required. Antibiotics are not usually indicated, but may be given if secondary infection is suspected or in a very ill child. Treatment of cardiac failure or mechanical ventilation is occasionally necessary. A nebulized antiviral agent, ribavirin, may be helpful in high-risk babies, such as those with congenital heart disease.

Asthma

Incidence

Very common; occurs in at least 1 in 7 children.

Aetiology

Allergens, particularly house dust mite, are always important in children. Often a family history of asthma, allergies or eczema.

Clinical features

Mild asthmatics may have only chronic cough, particularly nocturnal or exercise-induced. More severe symptoms include wheezing and respiratory distress. Children with chronic under-treated asthma may develop chest deformity (Fig. 260) and growth failure.

Management

Severity of attack best assessed by monitoring peak flow. Acute bronchospasm usually responds to inhaled beta-sympathomimetics or xanthines. Prophylaxis with inhaled sodium cromoglycate or corticosteroids is helpful in chronic asthma.

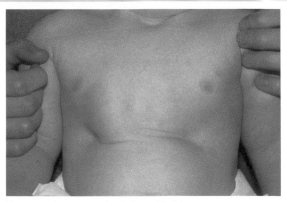

Fig. 259   Chest recession in bronchiolitis.

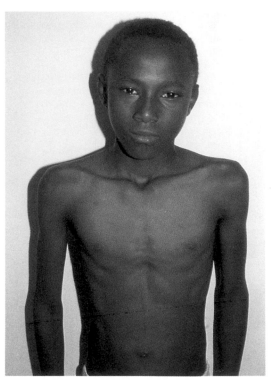

Fig. 260   Chest deformity in a chronic asthmatic.

Pneumonia

Aetiology

In infancy, bronchopneumonia is usually caused by *Haemophilus influenzae* or rarely by *Staphylococcus aureus*. Pneumococcal infection causes lobar pneumonia (Fig. 261) in older children. Mycoplasma pneumonia is also common.

Clinical features

Fever, tachypnoea, meningism and feeding difficulties. Localizing signs are often absent in infants, so chest X-ray is usually necessary in any ill child. Recurrent chest infections, wheeze or localized air-trapping is sometimes due to inhalation of a foreign body.

Management

Broad-spectrum antibiotics until specific organism and sensitivities identified. Erythromycin if Mycoplasma is suspected.

Cystic fibrosis

Incidence

The most common cause of suppurative chronic lung disease and pancreatic insufficiency in children in the UK, USA and Australia. Autosomal recessive inheritance; carrier rate in general population is 1 in 20. Cystic fibrosis affects 1 in 1600 live births.

Aetiology

Abnormality of exocrine and mucus-secreting glands; aetiology unknown. Heterozygote carriers are asymptomatic, but are detectable by genetic analysis.

Clinical features

Meconium ileus and neonatal gut obstruction. Recurrent chest infections (Fig. 262), failure to thrive and malabsorption. Clubbing of fingers and toes may occur.

Diagnosis

Sweat test is definitive diagnostic test. Elevated plasma immunoreactive trypsin in first few weeks of life in those with pancreatic insufficiency. Antenatal diagnosis is now possible in affected families using DNA analysis from chorionic villus sampling.

Management

Pancreatic supplements control malabsorption. Prompt and aggressive treatment of chest infections with antibiotics and postural drainage. Prophylactic antibiotics may be helpful. Long-term survival into adult life depends on severity of chest involvement. Chronic chest deformity and infections caused by antibiotic-resistant organisms frequently develop.

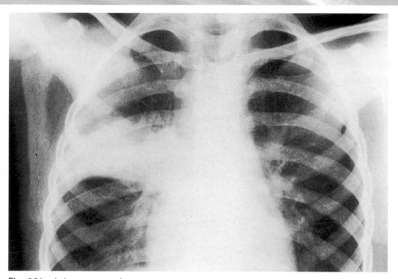

Fig. 261 Lobar pneumonia.

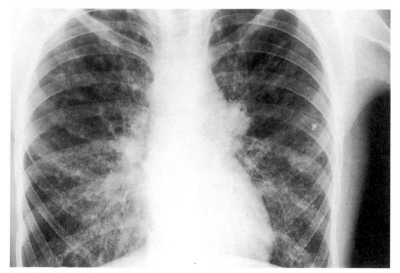

Fig. 262 Cystic fibrosis.

Congenital heart disease

Incidence

Common; at least 1 in 300 live births.

Diagnosis

Asymptomatic cardiac murmurs are often heard during routine examination. Cyanosis (Fig. 264) or heart failure usually indicate a serious structural defect. Clubbing of fingers (Fig. 263) and toes may develop in conditions such as Fallot's tetralogy. Echocardiogram and cardiac catheterization give precise detail of cardiac structure. Chest X-ray and electrocardiogram are helpful, but rarely diagnostic. Coarctation of aorta is suspected when there is inequality or delay of femoral pulses.

Management

Depends on underlying problem. Most common abnormality is ventricular septal defect which usually closes spontaneously. Surgery may be required for more serious defects.

Acute laryngo-tracheo-bronchitis (croup)

Incidence

Common under 4 years of age. Usually a viral illness.

Clinical features

Coryzal symptoms for a few days, then a characteristic barking cough and inspiratory stridor (croup). Symptoms often worse at night or when child is anxious or crying.

Management

Oxygen is often needed. Nebulized budesonide and oral dexamethasone reduce severity of symptoms. Occasionally, tracheal intubation may be required if there is severe airway obstruction.

Acute epiglottitis

Aetiology and incidence

Potentially fatal *Haemophilus influenzae* type B infection. Uncommon after HiB vaccination.

Clinical features

Sudden onset of stridor, toxicity and airways obstruction.

Management

Examination of throat is contraindicated unless there is immediate expert provision for tracheal intubation (Fig. 265) which is often difficult. Intravenous ampicillin or a cephalosporin usually controls oedema and inflammation of epiglottis within 48 h.

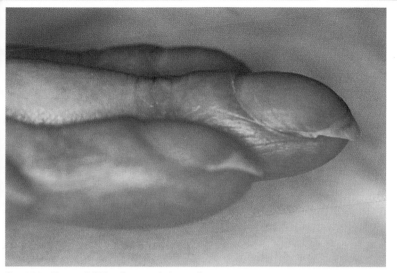

Fig. 263 Finger clubbing in cyanotic heart disease.

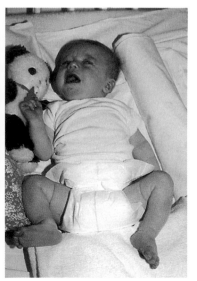

Fig. 264 Cyanotic congenital heart disease.

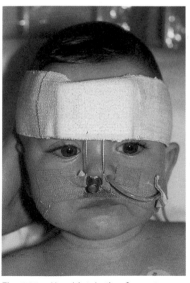

Fig. 265 Nasal intubation for acute epiglottitis.

Congenital anomalies

Acute glaucoma

Congenital condition producing increased pressure inside eye from lack of drainage at angle of anterior chamber. The eye becomes large (buphthalmos) and the cornea becomes cloudy (Fig. 266). Urgent referral to ophthalmologist for decompression and surgery.

Cataract

Usually congenital and sometimes familial. Secondary cataracts occur in rubella embryopathy, galactosaemia and diabetes. Opacity in the lens (Fig. 267) is seen. Other ocular anomalies such as nystagmus or visual disturbance are often present. Management depends on cause and likelihood of interference with vision. Early surgery within the first months diminishes the risk of subsequent amblyopia.

Microphthalmos

Developmental anomaly often associated with congenital rubella. Surgery may improve appearance if the palpebral fissure is short.

Ptosis

Often familial and usually unilateral. In the majority of cases, binocular vision is unaffected. Shortening of the levator palpebrae superioris may improve the cosmetic appearance, or improve vision if ptosis is severe and the eyelid covers the pupil.

Coloboma

Developmental anomaly of the iris (Fig. 268). Often familial. Vision is usually unaffected, unless there is a retinal anomaly.

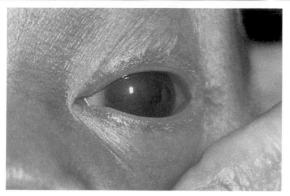

Fig. 266   Cloudy large cornea in congenital glaucoma.

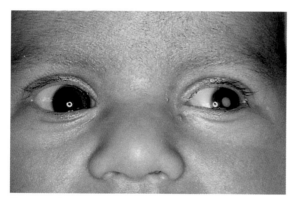

Fig. 267   Cataract.

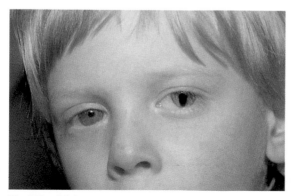

Fig. 268   Coloboma.

Strabismus (squint)

Incidence

Common in early childhood. All fixed squints and any squint persisting after 5–6 months of age require careful evaluation.

Clinical features

Usually obvious (Fig. 269). Symmetrical corneal reflection or occlusion testing may assist diagnosis in less obvious cases. Epicanthic folds may give rise to a false appearance of squint.

Management and prognosis

Suppression of vision (amblyopia) in the deviated eye may be permanent if squint is not detected and treated early. Correction of refractive error and occlusion of the non-squinting eye are mandatory. Surgery is sometimes necessary.

Malignancy

Incidence and inheritance

Retinoblastoma is the most common malignant intraocular tumour in childhood. Sometimes autosomal dominant inheritance.

Clinical features

Opacity of pupil, squint or poor vision in affected eye. Proptosis occurs with tumours involving the orbit, particularly metastatic neuroblastoma.

Management

Treatment of retinoblastoma includes surgery and radiotherapy. Metastases are rare and long-term prognosis is good.

External angular dermoid cyst

Commonly found around the orbit, usually above and lateral to the palpebral fissure. Surgery is usually necessary to improve appearance, because the cysts gradually increase in size.

Infection and trauma

Conjunctivitis is common in neonatal period. Recurrent mild conjunctivitis (Fig. 270) is usually due to non-patency of the nasolacrimal duct which resolves in the first year of life. In older children, painful corneal abrasions are usually caused by foreign bodies in the eye. Conjunctival haemorrhage may occur after birth or in association with direct trauma (Fig. 271).

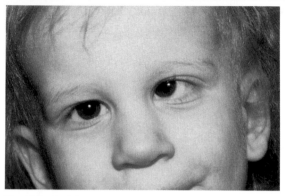

Fig. 269 Squint.

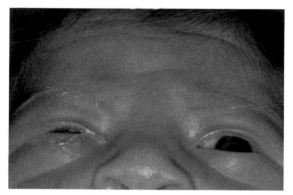

Fig. 270 Recurrent minor conjunctivitis.

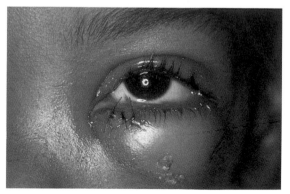

Fig. 271 Traumatic eye lesion with laceration and conjunctival haemorrhage.

Aetiology

Non-accidental injury (NAI) or child abuse usually occurs when parents or other adults caring for children injure the dependent but demanding child. Child abuse may also take the more subtle form of physical or emotional neglect or deprivation.

Clinical features

There is often a history of supposed accident. Suspicion should be aroused when history and injury are conflicting, inconsistent or repeated. Unexplained fractures or bruises, particularly multiple or of varying age, are often found. Rough handling or direct hitting may cause fractures of ribs or long bones. Gripping and shaking an infant may leave finger-mark bruises, posterior rib fractures, retinal and intracranial haemorrhage. Babies may suffer serious long-term neurodevelopmental disability as a result of shaken baby syndrome. Cigarette burns (Fig. 272) leave discrete punched out lesions. Whip marks (Fig. 273) are more common in older children. Dip-burns to the buttocks and feet (Fig. 274) occur when an infant is lowered into scalding water. Human bite marks (Fig. 275) are sometimes clearly seen. Careful measurement of the size of the teeth marks will determine whether an adult or child has inflicted the bite injury.

Management

If non-accidental injury is suspected, society has a responsibility to protect the child. In addition to medical treatment of the injuries, this will involve multi-disciplinary assessment of the family situation and possible contributing factors, and exclusion of alternative diagnoses. With careful supervision and sympathetic support, many children can continue to be cared for by their parents. Occasionally, the child may be safer in the care of others.

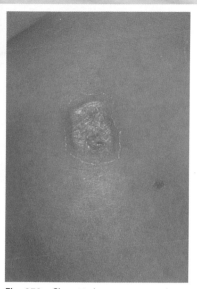

Fig. 272 Cigarette burn.

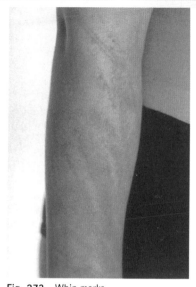

Fig. 273 Whip marks.

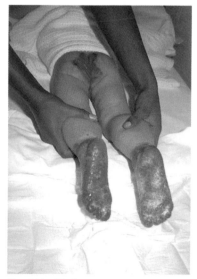

Fig. 274 Dip-burns.

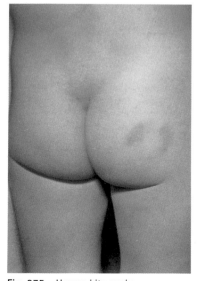

Fig. 275 Human bite marks.

Recognized with increasing frequency recently. Only a minority of cases are associated with a sudden or violent attack. In most cases, the children have been abused by somebody in the family or known to the child; therefore, acute injury is uncommon.

Presentation

It is important that a child who gives a suspicious history of abuse is believed. Children may present with many minor symptoms including vaginal discharge, vaginal bleeding, urinary tract infection, abdominal pain, or perineal soreness and irritation. A change in behaviour may be extremely significant.

Physical signs

The majority show no abnormal physical signs, but there are important pointers to the diagnosis even though they occur in only 10–30% of cases. Visible bruising in the perineal region and a torn hymen, although uncommon, may be diagnostic of violent abuse. Most vaginal discharge (Fig. 276) is not due to sexually transmitted infection, but occasionally gonorrhoea may be diagnosed on culture. Other infections, such as genital warts (Fig. 277) can be transmitted by sexual contact, but proving that this was due to child sexual abuse is difficult because there may be other methods of transmission of the human papilloma virus, particularly in very young children. An infant can become infected with papilloma virus during birth by normal vaginal delivery of an asymptomatic but infected mother, and the lesions in the child may take up to 2 years to develop. Whenever there is vulval bleeding or soreness, a careful inspection should be made to see if there are signs such as gaping vagina or anus. The limits of normality are difficult to define: always ask an experienced clinician to make an assessment if in doubt. Other medical conditions, lichen sclerosis et atrophicus (Fig. 278) or rare conditions such as vulval psoriasis (Fig. 279), may be mistaken for child sexual abuse.

Management

The management of suspected child sexual abuse requires great skill. A senior and experienced clinician must be involved and appropriate consultations made with police and social services. Long-term family therapy or individual counselling are often needed to support children and families. Occasionally, legal steps may need to be taken to protect the child.

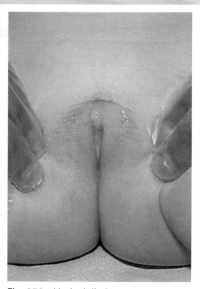

Fig. 276 Vaginal discharge.

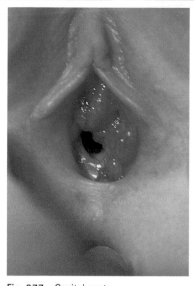

Fig. 277 Genital warts.

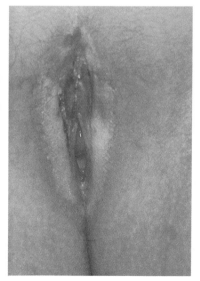

Fig. 278 Lichen sclerosus et atrophicus.

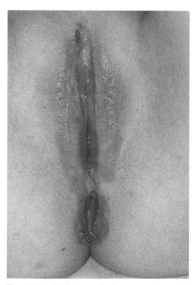

Fig. 279 Vulval psoriasis.

Guilt and a sense of failure often accompany the birth of a low birth weight infant. The appearance, behaviour and illness of a preterm infant may be difficult for the parents to accept and understand. Discussion and explanation of the infant's condition and management, including the awesome equipment of the modern neonatal unit, will help to alleviate some of the uncertainty faced by the family, even though an accurate prediction of outcome cannot be made in the early stages. Unnecessary admission of well, low birth weight infants to a specialized neonatal unit should be avoided whenever possible, as such admission always results in separation for some members of the family. Open visiting for all family members, including siblings (Figs 280 and 281) should be encouraged, and some contribution towards active participation in the infant's care is usually possible and is always satisfying. This may include nursing, cuddling, nappy changing, bathing and feeding all but the most ill preterm infant. Even in the event of the death of the baby, parents are often best supported by allowing them to participate in the final decisions and moments of the infant's life. With understanding and good support, many problems and parental anxieties can be overcome.

Admission to hospital is distressing for all of us, but it is worse for children. A child under 5 years may not only be frightened by the illness and painful procedures, but also may be even more upset by separation from the family. It is very important that someone already known to the child should stay with them in hospital; preferably this should be one of the parents. Parents, siblings and other relatives on the ward often add to the work of the staff because they naturally expect to ask questions about the tests and treatment that is happening to their child. Even so, their presence helps the staff to care for the ill child better, and makes the stay in hospital much less frightening for the child. After-effects, such as nightmares, clinging and a recurrence of enuresis, are less common in children whose mothers stay with them in hospital. Play allows children to bear the strain of the admission (Fig. 282) and often reveals information about their physical and emotional problems. It is very important that in a long chronic illness there should be help with schoolwork to minimize disruption to the child's daily life and educational progress.

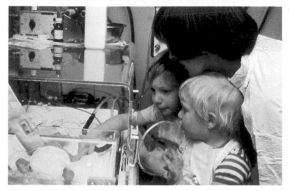

Fig. 280 Siblings visiting neonatal nursery.

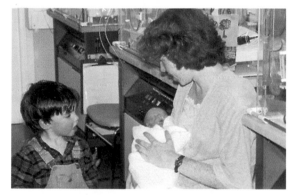

Fig. 281 Showing the baby to her brother.

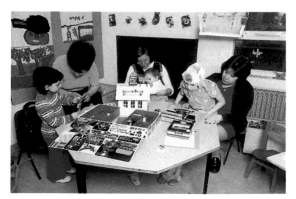

Fig. 282 Hospital playgroup with children and parents.

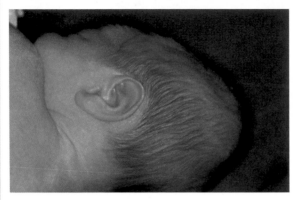

1. Head of a 2-day-old infant.

a. What is the differential diagnosis?
b. How can a specific diagnosis be made?
c. What is the significance and natural history of the conditions?

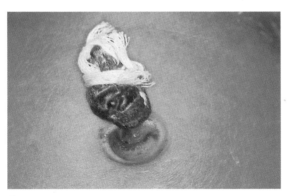

2. Umbilical cord of a 5-day-old infant.

a. What is the diagnosis?
b. What is the management of this condition?

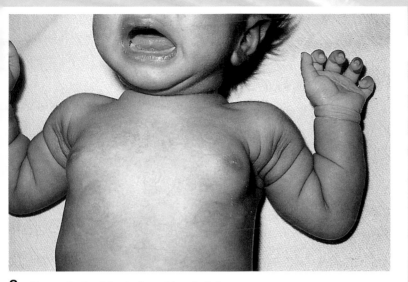

3. Chest of a healthy 3-day-old male infant.

a. What is the diagnosis?
b. Describe other associated conditions.
c. What explanation should be given to the parents?

4. Thigh of a healthy thriving
4-week-old infant.

a. What is the differential diagnosis?
b. How can they be differentiated
   clinically?
c. Describe the management of both
   conditions.

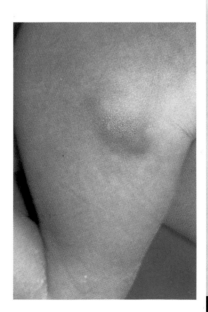

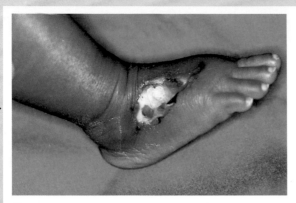

5. Ulceration of foot of a 6-week-old preterm infant.

a. What is the most likely cause of the ulceration?
b. How may long-term damage be limited?

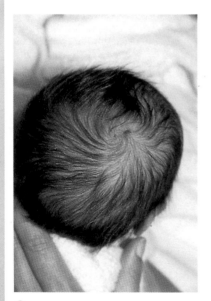

6. Lesion on scalp of newborn infant.

a. What is the differential diagnosis?
b. Name three procedures that may cause a similar lesion.
c. What is the purpose of the procedures?

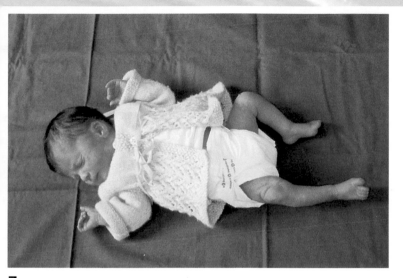

7. Newborn infant with head turned towards the right.

a. Which neonatal reflex is being demonstrated?
b. Name at least four other neonatal reflexes.
c. What is the relevance of neonatal reflexes?

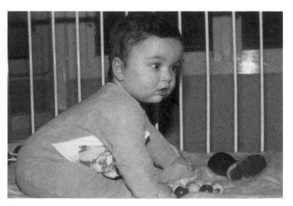

8. Infant sitting in tripod position.

a. What is the age of the infant?
b. What other motor milestones should be achieved by this age?

9. A 5-year-old child in the standing position.

a. What is the paediatrician doing?
b. What is the instrument called?
c. How is the test applied in younger infants?

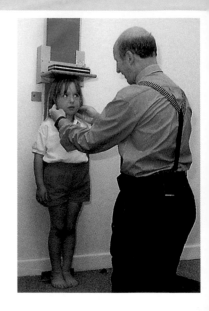

10. Face of an irritable, listless infant with poor appetite.

a. What features are shown?
b. What is the diagnosis and cause?
c. What is the treatment?

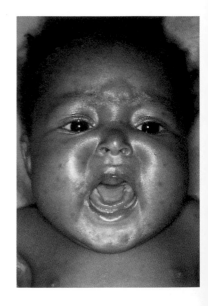

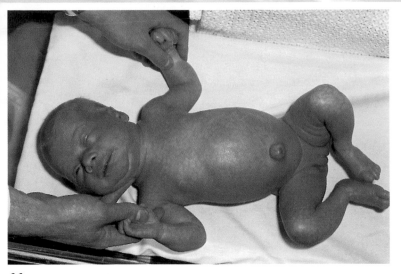

11. A 3-week-old infant.

a. Which clinical signs are shown?
b. What is the underlying diagnosis?
c. Name other associated signs and symptoms.
d. What is the prognosis of this condition?

12. Small white lesion on prepuce of a newborn male infant.

a. What is the diagnosis?
b. What is the underlying pathology?
c. Where may similar lesions occur?

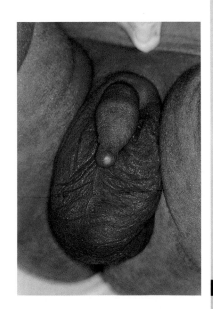

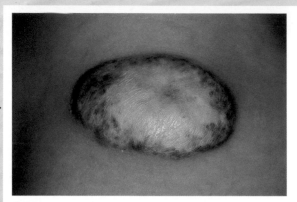

13. Skin lesion on a child now aged 2 years. The lesion developed a few weeks after birth and was bright red for about 18 months.

a. What is the diagnosis?
b. What is the natural course of this type of lesion?
c. What are the complications?

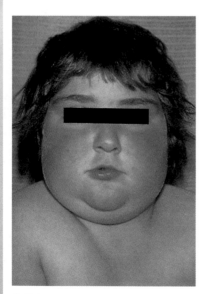

14. Face of a 10-year-old boy.

a. What is the differential diagnosis?
b. Which other clinical features would be helpful to support the diagnosis?
c. Which biochemical investigations will assist in diagnosis?

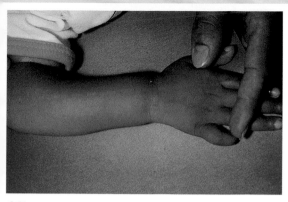

15. Hands and forearm of a 3-year-old child.

a. What is the diagnosis?
b. Name other clinical signs.
c. What are the classic biochemical and radiological changes?

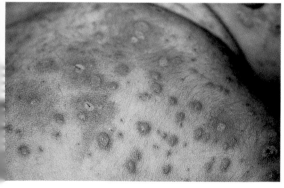

16. Itchy rash in an otherwise healthy 5-year-old child.

a. What is the diagnosis?
b. What is the incubation period of this infection?
c. What advice should be given to the child's mother who is 39 weeks' pregnant?

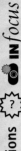

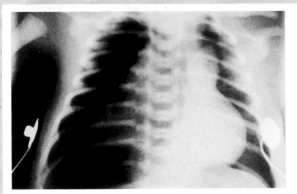

17. Chest X-ray of a 4-hour-old infant with respiratory distress.

a. What is the diagnosis?

a. Name associated clinical signs.

b. What are the predisposing conditions?

c. How should this condition be managed?

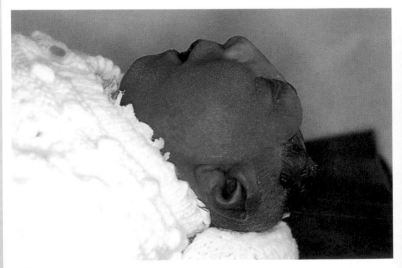

18. Newborn infant who died a few hours after birth.

a. What is the diagnosis?

b. Name other associated anomalies.

c. What is the prognosis and management of this condition?

19. Back of a newborn infant.

a. What is the diagnosis?
b. How can the diagnosis be confirmed?
c. What is the recurrence risk in future pregnancies?
d. How can the risk be reduced?

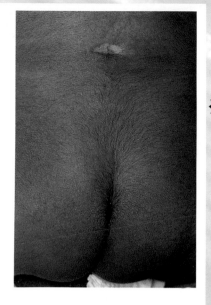

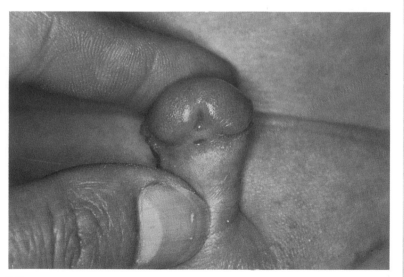

20. Phallus of a newborn infant.

a. What is the diagnosis?
b. What are associated conditions?
c. What is the management of this condition?

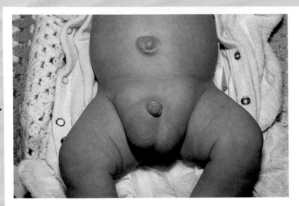

21. Abdomen and genitalia of a 6-month-old infant.

a. What are the diagnoses?
b. What are predisposing factors?
c. What is management of these conditions?

22. A 14-year-old girl with short stature.

a. Describe the clinical features shown.
b. What is the diagnosis?
c. Name associated problems.
d. What is the management of the condition?

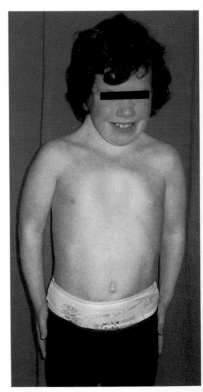

23. Neck swelling in a 6-month-old infant.

a. What is the differential diagnosis?
b. Which other clinical signs help to confirm the diagnosis?
c. What is the management of these conditions?

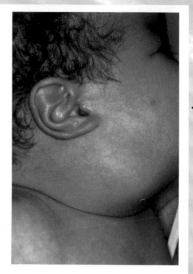

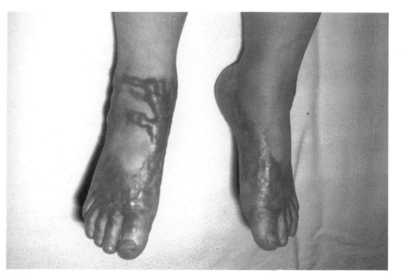

24. Feet of a 3-year-old child.

a. What is the diagnosis?
b. What are predisposing factors?
c. How can this condition be treated?

25. This is a 4-year-old boy with learning difficulties.

a. What is the diagnosis?
b. Name other associated features of this condition.
c. Which investigations will be helpful?

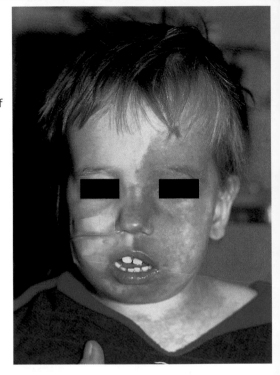

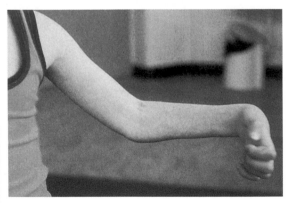

26. This 9-year-old boy had a fracture of the elbow some months previously.

a. What is the diagnosis?
b. What is the aetiology of the condition?

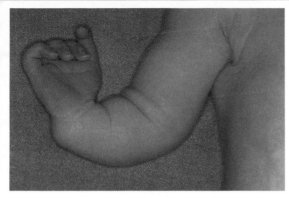

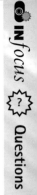

27. This is the forearm and hand of a young infant.

a. What features are shown?
b. Which investigations will be helpful?

28. Abdominal X-ray of a newborn infant.

a. What is the diagnosis?
b. How would this infant present?
c. Name other associated problems.

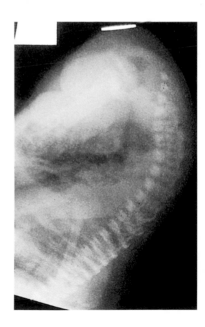

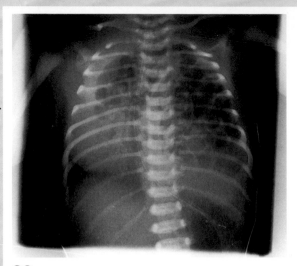

29. Chest X-ray of a neonate with respiratory distress soon after birth.

a. What is the diagnosis?
b. What is the emergency treatment of this condition?
c. What is the prognosis?

30. Abdomen of 3-month-old ex-preterm infant.

a. Describe the clinical features shown.
b. What is the treatment?
c. What is the prognosis?

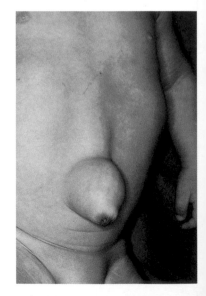

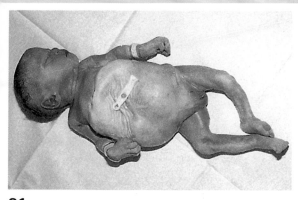

31. Newborn infant who could not be resuscitated at birth.

a. What is the diagnosis?
b. Describe the clinical features.
c. What is the likely cause of death?
d. How can this condition be diagnosed antenatally?

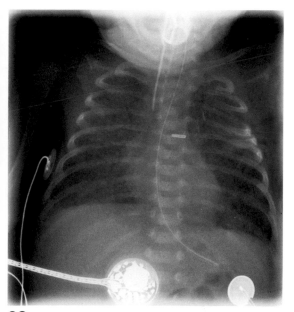

32. Chest X-ray of ex-preterm infant who required long term oxygen therapy.

a. What is the diagnosis?
b. What operative procedure has been performed?
c. What is the long term prognosis?

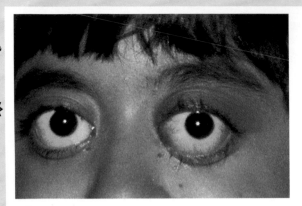

33. Eyes of a 12-year-old boy.

a. What clinical sign is shown?
b. What is the differential diagnosis?

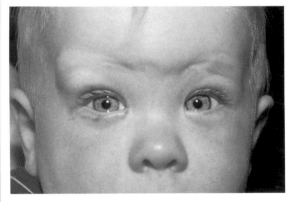

34. Face of a 9-month-old infant.

a. What is the diagnosis?
b. What is the aetiology?
c. What is the prognosis and management?

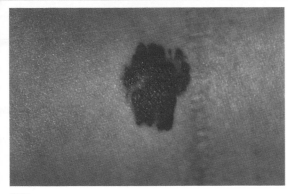

35. Skin lesion on a 9-month-old child.

a. What is the diagnosis?
b. Describe the clinical course of this type of lesion.
c. What are the complications?
d. What are the associations?

36. Perineum of a 4-day-old female infant.

a. What is the diagnosis?
b. What is the cause and significance of this condition?

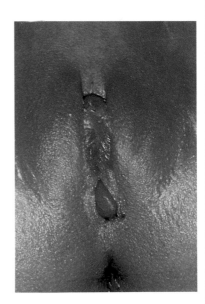

37. Breast-feeding.

a. What are the benefits of breast-feeding?
b. Are there any contraindications?

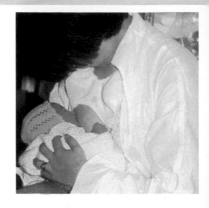

38. Back of a 2-year-old child who had collodion skin at birth.

a. What is the diagnosis?
b. What is the treatment?
c. What is the prognosis?

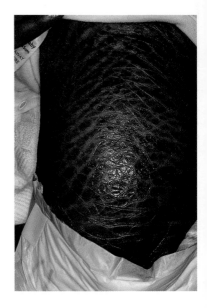

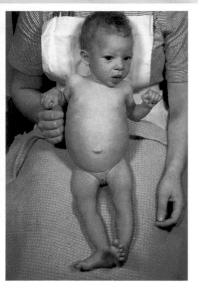
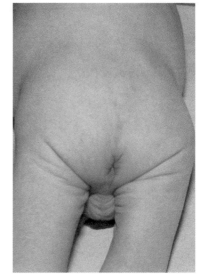

39. A 12-month-old infant with poor appetite and poor weight gain.

a. What is the most likely diagnosis?
b. What is the underlying cause?
c. What other clinical signs and symptoms may occur?

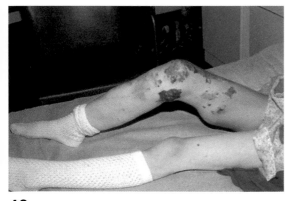

40. Legs of a 10-year-old girl.

a. Describe the clinical features shown.
b. What is the diagnosis?
c. What are the underlying pathology and associations?
d. What is the mode of inheritance?

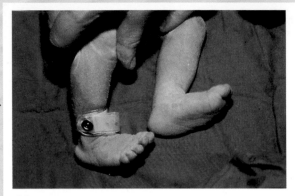

41. Feet of a newborn infant.

a. Describe the foot abnormality.
b. What is the differential diagnosis?
c. Name other associated clinical features.

42. Abdomen of a 10-day-old infant.

a. What is the diagnosis?
b. What is the aetiology of this condition?
c. What is the treatment?

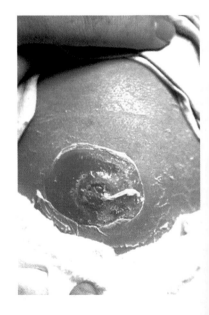

43. Leg of a newborn infant whose mother had an itchy rash in early pregnancy.

a. What is the diagnosis?
b. How is this condition treated in late pregnancy?

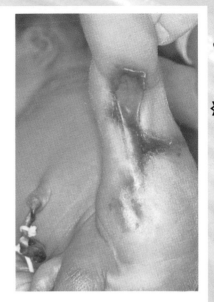

44. An 8-year-old child with generalized lymphadenopathy and poor growth.

a. What is the diagnosis?
b. What are the underlying causes?

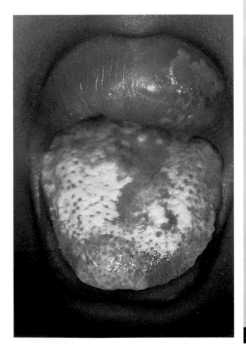

45. Head and ear of an 8-week-old infant.

a. What is the diagnosis?
b. Are there any other manifestations?
c. What is the treatment?

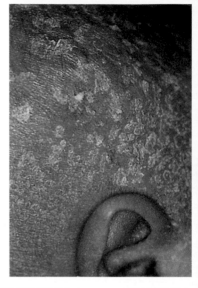

46. Chest of a breast-fed 10-month-old infant.

a. What is the diagnosis?
b. What is the usual management of this condition?
c. Are there any other underlying causes?

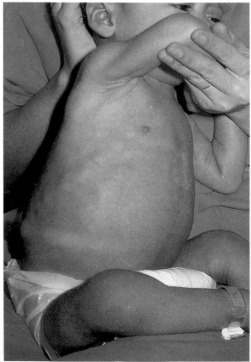

47. Limb of a 5-year-old child.

a. What is the diagnosis?
b. What are the associations?
c. What is the management?

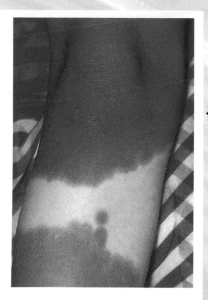

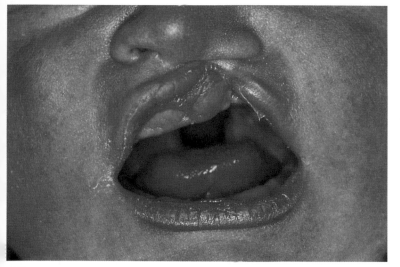

48. Face of a young infant.

a. What are the complications associated with this condition?
b. What is the risk of recurrence in future pregnancies?

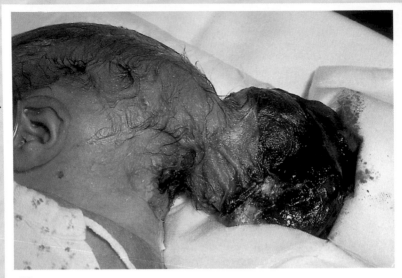

49. Head and neck of a newborn infant.

a. What is the diagnosis?
c. What are the complications?
d. What is the recurrence risk in future pregnancies?

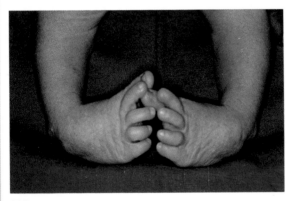

50. Feet of a newborn infant born to a mother with oligohydramnios.

a. What is the cause of this condition?
b. What is the management?
c. Are there any other associated anomalies?

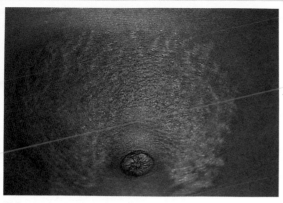

51. Abdomen of a 10-year-old boy.

a. What is the clinical sign?
b. Name two underlying causes and other associated clinical features.

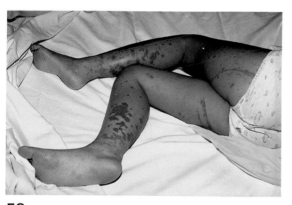

52. This 6-year-old child presented with difficulty in walking.

a. What is the diagnosis?
b. Which investigations will be helpful?
c. What is the prognosis?

53. Ear of an 8-year-old child with a pyrexia of unknown origin and abdominal pain.

a. What is the differential diagnosis?
b. What are the potentially serious complications of these conditions?

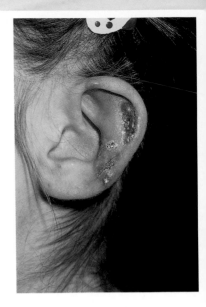

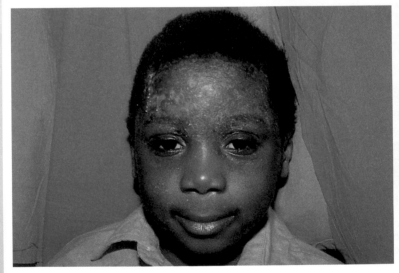

54. This 8-year-old boy has asthma.

a. What is the diagnosis?
b. Which other sites are commonly affected?
c. What are the complications of this condition?

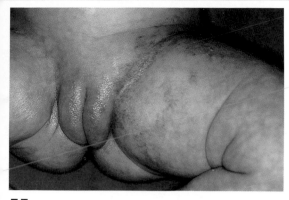

55. Thigh of a 4-week-old infant with poor feeding.

a. What is the differential diagnosis?
b. Which investigations will be helpful?
c. What is the treatment of this condition?

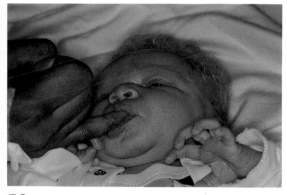

56. Child born to African parents.

a. What is the diagnosis?
b. What are the associated conditions?
c. What is the management of this condition?

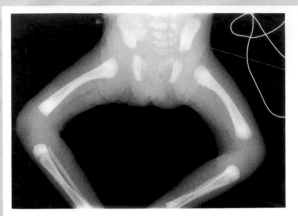

57. X-ray of a newborn with intra-uterine growth retardation and thrombocytopenia.

a. Describe the bony abnormality.
b. What is the diagnosis?
c. Name other clinical associations.

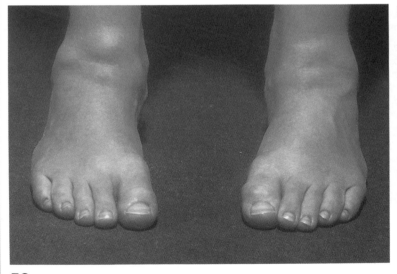

58. This 8-year-old has difficulty in walking.

a. What is the differential diagnosis?
b. Which investigations will be helpful?
c. What is the management?

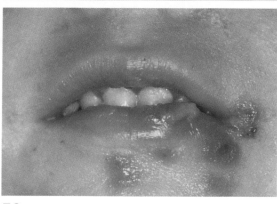

59. Mouth of a 2-year-old child.

a. What are the symptoms of this condition?
b. What is the diagnosis?
c. Describe the clinical course and complications.

60. A 4-year-old boy with a heart murmur.

a. What is the diagnosis?
b. What are the clinical signs?
c. What is the underlying cardiac condition?
d. What is the mode of inheritance?

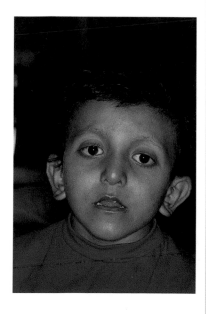

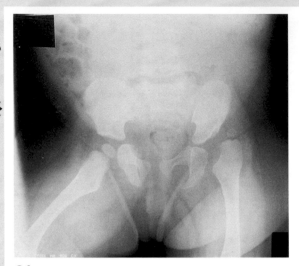

61. X-ray of the pelvis of a 16-month-old child with an abnormal gait.

a. What is the diagnosis?
b. What are predisposing factors?
c. How is the condition treated?

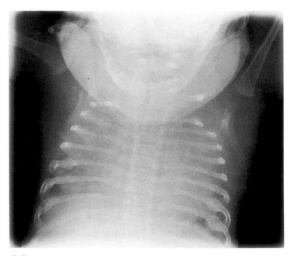

62. Chest X-ray of 3-month-old infant born at 25 weeks' gestation.

a. What are the abnormal radiological signs?
b. What are the causes of these conditions?
c. How can the risk of these conditions be reduced?

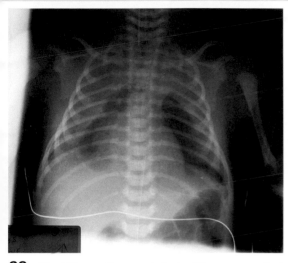

63. Chest X-ray of a term infant with severe respiratory distress.

a. What is the diagnosis?
b. What are predisposing conditions?
c. What is the management of this condition?

64. A 3-month-old ex-preterm infant.

a. Which clinical signs are shown?
b. Which investigations may be helpful?
c. What is the management of this condition?

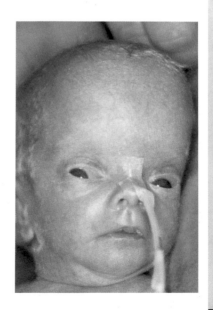

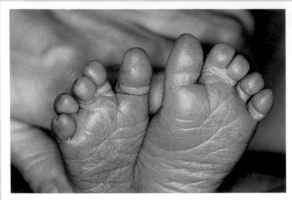

65. Feet of a newborn infant.

a. What is the diagnosis?
b. What is the significance of this condition?

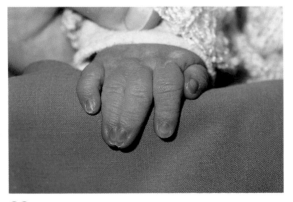

66. Hand of a young infant.

a. What is the diagnosis?
b. What is the management of this condition?

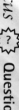

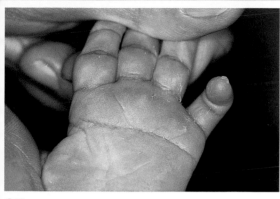

67. Hand of newborn infant.

a. What is the clinical sign?
b. What is the clinical significance of this sign?
c. What are other associated clinical features?

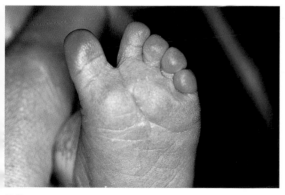

68. Foot of a young infant.

a. What is the clinical sign?
b. Which diseases are more common in children with this condition?

69. Anus and perineum of a 3-year-old male infant.

a. What are the lesions?
b. How are these lesions acquired?
c. Which investigations will be helpful?

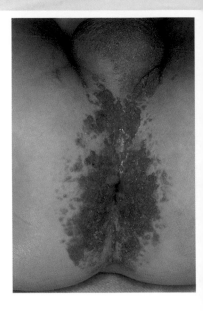

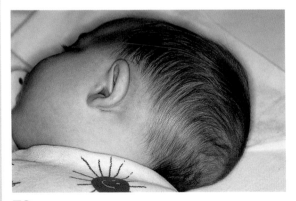

70. 10-month-old infant with a bluish swelling behind the right ear.

a. What is the diagnosis?
b. What is the management of this condition?

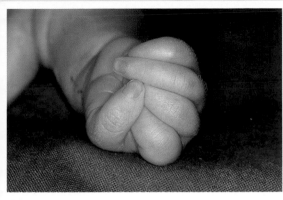

71. Hand of a term newborn infant of birth weight 1850 g.

a. What is the diagnosis?
b. What are other clinical features of this condition?
c. What is the life expectancy of infants with this condition?

72. Ear of a young infant.

a. What is the diagnosis?
b. Which investigations should be undertaken?
c. What is the inheritance of this condition?

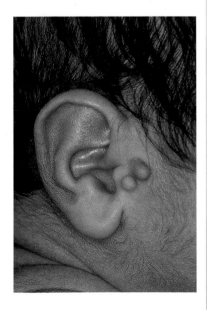

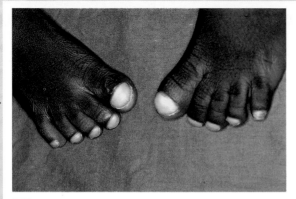

73. Toes of a 4-year-old child with failure to thrive.

a. What is the diagnosis?
b. What are the underlying causes?
c. Which investigations will be helpful?

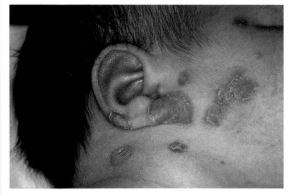

74. Face of a 6-week-old infant.

a. What are the lesions?
b. What is the underlying cause?
c. What is the management of this condition?

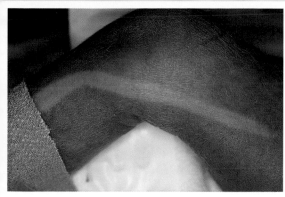

75. Leg of a sick preterm infant with an intravenous infusion in the foot.

a. What is the diagnosis?
b. What is the management of this complication?

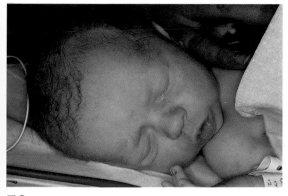

76. Newborn infant with Hb 3.5 g/dl.

a. What is the differential diagnosis?
b. Which investigations will be helpful?

77. Trunk of an 18-month-old child with seizures.

a. What are the clinical signs shown on the skin?
b. What is the diagnosis?
c. What is the inheritance of this condition?

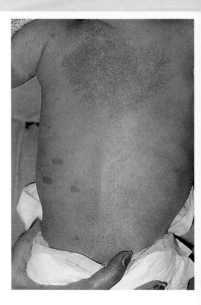

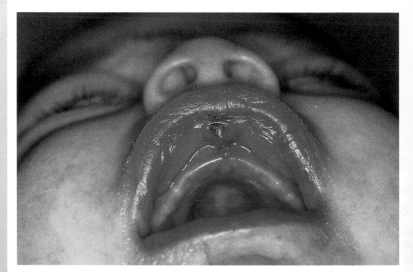

78. Mouth of an irritable young infant.

a. What is the diagnosis?
b. What is the underlying cause?
c. What is the management?

79. Legs of a 7-year-old boy who has difficulty running.

a. What is the clinical sign?
b. What is the diagnosis?
c. What other signs and symptoms occur in this condition?
d. How can the diagnosis be confirmed?

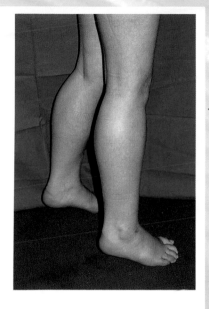

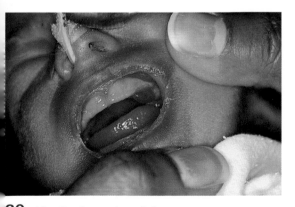

80. Mouth of a newborn infant.

a. What is the diagnosis?
b. What symptoms will occur?
c. What is the management of this condition?

81. Back of a newborn infant.

a. What are the clinical signs?
b. What are the differential diagnoses?
c. Which investigations will be helpful?

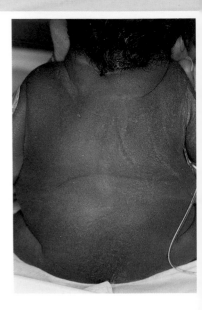

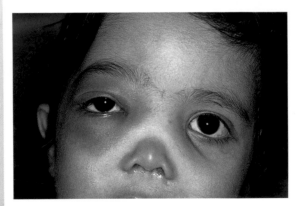

82. Face of a 2-year-old child.

a. What is the diagnosis?
b. What is the treatment of this condition?
c. What complications may occur?

83. A 4-month-old infant.

a. What is the clinical sign shown?
b. What is the likely diagnosis?
c. What is the aetiology of this condition?

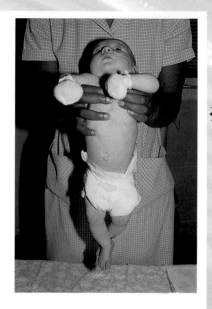

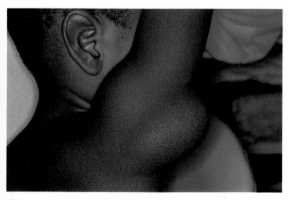

84. Painless swelling under the arm of a 2-year-old child.

a. What is the differential diagnosis?
b. What is the management of this condition?
c. What is the recurrence risk?

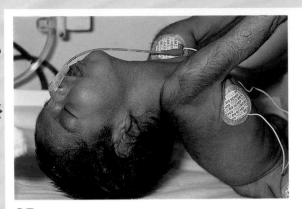

85. Newborn infant being pulled up by forearms.

a. What clinical sign is shown?
b. What is the differential diagnosis?
c. Which investigations will be helpful?

86. Chest of a 3-day-old neonate.

a. What is the diagnosis?
b. What is the treatment?
c. What is the prognosis?

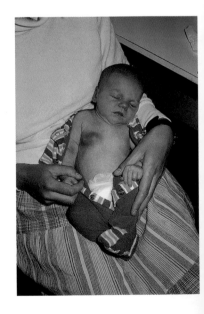

87. Neck of a newborn term infant.

a. What is the diagnosis?
b. Which investigations will be helpful?

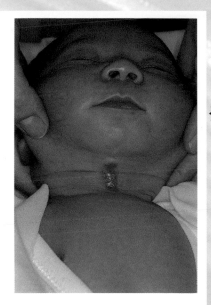

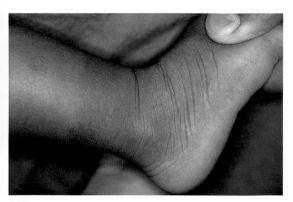

88. Foot of a 4-month-old infant.

a. What is the diagnosis?
b. Where is the lesion most commonly seen?
c. What is the course and prognosis?

89. Chest and axilla of a newborn male infant.

a. What is the diagnosis?
b. What is the management of this condtion?

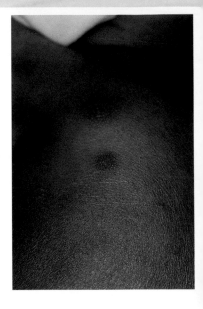

90. Postmortem examination of a pale, hydropic neonate born with Hb 2 g/dl.

a. What is the abdominal organ?
b. What is the differential diagnosis?
c. What maternal investigations will raise suspicion of the diagnosis antenatally?

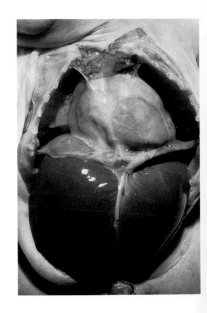

91. A 2-year-old child with a painful swelling in the neck.

a. What is the diagnosis?
b. Which organisms are commonly involved?
c. What is the management of the condition?

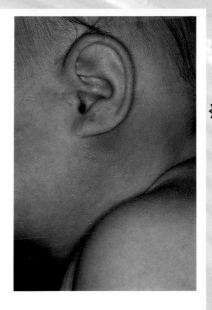

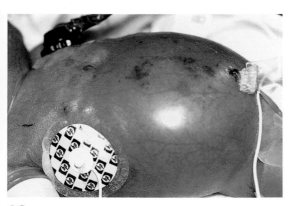

92. Abdomen of a 3-day-old born at 26 weeks' gestation.

a. Which clinical signs are shown?
b. What is the likely diagnosis?
c. Which signs are associated with a poor prognosis?

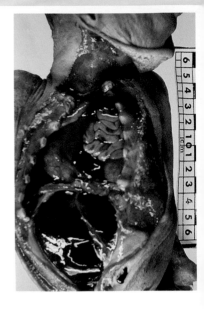

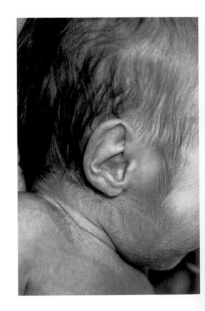

93. Postmortem of a newborn infant who did not respond to resuscitation.

a. What is the diagnosis?
b. Which clinical signs occur in this condition?
c. What is the emergency treatment?

94. Painful swelling in front of the ear of a baby.

a. What is the diagnosis?
b. What are the underlying causes?
c. What is the treatment?

95. Discoloration behind the ear of a 5-year-old child.

a. What is the diagnosis?
b. What is the underlying cause?
c. What is the management?

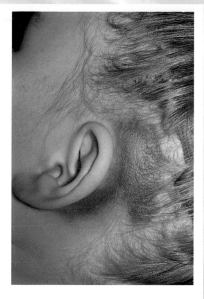

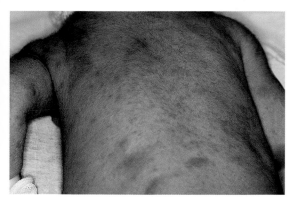

96. Erythematous rash on the trunk of a 10-day-old infant.

a. What is the diagnosis?
b. What symptoms occur in this condition?
c. What is the course and prognosis?

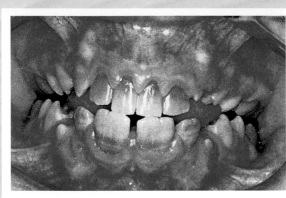

97. Teeth of a 12-year-old with a chronic cough.

a. What is the diagnosis?
b. Which other system will be affected?
c. How can the condition be prevented?

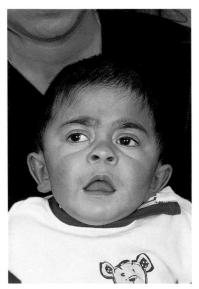

98. This 12-month-old child has delayed development.

a. What are the clinical features and differential diagnosis?
b. Which radiological changes occur in this condition?
c. How can the diagnosis be confirmed?

99. This is an 8-year-old boy with increasing head growth since infancy.

a. What is the diagnosis?
b. What signs and symptoms will he develop?
c. What is the inheritance of this condition?

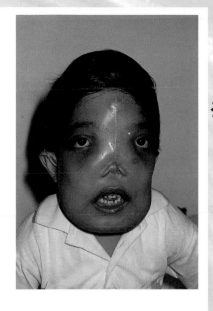

100. Scalp of a healthy young infant.

a. What is the differential diagnosis?
b. How can the diagnosis be confirmed?
c. What is the management?

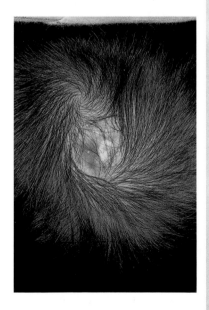

101. Newborn infant with anaemia and thrombocytopenia.

a. What is the diagnosis?
b. What are associated complications?
c. Which investigations will be helpful?

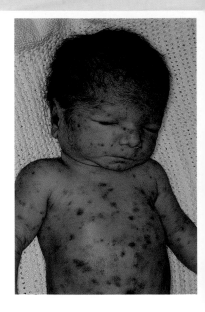

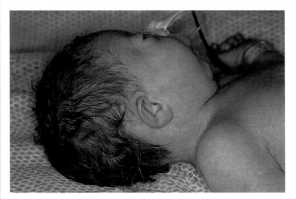

102. Head and neck of a young infant.

a. What abnormal features are shown?
b. What associated abnormalities may be found?
c. What investigations will help to identify associated anomalies?

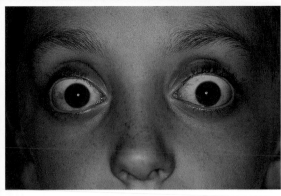

103. Eyes of a 12-year-old girl.

a. What is the clinical sign?
b. Which other signs and symptoms may be present?
c. What is the treatment of this condition?

104. Back of a newborn infant.

a. What is the lesion?
b. What is the significance of the lesion?
c. How can it be treated?

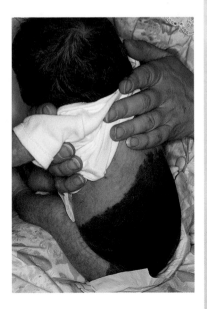

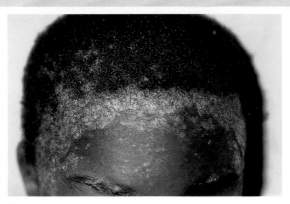

105. Forehead of a 12-year-old boy.

a. What is the diagnosis?
b. What are the complications and associations of this condition?
c. What is the treatment?

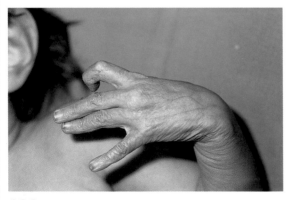

106. Hand of an infant with a high arched palate.

a. What is the differential diagnosis?
b. What are associated features?

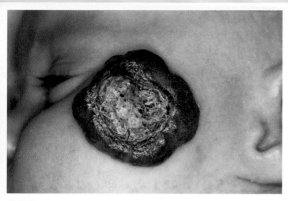

107. Lesion on the cheek of a healthy thriving 8-month-old infant.

a. What is the diagnosis?
b. What is the management?
c. What is the prognosis?

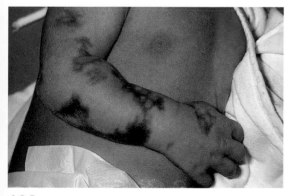

108. Arm of a healthy newborn infant.

a. What is the diagnosis?
b. Which investigations should be performed?
c. What are the long term complications?

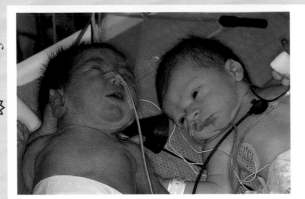

109. These newborn infants are twins.

a. What is the diagnosis?
b. What are the complications of this condition?

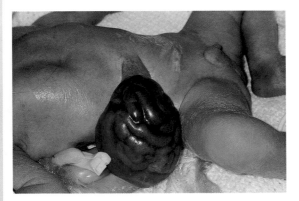

110. Abdomen of a newborn infant.

a. What is the diagnosis?
b. What is the management of this condition?
c. Which chromosome abnormality is associated with this condition?

111. This healthy 9-year-old girl has no history of trauma.

a. Which investigations will be helpful?
b. What is the most likely diagnosis?
c. What is the management of this condition?

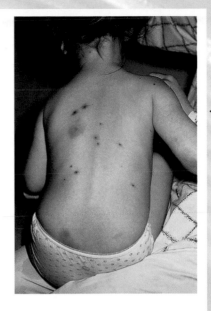

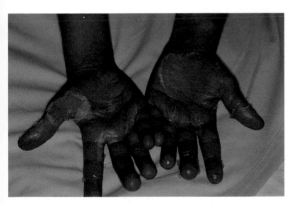

112. Hands of a 9-year-old boy several weeks after a febrile illness.

a. What is the most likely diagnosis?
b. What other signs and symptoms will help to confirm the diagnosis?
c. What is the prognosis of this condition?

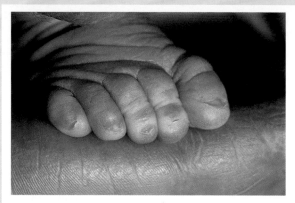

113. This infant has a dislocated knee.

a. What is the diagnosis?
b. What are the complications of this condition?
c. What is the inheritance of this condition?

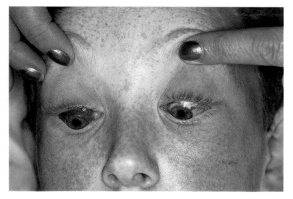

114. This boy developed a rash after being prescribed antibiotics for a urinary tract infection.

a. What is the diagnosis?
b. What are the clinical manifestations of this condition?
c. What is the management of this condition?

115. This toddler has an itchy rash.

a. What is the diagnosis?
a. What is the management of this condition?
b. What are common causes of this condition?

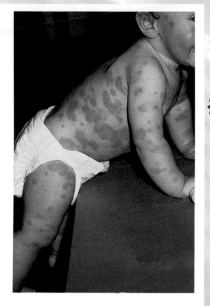

116. Hair of a child with severe developmental delay.

a. What is the diagnosis?
b. What is the biochemical abnormality?
c. What is the course and prognosis of this condition?
d. What is the recurrence risk in future pregnancies?

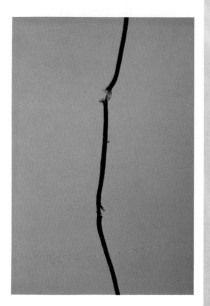

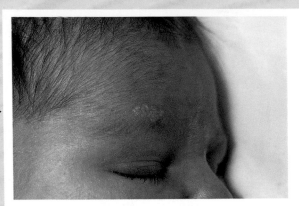

117. This skin lesion above the eyebrow has been present since birth.

a. What is the diagnosis?
b. What is the course and prognosis?
c. What is the management of this lesion?

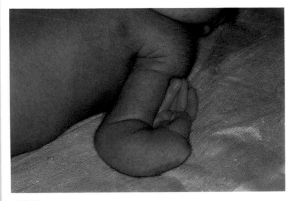

118. This 3-month-old infant has spontaneous bruising.

a. What is the most likely diagnosis?
b. Which investigations will be helpful?
c. What are associated abnormalities?

119. A 24-hour-old infant.

a. What was the presentation of this baby at birth?
b. What are the associated complications?
c. Which investigations should be undertaken?

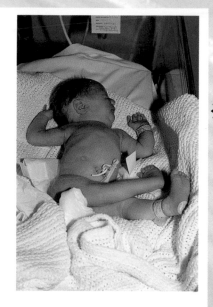

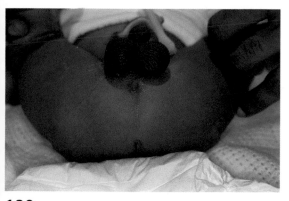

120. Perineum of a newborn male infant.

a. What is the diagnosis?
b. What are other associated abnormalities?
c. What is the management of this condition?

Answers

1.
   a. Moulding, cephalhaematoma, and caput succedanaeum.
   b. By palpation of the skull and soft tissue swelling:
- Moulding—overlapping of cranial sutures which occurs during normal vaginal delivery.
- Cephalhaematoma—Bleeding limited by periosteum and which does not cross suture lines. A distinct bony edge can be palpated around the circumference of the swelling.
- Caput succedanaeum—soft tissue induration, oedema and bruising of presenting part.

   c. All disappear spontaneously and are of no worrying significance. Cephalhaematomas resolve slowly and are occasionally accompanied by calcification.

2.
   a. Normal separation of the umbilical cord with a moist base. There is no sign of any surrounding erythema (cellulitis) or pussy disharge which would be suggestive of infection.
   b. Gentle cleaning with water or a spirit swab is all that is required until spontaneous separation occurs. Topical antibiotic powder may delay separation.

3.
   a. Normal physiological gynaecomastia.
   b. Discharge of a small amount of milk may occur in both male and female infants in the first few days after birth. Mucousy or blood-stained vaginal secretions are also common in female infants around 5-7 days of age.
   c. Parents should be reassured of the physiological nature of these events which are due to placental passage of maternal hormones.

4.
   a. Abscess or subcutaneous fat necrosis.
   b. An abscess is usually tender and becomes fluctuant over the course of a few days. Subcutaneous fat necrosis presents as an erythematous, indurated non-tender subcutaneous swelling, usually over a bony prominence.
   c. Management:
- Abscess—systemic antibiotics prevent local spread to other areas of skin, or dissemination to other sites (e.g. osteomyelitis, meningitis), and septicaemia.
- Subcutaneous fat necrosis—resolves spontaneously but if extensive may take several months. Occasionally associated with calcification and/or hypercalcaemia.

5.
   a. Extravasation of intravenous fluid probably containing an irritant (e.g. calcium).

b. Long term damage may be limited by:
- Care in siting peripheral intravenous infusions as contractures may occur with scarring after extravasation of fluid near joints.
- Intravenous fluids containing irritants should be delivered via central venous catheters whenever the risk of extravasation is worrying (e.g. total parenteral nutrition).
- Prompt irrigation of recent extravasation using large volumes of a diluent containing hyaluronidase and multi-puncture drainage may result in limitation of tissue damage.

6.
a. Traumatic lesion from obstetric procedure or small partial thickness scalp defect. Partial thickness scalp defect may occur as an isolated congenital anomaly or in association with trisomy 13—Patau syndrome.
b. Artificial rupture of membranes, fetal scalp sampling, fetal scalp electrode.
c. Obstetric procedures:
- Artificial rupture of membranes—facilitates descent of presenting part.
- Fetal scalp sampling—measurement of blood pH and base deficit, may assist in monitoring fetal well-being.
- Fetal scalp electrode—allows continuous monitoring of fetal heart rate.

7.
a. Asymmetric tonic neck reflex.
b. Moro or startle, sucking, rooting, grasp (palmar and plantar), glabellar tap, placing, walking, traction and Galant reflexes.
c. None have any particular anatomical significance but absence or delayed appearance may be an early sign of a neurological problem. The presence or absence of neonatal reflexes must be considered in association with gestational age, history and other aspects of the neurological examination.

8.
a. The age of the infant is 4–6 months.
b. Other motor milestones of infants of this age range include:
- In prone position can push up onto forearms and lift head and chest.
- Beginning to rise to standing position and weightbearing when supported under arms or around thorax.
- Starting to roll over, initially from front to side and then on to back.

9.
a. Obtaining an accurate measurement of the height of the child. It is important that the child's feet are flat on the ground with the heels touching the base of the measuring device and that the angle of the jaw is parallel to the weighted board touching the head.
b. Stadiometer.
c. A similar device is used with the infant in the horizontal position and the legs of the infant held straight (i.e. knees not flexed).

10. *a.* Pallor, patchy pigmentation or depigmentation, sparse friable hair, coated tongue, and oedema.

b. Kwashiorkor (protein energy malnutrition) due to inadequate dietary protein intake.

c. Treatment includes:
- Gradual reintroduction of a nutritionally adequate local diet.
- Vitamin supplementation.
- Treatment of associated infections.
- If the child is severely anaemic, very slow infusion of small volume red cell infusion may be beneficial.

11. *a.* Clinical signs shown are:
- Coarse facial features.
- Marbled appearance of the skin (cutis marmoris).
- Umbilical hernia.

b. Congenital hypothyroidism.

c. Other clinical features include a large protruding tongue, hoarse cry, constipation, hypotonia, prolonged jaundice, poor weight gain, poor feeding, and paucity of spontaneous activity.

d. Delay in diagnosis and treatment may result in developmental delay and long term intellectual impairment. Early thyroid hormone replacement improves the outlook but must be continued for life.

12. a. Epithelial pearl.

b. The lesions are epidermal cysts. They are asymptomatic and no treatment is required as they resolve spontaneously within a few days or weeks after birth.

c. Epithelial pearls most commonly occur as a cluster in the midline at the junction of the soft and hard palate (Epstein's pearls) in newborn infants. They also occur less commonly on the alveolar margin.

13. *a.* Resolving strawberry naevus which shows central pallor indicating involution.

b. Strawberry naevi grow rapidly over the first year of life and then regress over the next few years, leaving only a flat pale depigmented area.

c. Bleeding, ulceration, infection and consumption thrombocytopenia are rare complications. Occasionally if the naevus causes pressure on a vital organ (e.g. eyes or airway) oral steroids will help to hasten involution.

14. *a.* Simple obesity or Cushing's syndrome.

b. Clinical features:
- Truncal obesity, growth retardation, hirsutism, apnoea, striae, osteoporosis and muscle wasting are suggestive of Cushing's syndrome.
- Obese children have excess limb skin fold thickness as well as truncal fat and they are often quite tall for their age. Simple obesity has a genetic component.

c. Biochemical investigations. In Cushing's syndrome due to an adrenal adenoma or carcinoma, ACTH levels are suppressed and elevated urinary steroid metabolites fail to decrease after a dexamethasone load (suppression test).

15.
a. Swelling of the long bone metaphyses in rickets.
b. Bowing of the tibia, swelling of the costochondral junctions (rachitic rosary), craniotabes and delayed closure of fontanelle, bone tenderness, muscle weakness, irritability and fretfulness.
c. Biochemical changes include hypocalcaemia, hypophosphataemia, elevated alkaline phosphatase, low vitamin D levels.
Radiological signs of rickets include splaying of the metaphyses of long bones, delayed epiphyseal ossification, and pathological fractures.

16.
a. Chicken pox (varicella) caused by herpes zoster virus.
b. Incubation period is 12–21 days. The period of infectivity begins 2 days before the the rash appears and ends when all the lesions have crusted.
c. Exposed, non-immune mothers should be given hyperimmune zoster globulin (VZIG) to reduce the risk of severe varicella in the newborn baby. The baby should be given VZIG if the mother develops the rash between 7 days prior to delivery and 28 days post-delivery. Oral acyclovir is also recommended for infants who develop varicella within 48 h of birth as neonatal pneumonitis has a high mortality.

17.
a. Large right pneumothorax.
b. Reduced air entry, hyper-resonance and hepatomegaly. May be detected in preterm infants by transillumination with cold light.
c. Resuscitation, hyaline membrane disease, transient tachypnoea of the newborn, pulmonary hypoplasia, and mechanical ventilation including continuous positive-airways pressure. Spontaneous pneumothoraces occur in up to 1% of term babies.
d. Tension pneumothorax requires insertion of an intercostal drain after appropriate analgesia. Small spontaneous pneumothoraces usually resolve without drainage. A high oxygen environment will hasten resolution, but should not be used in preterm infants at risk of retinopathy of prematurity.

18.
a. Anencephaly—absence of forebrain and skull vault with secondary distortion of face.
b. Mid-line defects, (e.g. cleft palate and abnormal cervical vertebrae).
c. Incompatible with life, although may survive for several hours or days. Anencephaly is easily recognizable on antenatal ultrasound scan, and this enables parental choice over continuation of the pregnancy. After birth, the infant can be suitably wrapped for the parents to view the baby. Occasionally, when an anencephalic infant is liveborn and birthweight >2.2 kg, the heart may be suitable for organ donation.

19.
a. Small meningocele.
b. Plain X-ray of the spine will show a defect in the vertebral arch. Ultrasound scan will demonstrate a cystic lesion and usually an underlying connection with the spinal canal. Magnetic resonance imaging or computed tomography scan will help to demonstrate the full anatomy before surgery.
c. 1 in 20 risk of recurrence for subsequent pregnancies after one child with any neural tube defect.
d. Periconceptual maternal folic acid reduces the recurrence risk.

20.
a. Hypospadias with the urethral orifice on the shaft of the penis.
b. Redundant dorsal hooded prepuce due to failure of fusion of the ventral foreskin, ventral curvature of the penis (chordee), and renal tract anomalies.
c. Most will require surgery. Circumcision should be delayed until corrective surgery has been performed, as the prepuce may be required for the urethroplasty. Chordee should be assessed when the penis is erect and, if present, release of the tethering skin may be required. Renal ultrasonography will exclude other renal anomalies.

21.
a. Umbilical hernia, bilateral inguinal herniae and bilateral hydroceles.
b. Inguinal herniae occur in 30–40% preterm male infants. Umbilical herniae are more common in black infants.
c. The majority of umbilical herniae resolve within the first few years. Occasionally, cosmetic surgery at around 3 years of age may be required. Congenital hydroceles always resolve spontaneously. Inguinal herniae require surgical repair soon after diagnosis as there is a high risk of strangulation in infancy.

22.
a. Webbing of the neck, wide-spaced nipples, and absence of breast development.
b. Turner syndrome (XO).
c. Associated problems:
  • Coarctation of the aorta.
  • Ovarian dysgenesis leading to failure of secondary sexual development and infertility.
d. Management:
  • Recombinant growth hormone can be used to improve short stature.
  • Cyclical oestrogen replacement will promote secondary sexual characteristics in adolescence, but infertility is invariable.

23.
a. Differential diagnosis of neck swelling:
  • Cystic hygroma.
  • Lymphadenopathy.
  • Lymphadenitis (abscess formation).
b. Cystic hygroma will transilluminate.
An abscess/lymphadenitis will be tender and may become fluctuant.

c. Cystic hygroma—surgical excision but may be difficult.
   Abscess—systemic antibiotics and surgical drainage when it becomes fluctuant.
   Lymphadenopathy—investigation will depend on the most likely underlying cause (e.g. tuberculosis, lymphoma).

24. a. Keloid—excessive scar formation often following minimal trauma.
   b. Keloid scar formation is more common in people with black skin.
   c. There is no satisfactory treatment for established keloid scars and no way to limit the development of further keloid. Surgical excision is difficult because of the tendency to increasing keloid formation.

25. a. Sturge–Weber syndrome with extensive facial haemangioma or port-wine stain, characteristically in the distribution of the trigeminal nerve.
   b. Epilepsy, macrocephaly, meningeal haemangioma on the same side as the facial haemangioma which may occasionally cause a contralateral hemiplegia, cerebral atrophy, and cerebral calcification.
   c. Electroencephalogram will often show an irritable focus. Neuro-imaging (e.g. computed tomography with contrast or magnetic resonance imaging angiogram brain scan) will confirm the presence of a meningeal haemangioma.

26. a. Volkmann's ischaemic contracture with wasting of forearm, flexion deformity of wrist and claw deformity of the hand.
   b. The deformity is secondary to arterial ischaemia secondary to supracondylar fracture of lower end of humerus. Reduction of a supracondylar fracture should always be undertaken with appropriate anaesthesia and by an experienced paediatric orthopaedic surgeon. Careful monitoring of the circulation of the limb distal to the elbow will alert clinicians to early signs of ischaemia post-reduction of the fracture.

27. a. Absent thumb and short forearm.
   b. X-ray of the forearm will confirm presence or absence of the radius. A full blood count and blood film—absent thumb and radius is sometimes associated with thrombocytopenia and/or anaemia. Thrombocytopenia associated with absence of the radius is TAR syndrome. There are also other syndromes associated with anaemia and absent thumb and radius (e.g. Fanconi anaemia). Absence of the thumb may also occur as an isolated anomaly.

28. a. Imperforate anus and high rectal atresia with a radiopaque marker demonstrating the external anal sphincter or skin tag.
   b. Usually diagnosed on routine neonatal examination soon after birth. If there is a high rectal atresia, and the external anal sphincter is present, may occasionally present later as intestinal obstruction or delayed passage of meconium.

c. Recto–genito–urinary fistulae are common, particularly with high rectal lesions. Prophylactic urinary antisepsis will help to prevent urinary tract infections until the anatomy is clarified by further radiological investigations.

29.
a. Diaphragmatic hernia with herniation of bowel into left hemi-thorax. Heart and mediastinum are displaced to the right.
b. Resuscitation, including mechanical ventilation, is usually required. Continuous decompression of the gut with a large bore nasogastric tube (Ryle's tube). Stabilization prior to surgical repair is essential, including management of pulmonary hypertension with vasodilators, including nitric oxide.
c. Definitive surgery is not usually technically difficult. Survival depends on severity of pulmonary hypoplasia and pulmonary hypertension. Despite advances in pre-surgical stabilization, survival rate is still only around 60%.

30.
a. Umbilical hernia and divarication of the recti.
b. Nil required.
c. Both conditions improve over the first 3 years of life. Umbilical herniae do not become trapped or result in incarceration of the bowel, but they often increase in size on crying. Strapping of the abdomen or umbilicus does not hasten resolution. Cosmetic surgery is only occasionally required if an umbilical hernia has not resolved by 3 years of age.

31.
a. Prune-belly syndrome.
b. Clinical features include laxity or absence of the abdominal wall musculature, low set ears, genital anomalies and arthrogryposis (flexion contractures of the joints and limbs) secondary to oligohydramnios due to reduced fetal urine output.
c. Respiratory insufficiency due to pulmonary hypoplasia.
d. Obstructive uropathy can be diagnosed by antenatal ultrasound when there are dilated renal pelves and oligohydramnios.

32.
a. Bronchopulmonary dysplasia (BPD) or chronic lung disease.
b. There is a radio-opaque clip in the left hemithorax indicating surgical ligation of a patent ductus arteriosus (PDA).
c. Ligation of PDA may hasten weaning from mechanical ventilation. Most infants with BPD who can be weaned survive, but many have recurrent lower respiratory tract infections and wheezing in the first few years of life. Long-term respiratory prognosis is uncertain as survival of low birth weight infants is relatively recent, but respiratory function appears to be normal in adolescence.

33.
a. Bilateral proptosis (protrusion of the eyes).
b. Differential diagnosis of proptosis includes Graves' disease (thyrotoxicosis or hyperthyroidism), tumours involving the orbit

(e.g. metastatic neuroblastoma, and retinoblastoma, which usually presents in the first few years of life). Cerebral tumours may also cause pressure on the optic pathway or cavernous sinus resulting in proptosis, visual field defects and other visual disturbance.

34.
 a. External angular dermoid—there is a swelling superior and lateral to the right eye.
 b. Cystic developmental anomaly found along the suture line of the skull, typically around the orbit or midline from the occiput to the base of the nose.
 c. Usually increase slowly in size and sometimes become infected. Surgery to remove the dermoid cyst is usually done for cosmetic reasons or because of recurrent infection.

35.
 a. Strawberry naevus (capillary haemangioma).
 b. Not present at birth, but appear as a bright red lesion within first few months. Grow rapidly into protuberant, pitted, lesions over the first year, then spontaneously regress slowly leaving only a smooth, pale, depigmented area by 3–4 years of age.
 c. Occasionally may ulcerate, bleed or develop consumption thrombocytopenia or secondary infection. Systemic steroids may help to reduce size of lesions encroaching on vital organs (e.g. airway or eyelids).
 d. Prematurity—occurs in approximately 30% preterm infants.

36.
 a. Posterior vulval or hymenal tag —a fleshy protuberance in the genital area of female infants which is sometimes associated with a mucousy or watery, blood stained discharge in the first few days after birth.
 b. Hypertrophy of the newborn hymen resulting from placental transfer of maternal hormones. It is a normal physiological phenomenon which is of no worrying significance. No treatment is necessary and spontaneous involution always occurs within a few days or weeks after birth.

37.
 a. Breast-feeding is nutritionally appropriate unless the infant is extremely premature, when supplementation, especially of protein, calcium, sodium and phosphate may be required. Breast-feeding provides protection against infection, especially *Escherichia coli* and gastroenteritis, reduces the risk of cot death, facilitates development of healthy maternal/infant relationship, and is convenient and economical.
 b. There are very few contra-indications to breast-feeding which include occasional maternal drugs (e.g. tetracycline, or cancer chemotherapy).

38.
 a. Ichthyosis—an inherited skin condition with abnormal keratinization characterized by visible scaling.
 b. Mild forms may be treated with simple emollients or mild keratolytics (e.g. salicylic acid in aqueous cream). More severe forms may present

as collodion skin in the neonatal period, and careful nursing and medical care will be required to prevent secondary infection and to compensate for losses of water, electrolytes and protein.

c. Ichthyosis usually persists throughout life, but not all infants with collodion skin in the newborn period develop ichthyosis in later childhood.

39.
a. Coeliac disease or gluten sensitivity.

b. Permanent intolerance of dietary wheat, rye and sometimes barley and oats.

c. Most children present before 2 years of age with chronic diarrhoea, vomiting, abdominal distension, wasted buttocks, irritability and hypotonia. The stools are pale, frothy, foul-smelling (steatorrhoea) and difficult to flush away in the toilet. There may also be mouth ulcers, smooth tongue, finger clubbing, peripheral oedema and signs of rickets.

40.
a. Cutaneous and subcutaneous hemangiomata and asymmetric limb hypertrophy.

b. Klippel–Trenaunay–Weber syndrome.

c. Associated arteriovenous fistulae are common and lymphangiomatous anomalies sometimes occur. Surgical excision of the haemangiomata and fistulae is often difficult, but embolization of connecting vessels is sometimes successful. The aim of treatment is usually to limit abnormally rapid growth of the affected limb.

d. Sporadic occurrence.

41.
a. Rocker-bottom feet with protuberant heel and convex dorsum of the feet.

b. Chromosomal abnormalities, particularly trisomies (e.g. trisomy 18, Edward's syndrome; trisomy 13, Patau syndrome).

c. Low birth weight and intrauterine growth restriction, microcephaly, midline facial defects, flexion deformities of the limbs, abnormal posture of the hands with overlapping fingers, pulmonary hypoplasia and congenital heart disease. Epilepsy and severe neurodevelopmental delay are inevitable in the few infants who survive beyond the neonatal period.

42.
a. Periumbilical cellulitis—erythema and desquamation of the skin surrounding the umbilicus. There is sometimes a purulent, yellowish discharge.

b. Bacterial infection most commonly due to *Staphylococcus aureus*.

c. Prompt intravenous broad spectrum antibiotics (e.g. cefuroxime, or flucloxacillin and gentamicin) after appropriate swabs and cultures. Inadequate or delayed treatment can lead to disseminated sepsis including septicaemia, osteomyelitis or toxic epidermal necrosis (staphylococcal scalded skin syndrome).

43.   *a.* Scars of intrauterine herpes zoster (chickenpox).

     b. The non-immune mother should be given hyperimmune zoster globulin (VZIG) to limit the effects of the infection on the developing fetus. If the maternal rash occurs within a week of delivery, the newborn infant will also require VZIG. Acyclovir should be given to newborn infants when maternal chickenpox develops within a week of birth in order to reduce the risk of life-threatening neonatal complications (e.g. pneumonitis).

44.   *a.* Severe oral candidiasis (thrush, moniliasis).

     b. Thrush in infancy is an extremely common and usually benign condition. It is more common after the administration of antibiotics. If thrush is recurrent or is difficult to eradicate, an underlying immunodeficiency disorder should be suspected. Beyond infancy, oral candidiasis is usually associated with an immunodeficiency disorder (e.g. HIV or severe combined immunodeficiency disorder or immuno-suppressive treatment for malignancy). Inhaled corticosteroids may also cause troublesome oral thrush in older asthmatic children.

45.   *a.* Seborrhoeic dermatitis—on the scalp it is called cradle cap.

     b. Greasy plaques or scaly rash around eyebrows, ears, hairline and in the perineum. Occasionally discoid lesions spreading up the trunk from the napkin area (napkin psoriasis).

     c. Cradle cap usually responds to a simple keratolytic shampoo. Seborrhoeic dermatitis always improves spontaneously towards the end of the first year of life. A mild corticosteroid cream (e.g. 1% hydrocortisone cream) may be helpful in more troublesome seborrhoeic dermatitis, but should be used sparingly, particularly on the face.

46.   *a.* Swelling of the costo-chondral junctions in rickets (rachitic rosary).

     b. Oral vitamin D supplementation will be necessary to correct the biochemical and radiological abnormalities and to prevent long-term bony deformity, particularly of weight-bearing limbs. Dietary education of the family and improved long-term dietary intake of vitamin D will be important to prevent recurrence of rickets and to protect other family members, especially future infants.

     c. Malabsorption, liver disease, renal tubular dysfunction, long-term anticonvulsants and hereditary X-linked hypophosphataemic rickets.

47.   *a.* Vitiligo—areas of pigmented and depigmented skin.

     b. Vitiligo is sometimes associated with Waardenburg syndrome—white forelock and sensorineural hearing loss. Waardenburg syndrome is often inherited as an autosomal dominant condition. Adults with Waardenburg syndrome may be difficult to recognize as they often dye the white forelock. Underlying autoimmune disorders are much less common in children with vitiligo than adults.

     c. Cosmetic creams may be used to disguise the depigmented skin, but the result is often unsatisfactory.

48. a. Complications of cleft lip and palate include feeding difficulties, poor weight gain and orthodontic problems. Regurgitation of milk into the nasopharynx may lead to recurrent middle ear infections and hearing deficit. Speech problems, especially nasal voice, occur if palate closure is after 9–12 months of age.

b. Cleft lip and palate occur in approximately 1 in 600 livebirths. After one affected sibling, there is a higher risk of recurrence in future children.

49. a. Occipital encephalocele.

b. Complications include meningitis and epilepsy. The severity of the neurological deficit will be dependent upon the amount and part of brain which has to be excised to allow skull closure.

c. In the absence of peri-conceptual maternal folic acid supplementation, there is a 1 in 20 risk of recurrence of a neural tube defect in each subsequent pregnancy.

50. a. Postural talipes is due to intrauterine compression.

b. In mild postural talipes, there is a full range of passive movement of the foot and ankle and spontaneous resolution will occur. Occasionally, splinting of the feet is used for more severe postural talipes, although there is no evidence for efficacy of this treatment.

c. Associated anomalies:
- Congenital dislocation of the hip.
- Meningomyelocele.

51. a. Striae or stretch marks on the abdomen.

b. Striae are uncommon in children. Underlying causes in childhood include Cushing's syndrome and simple obesity. Cushing's syndrome should be suspected in those with moon facies, truncal obesity, hirsutism, acne, muscle wasting, and slow growth. Cushing's syndrome may be due to excessive cortisol produced by adrenal hyperplasia caused by pituitary adenomata (Cushing's disease) or secondary to excessive exogenous corticosteroid administration.

52. a. Henoch–Schönlein purpura (HSP).

b. Investigations:
- Test urine for haematuria and proteinuria.
- Renal function tests including serum creatinine.
- Monitor blood pressure.
- Platelet count and clotting studies to exclude thrombocytopenia and bleeding disorders, although distribution of rash in HSP is usually characteristic.

c. HSP usually runs a self-limiting course over weeks. Relapse or recurrence occurs in approximately 30% cases of HSP. Glomerulonephritis occurs in a minority of cases (<1%), but there is a low risk of long term chronic renal failure.

53.
   a. The differential diagnosis of necrotic inflammatory skin lesions include polyarteritis nodosa and severe Henoch–Schönlein purpura (HSP).
   b. Polyateritis nodosa is rare in childhood, but should always be suspected when HSP is severe, recurrent or presents with atypical lesions or symptoms. The most worrying long-term complications of both polyarteritis nodosa and HSP are renal failure and bowel infarction.

54.
   a. Eczema.
   b. Flexures particularly the popliteal and antecubital fossae, wrists and trunk are most commonly affected.
   c. Eczema is intensely itchy and secondary infection often occurs after there has been excoriation of the skin from scratching. Eczema herpeticum (herpes simplex virus) is an uncommon complication which is sometimes difficult to distinguish clinically from bacterial infection, but once diagnosed responds rapidly to oral acyclovir. Chronic untreated eczema may result in lichenification and hyperpigmentation of the skin which can be difficult to eradicate.

55.
   a. Osteomyelitis or bone tumour. Osteomyelitis presents insidiously in neonates and may be quite extensive before clinical signs become apparent.
   b. Full blood count, blood cultures, erythrocyte sedimentation or C-reactive protein usually confirm infection/inflammation.
MRI bone scan will assist the orthopaedic surgeon in obtaining a tissue diagnosis by needle aspirate or bone biopsy. Technetium bone scan will show a hot spot at an early stage in acute osteomyelitis but may be difficult to interpret in very young infants.
   c. Broad-spectrum systemic antibiotics including anti-staphylococcal cover for at least 3 weeks.

56.
   a. Albinism—absence of pigmentation in the skin and hair.
   b. Hypopigmentation of the iris and retinal abnormality leading to extreme sensitivity to bright light including sunlight.
   c. Some children with albinism have lack of pigmentation only in the skin. If the retina is affected, protection from bright sunlight will help to limit damage, but visual impairment is common, progressive and often severe in later life.

57.
   a. Metaphyseal streaking of the long bones ('celery stalk appearance').
   b. Congenital rubella syndrome (rubella embryopathy).
   c. Infants infected with the rubella virus in early gestation (<12 weeks) will be most severely affected. Microcephaly, congenital heart disease, intra-cranial calcification, hepatosplenomegaly, lymphadenopathy, failure to thrive, neurodevelopmental delay, epilepsy, deafness and cataracts may occur. Infection later in pregnancy may still cause sensorineural hearing loss which is progressive, even after birth.

58.
  a. Bilateral swollen ankles–reactive arthritis, juvenile chronic arthritis (JCA), Henoch–Schönlein purpura, rheumatic fever, systemic lupus erythematous (SLE) and inflammatory bowel disease.
  b. Investigations–full blood count, throat swab, blood cultures, inflammatory markers e.g. CRP, ESR, antistreptolysin titre (AST), and autoantibody tests.
  c. Non-steroidal inflammatory drugs e.g. aspirin and ibuprofen help to relieve symptoms. Activity should be maintained whenever possible. Physiotherapy, hydrotherapy, and splinting provide symptomatic relief and reduce disability in chronic arthritis. Sometime immunosuppressive drugs or corticosteroids are required in severe cases.

59.
  a. Ulcers and blisters in and around the mouth are likely to be extremely painful and will cause difficulty in eating and drinking, excessive salivation and dribbling, mild fever, and irritability. Analgesia and adequate hydration will be important in the management.
  b. Herpes simplex stomatitis.
  c. Herpes simplex stomatitis is usually a self-limiting condition, but if the child is very young or immunocompromised, encephalitis or disseminated herpes infection can be life-threatening.

60.
  a. Noonan syndrome—phenotypic features of Turner syndrome, but normal karyotype. Children with Noonan syndrome are usually male, but occasionally females also affected.
  b. Clinical signs of Noonan syndrome are slow growth, short stature, webbed neck, low-set ears and hypertelorism (widely-spaced eyes).
  c. Pulmonary stenosis is the most common cardiac abnormality in Noonan syndrome. Coarctation of aorta is the most common cardiac lesion in Turner syndrome.
  d. Usually sporadic, but occasionally may be inherited as an autosomal dominant.

61.
  a. Dislocation of the left hip. The acetabulum of the left hip is shallow and the head of the left femur is displaced upwards and laterally.
  b. Congenital dislocation of the hip is more common after breech presentation, and in infants with talipes, spina bifida, arthrogryposis and in those with a family history of developmental dysplasia of the hip.
  c. Abduction splinting in a harness or plaster cast for at least 6 weeks. If the diagnosis is not made in the newborn period, surgery is more likely to be required.

62.
  a. Widespread parenchymal lung disease.
     Bilateral posterior fractures of 6,7 and 8th ribs.
  b. Chronic lung disease (CLD) or bronchopulmonary dysplasia which occurs in up to 40% extremely low birth weight infants. Osteopenia of prematurity which is usually due to phosphate or vitamin D deficiency.

c. The cause of CLD is multi-factorial and there is no clear method of prevention as yet. Adequate intake of phosphate and vitamin D, particularly in babies requiring prolonged parenteral nutrition, will reduce the risk of osteopenia of prematurity.

63.
a. Pneumomediastinum—central collection of air in the thorax.
b. Mechanical ventilation including continuous positive airways pressure, hyaline membrane disease, and meconium aspiration syndrome are predisposing factors. Occasionally a newborn infant who has established spontaneous onset of respiration at birth may develop an air leak (e.g. pneumomediastinum or pneumothorax).
c. In a term infant, a high inspired oxygen concentration will hasten resolution of air leaks, including pneumomediastinum. Surgical drainage is rarely required.

64.
a. Hydrocephalus—large head with a prominent forehead and setting sun eye sign.
b. Cranial ultrasound scan or computed tomograph brain scan will show dilatation of the lateral ventricles. Enlargement of the third and fourth ventricles will depend on the level of the obstruction.
c. Management depends on the underlying cause. When there is a rapid increase in head circumference or symptoms of raised intracranial pressure, a ventriculoperitoneal shunt may be required. After intraventricular haemorrhage in a preterm infant, ventriculomegaly may be transient and resolve sponateously.

65.
a. Syndactyly—webbing of the second and third toes of the left foot.
b. Syndactyly of the toes is a common minor cosmetic congenital anomaly and is of no functional significance. It is often inherited as an autosomal dominant.

66.
a. Syndactyly—webbing of the second and third fingers of the left hand.
b. Unlike syndactyly of the toes which is a common minor cosmetic congenital anomaly of no functional significance, syndactyly of the fingers will require plastic surgery to improve hand function as well as cosmetic appearance. Syndactyly of the fingers is much less common than syndactyly of the toes.

67.
a. Simian crease—a single transverse palmar crease.
b. Often associated with trisomy 21 (Down syndrome). Simian creases are also found in 18% normal children.
c. Hypotonia, flat moon shaped facies, broad nasal bridge, epicanthic folds, upward slanting eyes, Brushfield spots, third fontanelle, short neck, low hairline, flattened occiput (brachycephaly), small ears with an immature helix, broad spade-shaped hands, short incurved middle phalanx of the little finger (clinodactyly), and a wide gap between first and second toes (sandal gap).

68. *a.* Sandal gap—deep, wide crease on the plantar surface of the foot, between the first and second toes.

 b. Congenital heart disease, hypothyroidism, Hirschsprung's disease, duodenal atresia, cataracts, transient abnormal myelopoiesis and myeloid leukaemia are more common in children with Down syndrome. Infants with Down syndrome should have an echocardiogram in the neonatal period even if there are no clinical signs of cardiac disease as approximately 30% will have an atrio-ventriculo-septal defect.

69. *a.* Anogenital warts (condyloma acumanta) caused by human papilloma virus.

 b. Warts may develop up to 2 years after exposure and young children may acquire the virus from the genital tract of the mother during delivery. In children >2 years of age, sexual abuse should always be suspected.

 c. Tests for other sexually transmitted diseases should be performed and, if positive, the diagnosis of sexual abuse is confirmed. A multi-disciplinary approach with inter-agency collaboration will be necessary to assess the child and family.

70. *a.* Subaponeurotic or subperiosteal haematoma which may be associated with an underlying fracture of the skull.

 b. Skull X-ray will confirm the diagnosis of fracture. The infant should remain under observation in hospital for at least 24 h to ensure that there are no signs or symptoms of intracranial haemorrhage resulting in a subdural or extradural collection. Skull fracture in a young infant results from significant trauma. The history and circumstances of the injury will be important in assessing whether the injury was accidental.

71. *a.* Trisomy 18 (Edward syndrome)—clenched hand with overlapping of the fingers.

 b. Small for gestational age, microcephaly, pulmonary hypoplasia, flexion deformities of the hips and limbs, rocker-bottom feet, cryptorchidism, hirsutism, micrognathia, short palpebral fissures, low-set ears, microstomia, facial plasy and congenital heart disease.

 c. Most die within the first few months after birth. Fewer than 10% survive beyond the first year of life and they are always severely mentally and developmentally delayed.

72. *a.* Pre-auricular skin tags.

 b. Single skin tags are usually an isolated congenital anomaly and of cosmetic significance only. Multiple skin tags may be associated with other congenital anomalies of the head and neck. Patency of the external meatus and presence of the middle ear should be confirmed using an auriscope. Hearing tests should be undertaken as multiple skin tags are associated with hearing deficit in a small proportion of children.

   c. Sporadic occurrence.

73.   *a.* Clubbing of the toes.

   b. Cyanotic congenital heart disease, cystic fibrosis, bronchiectasis, inflammatory bowel disease, liver disease, gastrointestinal malabsorption and infective endocarditis.

   c. Cystic fibrosis—chest X-ray and sweat test. CT scan—bronchiectasis. Echocardiogram—heart defects and endocarditis. Fever, raised inflammatory markers (e.g. C-reactive protein)—endocarditis, ulcerative colitis and Crohn's disease. Colonoscopy, barium meal and follow-through or bowel biopsy will be necessary to make a definitive diagnosis of inflammatory bowel disease or malabsorption.

74.   *a.* Impetigo—discrete blisters with a surrounding flare and which later become crusted. It is highly infectious and transferred by hands or close contact.

   b. Bacterial infection caused by *Staphylococcal aureus*.

   c. Systemic antibiotics for at least 7 days, after taking superficial swabs and blood cultures. A combination of at least two anti-staphylococcal antibiotics (e.g. flucloxacillin and gentamycin or vancomycin) should be used until sensitivities of the organism are known.

75.   *a.* Intense pallor around the vein due to the effects of vasoconstriction in the surrounding subcutaneous tissue. The intravenous infusion contains an inotropic drug (e.g. dopamine or dobutamine).

   b. The peripheral infusion containing the inotrope should be ceased immediately to prevent tissue necrosis. Infusions of inotropes should always be given through a central venous catheter.

76.   *a.* Severe anaemia may be due to a feto–maternal transfusion, acute blood loss from the umbilical cord (e.g. velamentous insertion or unclamped cord), severe haemolytic disease, haemoglobinopathy (e.g. alpha thalassaemia major), intra-uterine viral infection, congenital leukaemia or erythroid dysplasia.

   b. A Kleihauer test for fetal cells in maternal blood within 48 h of delivery. Maternal and infant blood group and an indirect antiglobulin (Coomb's) test. IgM or PCR tests for viral infections. Bone marrow aspirate will be necessary to diagnose leukaemia or the underlying cause of transfusion-dependent anaemia.

77.   *a.* Large irregular pigmented naevus or shagreen patch on the upper back, 3 café au lait patches >1 cm diameter on the left lower back, numerous other smaller pigmented naevi and a Mongolian blue spot in the lumbosacral region.

   b. Neurofibromatosis (von Recklinghausen's disease).

  c. Autosomal dominant inheritance, but many cases occur as a new mutation.

78.
  a. Torn frenulum of the upper lip.
  b. Caused by aggressively forcing a teat or other object into the infant's mouth. A history of poor feeding by the infant is sometimes given by the carers.
  c. Non-accidental injury should be suspected. The family and social circumstances should be investigated by a multi-disciplinary child protection team.

79.
  a. Hypertrophy of the calf muscles.
  b. Duchenne muscular dystrophy.
  c. Gower sign on rising from the floor, proximal muscle weakness including shoulder girdle, increasing muscle weakness and atrophy, cardiomyopathy, and variable speech and educational delay.
  d. Serum creatinine phosphokinase will be markedly elevated. Electromyography, muscle ultrasound will be abnormal. Muscle biopsy will show absent or abnormal dystrophin. The dystrophin gene has been identified at Xp21.

80.
  a. Epulis—a rare, granulomatous lesion on the alveolar margin in the newborn period.
  b. The lesion is asymptomatic and does not interfere with feeding.
  c. No treatment is required as spontaneous resolution always occurs within a few weeks.

81.
  a. Short neck with redundant skin folds and a low hairline.
  b. Short neck and low hairline is often found in association with chromosomal abnormalities (e.g. Down syndrome, Turner or Noonan's syndrome, and Klippel–Feil syndrome).
  c. Chromosome analysis. X-ray of the neck and back may reveal skeletal anomalies (e.g. hemivertebrae or scoliosis).

82.
  a. Peri-orbital cellulitis.
  b. Broad spectrum systemic antibiotics for at least 7 days, after taking superficial swabs and blood cultures. Analgesia will be required.
  c. Systemic spread may result in bacteraemia or septicaemia. Local spread can lead to abcess formation in the orbit, resulting in ophthalmoplegia, loss of vision, proptosis, cavernous sinus thrombosis and cranial nerve palsy. The advice of a paediatric ophthalmologist should be sought immediately if the cellulitis does not respond rapidly, or if any new eye signs develop.

83.
  a. Scissoring of the legs.
  b. Cerebral palsy.
  c. The precise cause is usually not identifiable. In approximately 10%, it is due to hypoxic brain damage in fetal or early neonatal life. Spastic

diplegia is more common in preterm infants. Cranial ultrasound or a magnetic resonance imaging (MRI) brain scan in the first few weeks after birth will identify most preterm infants at high risk of cerebral palsy. Children with a hemiplegia or hemiparesis may have a cerebral infarct on computed tomography or MRI brain scan and, in some, an underlying coagulopathy will be identified.

84. a. Lipoma, neuroma or cavernous haemangioma.
b. Surgical excision will usually become necessary for cosmetic reasons and to make a precise diagnosis.
c. Recurrence risk is low, but will depend on the completeness of surgical excision and the nature of the lesion. Cavernous haemangiomas are often difficult to excise completely.

85. a. Marked head lag.
b. Hypotonia of neck muscles may be due to a congenital muscular dystrophy or myopathy, cerebral palsy, or metabolic disorders.
c. Cranial ultrasound or a magnetic resonance imaging brain scan, thyroid function tests, muscle biopsy and ultrasound scan, electromyography, routine biochemical tests including liver and renal function, plasma ammonia and lactate, serum creatinine phosphokinase, and urinary amino and organic acids.

86. a. Neonatal mastitis due to bacterial infection.
b. Broad spectrum systemic antibiotics for at least 7 days, after taking superficial swabs and blood cultures. Occasionally, surgical incision may be required to drain the pus if a fluctuant abscess develops. Care should be taken to avoid damage to the breast tissue during surgical incision.
c. Complete resolution occurs with prompt antibiotic treatment.

87. a. Midline neck lesions are usually thyroglossal cysts or fistulae.
b. Thyroid function tests should always be performed. An ultrasound scan of the neck may help to identify a fistula or cyst. A radio-isotope scan will show the precise location of functioning thyroid tissue. Surgical exploration and excision will usually be necessary for a definitive histological diagnosis and for cosmetic reasons, but surgery should always be delayed until the results of thyroid investigations are known.

88. a. Mongolian blue spot.
b. Mongolian blue spots most commonly occur over the lumbosacral region of the back.
c. The slate-grey or bluish pigmented area of skin gradually becomes less obvious as the infant grows older and the rest of the skin becomes darker with age. Mongolian blue spots are particularly common in Asian infants and almost universal in non-Caucasian neonates, but are rarely seen beyond the first year of life.

89. *a.* Accessory nipple, below and in line with the normally placed nipple and breast bud. Sometimes mistakenly diagnosed as a pigmented naevus.

  b. No treatment is necessary, but surgical excision can be performed for cosmetic reasons if the lesion causes the child embarassment when he is older. Occasionally, accessory nipples may also have an underlying breast bud which will enlarge in response to placental transfer of maternal oestrogen during gestation or normal physiological oestrogen production at puberty.

90. *a.* Massive hepatomegaly, which in association with profound congenital anaemia, is most likely to be due to extra-medullary haemopoiesis and heart failure.

  b. Alpha thalassaemia major, or severe haemolysis (e.g. rhesus haemolytic disease).

  c. A microcytic, hypochromic maternal blood film which is likely to be due to either iron deficiency anaemia or alpha thalassaemia trait. The father should also be screened to allow antenatal testing of the fetus if he is also a carrier. Maternal blood group and antibody testing will alert to the possibility of rhesus and other haemolytic disease.

91. *a.* Cellulitis, probably due to an underlying lymphadenitis or lymph node abscess.

  b. *Staphlyococcal aureus*, *Haemolytic streptococcus*, *Haemophilus influenzae*, and any bacteria which colonize the nasopharynx or upper respiratory tract.

  c. Broad-spectrum systemic antibiotics for at least 7 days, after taking superficial swabs and blood cultures. Occasionally, surgical incision may be required to drain pus if a fluctuant abscess develops.

92. *a.* Shiny distended abdomen with purpura/bruising of skin, prominent superficial veins and faint bluish discoloration of bowel visible through the abdominal wall.

  b. Necrotizing enterocolitis.

  c. Poor prognosis:
  • Perforation.
  • Persistent thrombocytopenia.
  • Persistent metabolic acidosis.
  • Abnormal blood clotting.
  • Failure of abdominal distension to improve within 48 h of commencing conventional mangement—ceasing enteral feeds, starting broad-spectrum antibiotics including metronidadazole to cover invasion of the bowel mucosa by anaerobic organisms, and circulatory support.

93. *a.* Diaphragmatic hernia with bowel in left hemithorax and heart displaced to the right.

  b. Clinical signs will include respiratory distress, cyanosis, a scaphoid abdomen, dextrocardia and reduced air entry in left hemithorax.

c. Emergency treatment will be intubation and ventilation. A large bore naso-gastric (Ryle's) tube on continuous drainage is essential to deflate the stomach.

Pulmonary hypertension is common and will need to be treated before definitive surgery is undertaken. Pulmonary vasodilators (e.g. prostacyclin, magnesium sulphate and nitric oxide) may be helpful.

94.
a. Swelling of the parotid gland (parotitis).
b. Acute bacterial or viral infection, most commonly mumps virus. Chronic or recurrent parotitis is often found in children with HIV infection before they develop other immunodeficiency-related infections.
c. Mumps is now uncommon in communities where the MMR vaccine is given at 12–18 months of age. Bacterial parotitis will respond to broad spectrum antibiotics. An HIV test should be considered in children with recurrent parotitis.

95.
a. Bruising behind the ear of a child beyond infancy is very rarely related to accidental trauma.
b. Non-accidental injury caused by repeated hitting of the ears with a closed fist (boxing) is the most likely cause.
c. Clotting studies and a platelet count will exclude the unlikely possibility of a bleeding disorder giving rise to spontaneous bleeding. The child may reveal the nature of the assault if he is interviewed by an experienced, sympathetic paediatrician. The family and social circumstances should be investigated by a multi-disciplinary team.

96.
a. Erythema toxicum (urticaria of the newborn, toxic erythema, eosinophil rash).
b. The infant will have no symptoms attributable to this rash.
c. The rash is extremely common towards the end of the first week and in the second week of life. It is usually widespread and fluctuating and disappears spontaneously. It is of no clinical significance and can usually be distinguished from septic spots on clinical examination by an experienced clinician.

97.
a. Staining of the teeth most likely due to the administration of the antibiotic tetracycline in early childhood.
b. The bones of the skeletal system.
c. Oral tetracycline is contra-indicated in children in whom full permanent dentition has not erupted i.e. under the age of 10 years. There is always an alternative antibiotic which can be prescribed, even in those who have known drug allergies.

98.
a. Coarse facial features with a high protuberant forehead (frontal bossing), broad cheek bones and an enlarged mandible most likely to be due to a neurodegenerative or storage disorder (e.g. mucopolysaccharidosis or mucolipidosis).

b. X-rays may show characteristic features including beaking of the vertebral bodies of the spine, broad ribs, osteolucent whirls in the iliac crest of the pelvis and thickening of the skull bones.
c. The diagnosis is made by identifying the specific enzyme defect in leucocytes, and the excretion of glycosaminoglycogans in the urine in mucopolysaccharidoses.

99.
a. Craniodiaphyseal dysplasia, a severely disfiguring and progressive disorder of bone, mainly affecting the skull, clavicles and sternum. Craniometaphyseal dysplasia is a similar, but much less severe, more slowly progessive disorder.
b. Cranial nerve palsies, deafness, visual disturbance, bone pain, difficulties with dentition and jaw opening, mastication and eating. Neurological symptoms and brain stem dysfunction may develop in the terminal stages when the foramen magnum is narrowed by bony overgrowth.
c. Autosomal recessive inheritance. There will be a 1 in 4 risk of recurrence.

100.
a. Cutis aplasia of the scalp or a small encephalocele.
b. The diagnosis can usually be readily distinguished by an experienced clinician. If an encephalocele is present, there will be a bony defect visible on skull X-ray. Cranial ultrasound, computed tomography or magnetic resonance imaging brain scan will define the extent of the brain protrusion.
c. Cutis aplasia heals by spontaneous granulation even when the lesion is large. Surgical repair is rarely required. Encephaloceles require excision and skin closure after appropriate neuro-imaging.

101.
a. Purpura and blueberry muffin spots—intrauterine viral infection (e.g. rubella, CMV or toxoplasmosis).
b. Growth restriction, microcephaly, hepatosplenomegaly, lymphadenopathy, microphthalmia, cataracts, chorioretinitis, hearing deficit, osteolytic bone lesions, intracranial calcification, and epilepsy.
c. Blood for specific IgM or PCR testing. Positive antibody tests (IgG) in young infants are not diagnostic of infection and may be maternal antibodies. Ophthalmological examination and hearing tests will be helpful. X-ray of long bones may show a celery-stalk appearance which is diagnostic of congenital rubella. Cranial ultrasound scan will demonstrate intracranial calcification.

102.
a. Micrognathia and low-set ears.
b. Examination of the palate is important when an infant has micrognathia. The Pierre–Robin syndrome is cleft palate in association with microcephaly.
c. Ultrasound scan of the renal tract will reveal renal tract anomalies in approximately 10% of infants with low-set ears. Hearing tests should

be done whenever there is an abnormality of the ears or multiple accessory auricles (skin tags).

103.
a. Graves disease—bilateral proptosis due to thyrotoxicosis (hyperthyroidism).
b. Symptoms of hyperthyroidism include persistent tachycardia, recurrent supraventricular tachycardia, tremor, irritability, sweating, weight loss and goitre.
c. Antithyroid drugs (e.g. carbimazole) until spontaneous remission occurs, usually within a few years of onset of symptoms. Occasionally, thyroidectomy may be necessary, and then life-long thyroid hormone replacement therapy will be required.

104.
a. Giant pigmented naevus in the bathing trunk distribution.
b. The untreated naevus will be of cosmetic significance. There is also a high risk of malignant transformation before puberty.
c. Dermabrasion or laser therapy will remove superficial naevus cells and improve the appearance. Surgical excision is necessary to reduce the risk of malignant transformation, but is often difficult and may require multiple procedures, skin grafting and blood transfusions.

105.
a. Psoriasis—erythematous pearly plaques most commonly around the hairline, and on the trunk, elbow and knees.
b. Pitting of the nails, oncholysis, and arthritis but not usually affecting the distal interphalangeal joints.
c. Topical salicylic acid, dithranol, coal tar, or vitamin D analogues (e.g. calcipotriol) are helpful in keeping psoriasis under control. Occasionally, a course of ultraviolet light may induce remission in severe cases.

106.
a. Long thin digits (arachnodactyly) of Ehlers Danlos or Marfan's syndrome.
b. Collagen disorders resulting in hypermobility of joints—the thumb and little finger can be hyper-extended onto the forearm. Tall stature, high arched palate, severe myopia, dislocation of the lenses of the eyes, chest deformity, scoliosis, aortic aneurysm, and aortic and mitral valve prolapse and regurgitation also occur in Marfan's syndrome.

107.
a. Strawberry naevus which is showing signs of spontaneous involution. The centre of the lesion has become necrotic.
b. No active management is required unless there is secondary infection or excessive bleeding.
c. The naevus will resolve completely over a period of months and will leave only a faint white mark on the skin. Natural involution provides the best cosmetic result and surgery is never indicated. Oral steroids will hasten resolution if there is troublesome bleeding.

108.
a. Ischaemic necrosis of the fat and skin of the forearm caused by arterial thrombosis or severe prolonged spasm.

b. A thrombophilia screen should be performed as many infants with ischaemic necrosis have protein C or S, anti-thrombin 3 or factor V Leiden deficiency.

c. There may be scarring of the affected tissue and limb, but usually normal function, as muscle is rarely involved. If a thrombotic tendency is identified, there will be a risk of venous thrombosis in adult life and in association with surgery.

109. a. Twin-to-twin transfusion in monozygotic twins; one is plethoric and one is pale.

b. Approximately 15% monozygotic twins have shared placental blood vessels. An acute transfusion may cause anaemia and hypovolaemia in the donor, and polycythaemia in the recipient. Symptoms depend on the volume and rate of transfusion. Slow chronic feto-fetal transfusion may result in intra-uterine growth restriction in the donor. The recipient will be at risk of heart failure and hydrops. Polyhydramnios is common and both twins are at risk of morbidity and mortality.

110. a. Exomphalos (omphalocele)—an abdominal wall defect at the umbilicus covered by a sac of peritoneum, or herniation of abdominal contents into the umbilical cord.

b. Surgical closure after careful inspection to exclude bowel atresias and stenoses. With large defects, the bowel is suspended in an artificial membrane and the contents are slowly returned into the abdominal cavity over a period of weeks.

c. Trisomy 13 (Patau syndrome).

111. a. Full blood count, including platelet count and coagulation studies.

b. Idiopathic thrombocytopenic purpura is the most common cause of spontaneous bruising and purpura in healthy children.

c. Most will resolve spontaneously. Oral steroids and intravenous immunoglobulin administration will cause a slightly faster rise in platelet count, but does not affect the prognosis. Treatment should be considered if there is mucosal bleeding, neurological signs or a history of recent head injury. Splenectomy is usually curative and performed in those with prolonged, persistent thrombocytopenia.

112. a. Kawasaki disease (mucocutaneous lymph node syndrome).

b. Fever persisting for 5 days and at least 4 of 5 of the following:
  • Marked cervical lymphadenopathy.
  • Erythema and oedema of palms and soles, and desquamation of the skin.
  • Polymorphous rash.
  • Bilateral conjunctival congestion.
  • Reddening and cracking of the lips.
  Thrombocytosis is common in the second week.

c. Aspirin and intravenous immunoglobulin reduce the risk of coronary aneurysms if given in the early stages of the disease.

113. *a.* Nail-patella syndrome—a rare condition which can usually be diagnosed at the time of the routine neonatal examination. The infant will have absent or hypoplastic finger and toe nails and there will be an absence of the prominence of the knee or sometimes even congenital dislocation. X-ray of the knee will confirm the absence of the patella.

b. Absent patella predisposes to recurrent dislocation of the knees. Osteoarthritis of the knees is common in adult life.

c. Sporadic occurrence.

114. *a.* Bilateral conjunctival hyperaemia—Stevens–Johnson syndrome.

b. Erythema multiforme, widespread vesiculo-bullous lesions of the skin and mucous membranes of the mouth, rectum, vagina, or conjunctiva. Extensive skin and fluid loss occurs and there is a high risk of secondary infection.

c. Discontinue the offending antibiotic. Barrier nursing to prevent infection and adequate fluid and electrolyte replacement therapy is the mainstay of treatment. Severe cases have a high mortality from septicaemia.

115. *a.* Erythema multiforme—widespread urticaria.

b. Systemic antihistamines reduce itching and limit the course if commenced early. Subcutaneous adrenaline may be life-saving in the few who develop severe respiratory obstruction with associated oedema of the mouth and tongue.

c. The offending allergen is often not identifiable, but drugs (e.g. penicillin) are a common cause. Recurrent urticaria may be due to food additives or coloring sensitivity. Rarely, there may be a familial acetylcholinesterase deficiency.

116. *a.* Menkes kinky hair syndrome—characteristic sparse, twisted kinky hair with partial breakages and twists on microscopic examination. All body hair is abnormal.

b. Probably a defect of copper-binding metalloprotein.

c. There is also profound neurological deterioration and failure to thrive. Death occurs in early childhood.

d. Menkes syndrome is an X-linked recessive condition. Male infants of a carrier mother have 50% chance of inheriting the syndrome.

117. *a.* Sebaceous naevus—an uncommon congenital lesion with a yellowish, waxy, pitted, hairless surface. Usually found on the scalp or around the hairline.

b. Malignant transformation occurs in some of these lesions in adult life, but the risk of this complication is difficult to determine.

c. Excision is advisable if the lesion persists into adolescence.

118. *a.* TAR (thrombocytopenia and absent radius) syndrome.

b. X-ray of the arm will confirm the presence or absence of the radius, and a full blood count, including platelet count.

c. Associated abnormalities include cardiac anomalies (Holt–Oram syndrome), the Fanconi pancytopenia syndrome, and the VACTERL association (**V**ertebral abnormalities, **A**nal atresia, **C**ongenital heart disease, **T**racheal defects, **R**enal anomalies, absent **R**adius, and **L**ung hypoplasia).

119. a. Breech presentation with extended legs.

b. Associated complications include traumatic delivery, oedema and bruising of the genitals and buttocks, and an increased risk of developmental dysplasia and congenital dislocation of the hips.

c. The hips should be carefully examined during the routine neonatal examination at around 24 h of age. After breech presentation, ultrasound examination should be always be performed to exclude congenital dislocation even if the hips appear normal on clinical examination.

120. a. Imperforate anus (anal atresia).

b. Renal tract anomalies (e.g. perineal, rectovaginal fistula and atresias), vertebral abnormalities, other atresias (e.g. tracheo-oesophageal atresia), and urinary tract infections.

c. High lesions require a preliminary colostomy and later surgical repair (anorectoplasty or pull-through procedure). Low lesions may have a simple skin flap over the anus and incision will be curative. Continence is rarely achieved in high lesions because of hypoplasia or damage to the internal sphincter.

Index

Invisible River

HELENA McEWEN grew up in Scotland and trained as an artist at Chelsea School of Art and Camberwell School of Art. She is the acclaimed author of *The Big House* and *...irl*. She lives in Scotland.

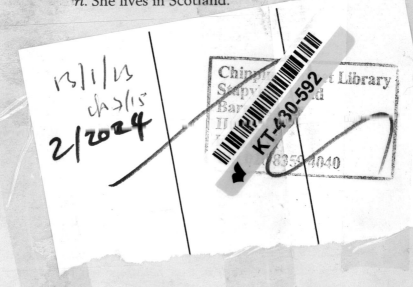

Invisible
River

Helena McEwen

BLOOMSBURY

LONDON · BERLIN · NEW YORK · SYDNEY

First published in Great Britain 2011
This paperback edition published 2012

Copyright © 2011 by Helena McEwen

The moral right of the author has been asserted

Bloomsbury Publishing, London, Berlin and New York

50 Bedford Square, London WC1B 3DP

A CIP catalogue record for this book is available from the British Library

ISBN 978 1 4088 2167 1
10 9 8 7 6 5 4 3 2 1

Typeset by Hewer Text UK Ltd, Edinburgh
Printed in Great Britain by Clays Limited, St Ives plc

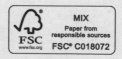

MIX
Paper from
responsible sources
FSC® C018072

www.bloomsbury.com/helenamcewen

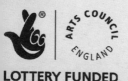

LOTTERY FUNDED

To my parents,
with love and thanks

Part One

1

I just wanted him to turn round and wave as the train went out, instead of walking up the platform with that gloomy stooped back. Turn round and wave and say, 'It's all right, you can leave, I'm all right.'

But he didn't, because he's not.

And when I walked along the moving carriage to look out the open window, the train threw me around against the knobs, like it was angry.

He didn't turn round, so part of me went with him up the platform. Went with him up to the house, where he'd be bound to get the bottle out, doesn't matter it's before breakfast.

That's why he didn't turn round. So part of me would go back with him, up to the house, into the kitchen.

And I saw St Michael's Mount slip away behind the hedges, with the sun glinting on the sea.

'Let me go!' I shouted at the sea, and then at the hedges, and into the marshes at Marazion.

And all the way through Cornwall past Redruth and Cambourne and Bodmin Moor and St Austell I could feel the pull of my father left alone.

I was halfway into Devon before it happened.

It was because of those tunnels cut in the red rock; you plunge into them after the miles of sealight, and the tentacles couldn't hold on. They had to let go, and then the city of London began to hum like a magnet, pulling me towards it.

It was telling me my future with promising feelings.

I arrived, and London splashed me all over. A big wave. Lots of experiences all at the same time, colours and loud noises. Women in patterned headscarves asking for money, and men in dark jackets calling out words, and many signs pointing you along bridges and upstairs and down walkways, and old ladies looking bewildered and men in uniform having an argument, and blaring traffic noise and electric skies shining dark and light at the same time and lights changing colours, and so many faces.

And after a lonely night in the hall of residence, at the end of a long grey corridor lit with striplighting that flickered and made the air tremble, and the strange dislocated not-here feeling in that little room that smelt of gravy, I walked out into the autumn morning and smelt a bonfire behind the exhaust fumes. I only had to cross the road to walk into the tall glass cube that would be my art school for the next three years.

I've brought my canvas bag with my brushes wrapped up in a tea towel, sticks of charcoal wrapped in tissue paper, a bottle of linseed oil and twenty-two tubes of paint, as though I am going to start painting straight away. But the girl who consults a list, and tells me we have been specifically told *not* to bring materials on Induction Day, sends me up in the lift to the third floor.

I find my way along the corridor to my name on a piece of paper taped to the wall, and put my bag down next to an easel. I am gazing at my white space.

'Who are you? I am Bianca,' says an Italian voice.

I turn round.

'Hello, I'm Eve.'

Bianca has also brought a canvas bag full of materials, gold paper and different coloured glass pots, which she begins to unpack.

'They have forgotten the TRO! In-TRO-duction,' she says. Her voice has a bell in it, a ting-a-ling sound. She is unusually thin, but she has a glitter about her.

'It's because they're inducing us, like babies being induced into the world of the art school,' says a voice from the corridor.

Bianca laughs.

'I'm Roberta,' she says, coming into the studio and putting her basket on the locker and two plastic bags on the ground, which both fall over, so paint-spattered tubs of acrylic roll over the floor. 'But call me Rob.'

She has a round face and dark curly hair.

'Hello, Rob.'

'I recognize you from the interview,' she says to me.

'Yes!' I say. 'What was yours like?'

'Oh, hellish. One of them was drunk!'

'I didn't like the head of painting much.'

'Oh, the small one who kicks your pictures about?'

'Yes!'

'No, me neither.'

'Where are you from?'

'Near Nottingham, and you?'

'Cornwall.'

'I'm from Rome,' says Bianca.

'Have you come all the way from Italy?' says Rob.

'I am escaping.'

'What from?'

'Bad people.'

'There are bad people here, you know.'

'Yes, but I don't know them!'

In the lift we discover that Rob's boyfriend, Mick, is doing metalwork at Camberwell.

The induction tutor glares at us, tapping her clipboard with her biro, as we join the first-years at the bottom of the stairs.

We are divided up. In our group there is a blonde girl from Ulster, a pretty and delicate-looking girl from Liverpool, slender as a bird, with pale skin. She wears a pair of enormous boots so she looks like a doll. Two girls from Manchester who titter together, a girl with long red hair, a Japanese boy and a young man with a black beard but no moustache who says 'fuck this' and 'fuck that' all the time.

'We will begin in Sculpture!' says the tutor, pointing her biro.

We walk through the doors into the noise of banging and welding and the screech of the circular saw. Sparks are flying, there is a smell of metal, sawn wood and plaster. A student in a blue overall is cutting through metal.

'Fuck this!' shouts the young bearded man into the noise.

We are shown how to use the lathe, what precautions to take with the welder, where the plaster of paris is kept, and how to use the glue-gunning machine.

We walk away from the screeching sound, past partitioned spaces with drawings taped to the walls and stacks of sketchbooks, into a room that is quiet.

Five people are in a kind of meditation, putting layers of white gauze soaked in plaster of paris on to armatures made of wood and wire. Their hands and fingers are white, and I like watching the white fingers smoothing the soaked gauze. They stand back patiently while we look at the ghostly forms.

Outside, next to the enormous kilns, are sheds full of bags of clay, huge pieces of stone, tree trunks, prams, bicycles, bits of rusty wrought iron and some old windows.

'Isn't it beautiful!' says Bianca.

We walk through large studios where students stand about in the midst of their work, gathered round kettles, smoking cigarettes, or look up from their absorption as though we are barely visible.

Rob says 'Hello!' to a blonde girl, who looks at her blankly and turns away.

We walk into the ground-floor studio for enormous canvases, large as the side of houses. 'Fuck that,' says the young man, with admiration.

'Who was she?' asks Bianca.

'She goes out with a friend of Mick's,' says Rob. 'She's a third-year and, well . . . I'm a first year. That's Suzanne! Stuck-up cow.'

'Porca miseria!' says Bianca. 'I can't bear these cool English cucumber types!'

Rob and I both laugh. 'What? What is funny?' says Bianca.

2

We are shown round the lecture theatre on the first floor, the art history department and the secretary's office. We are introduced to Miss Pym, the secretary, and Tom, the first-year tutor.

At last it is time for lunch.

Roberta and Bianca and I sit together with the red-haired girl, and discover things about each other. One wall of the canteen is made of glass, so we are in the courtyard along with the pigeons.

Cecile is a ballerina who has been dancing for the Royal Ballet, but received an injury and decided to change her career. She sits with a perfectly erect spine.

Rob is going to marry Mick. He is a blacksmith and they've known each other since they were five. We all say ooh! because childhood sweethearts make people say ooh! along with the vision of horseshoes, and cold autumn mornings, and a young man with a pinkish face holding the hind leg of a horse and tapping it.

We find out that Rob lives near London Bridge with Mick, that Bianca lives in Brixton with two Italian girls who are doing textiles at Goldsmiths, and the ballerina lives in Kensington with her husband, who is twenty-two years older.

'And I live in a soulless room down a long corridor in the Halls of Residence,' I say gloomily.

'I will ask around for you,' says Bianca.

'Thanks,' I say.

The stairwell winds up the centre of the building, lit by a huge skylight. The rooms and studios are arranged around the landings, and lit by walls of windows. The further up the building you go, the more London spreads out before you.

The print rooms on the second floor overlook the King's Road and St Stephen's, and are filled with printing presses for wood cut, lino cut and etching.

There are baths for soaking paper and lines to dry it on. There are racks for newly printed prints and acid baths for placing the etching plates. There are shelves with tins of ink, and a long wooden desk under the windows.

Round the corner, where the screen-printing press stands, the windows look over treetops towards the Fulham Road, and two girls stand at big basins in black plastic aprons, hosing ink out of the screen-printing mesh. The jet of water shoots out of the hose and turns red and yellow before coiling into the drain.

We look round Photography and the dark room, with the red light, and white baths of chemicals that flavour the air.

'I can't take any more!' says Bianca. 'I can't remember all these processes!'

Rob laughs. 'You don't have to, don't worry. It's just if you want to use this stuff, you have to have a vague idea.'

On the third floor we meet Steve, the head of film. He has long greasy hair that he smooths back from his forehead every now and then, slowly, with his whole hand, while looking sideways.

Bianca mimics his gesture and we get the giggles. He wears a jacket made of leather.

A tall girl with a scarf around her head strides out of a studio, saying, 'Who has stolen the red heads?' Steve tells us proudly that this girl is in the third year and has just been commissioned to make her *second* short film for Channel Four, and that red heads are spotlights.

There is a buzzing sound in the video rooms, and we watch a video of someone's hand putting pig's guts in a bucket, that goes round and round on a loop. Cecile pulls a disgusted face. Steve says, 'It makes a strong statement.'

In the editing suite Steve shows us how to use the projector and splice the film, the video equipment and where the spotlights are kept.

'I'm worn out!' says Bianca, as we come out on to the landing. 'I have to lie down,' and she lies down on the floor and closes her eyes.

We walk round the figurative studios, divided by a maze of white-painted partitions.

I walk past paintings of fossils and shells, screaming people and grey empty landscapes. The studios smell of oil paint, turpentine and white spirit. There is a quietness here.

In the life room the model is taking a break, wrapped in a blue curtain and drinking coffee from a plastic cup. She sits on the edge of the mattress, her pink toes stroking each other. The students are standing around and looking at each other's work. They turn to look at us with dazed expressions.

The technician's workshop is on the top floor. It smells of wood, and we meet Geoff, the technician, in a brown coat with a pencil behind his ear. He has a friendly open face and nods at each of us in turn and explains how to cut the stretchers, saw the angles, and nail them with corrugated nails, how to stretch the canvas over the stretchers, and melt the rabbit-skin glue to prepare the size. The ballerina asks him if you can make size without using animal products.

Sinéad, from Ulster, flicks her eyes up to the ceiling.

There are woodshavings on the floor and the circular saw makes a whirring sound as he shows us how to slice through the plank without cutting your hand off.

On the landing we meet Terry, the abstract tutor, who has bloodshot eyes.

'I've heard he has a drink problem,' whispers Sinéad, with a snort.

'This way,' he says.

Through the windows on the abstract floor, you can see all the way past the bend in the river to Westminster and the far-away blue buildings on the horizon.

The rooms are also lit from skylights in the roof, and I think that even this building, with all its light pouring in, began as a drawing; and before that it was a thought. And I'm glad the architect put so much light into his thought.

And I like wandering through the studio spaces full of abstract forms and sketchbooks bursting with ideas, stacked up on the floor or leaning against each other along makeshift shelves.

Sometimes the canvases are huge and fill a whole wall; cadmium-red singing on grey, with cobalt violet and sienna.

Sometimes they are small; collages made of feathers and corrugated cardboard and grey paint the colour of the sky and pigeons.

I sneak a look into a sketchbook and see pages of colour variations, like looking at different musical chords made visible and singing on the page.

Students begin to go downstairs for tea.

But when everyone leaves, the studios are not empty. The ideas are everywhere. They make the air hum. And I stand in the darkening space and see the twilight falling all the way to Westminster.

3

I take the silver lift down to the ground floor and feel a blast of cold wind from the open front door as I walk into the canteen. Through the wall made of glass, the big tree and the Henry Moore sculpture in the courtyard are turning blue. People are reflected in the glass.

I stand in the queue behind a tall young man in a tartan shirt that has dots of white paint spattered over it in an arc, that match up with the splashes on his trousers.

He has long black hair tied with an elastic band, blue-black like a crow. He turns his head. He smiles at me then frowns a funny frown and peers unexpectedly towards my eyebrows.

I have a spot on my forehead.

'It's about to pop!' he says, nodding at it.

'I know!' I say, laughing at his rudeness. We don't say anything else.

I get my mug of tea served from a big silver teapot by a lady in a white bath-cap.

'There you are, duck,' she says.

Bianca turns and waves at me. I sit down with her and Rob.

They are examining a list of options: etching, lithography, photography, animation, life drawing, painting: media and supports, sculpture: plaster/clay.

I look across to see where the dark-haired man went.

'Who's *that?*' says Bianca, looking round and seeing him too. He is leaning against a table, talking to someone. I like his easy way of moving.

'Oh, I know him. That's Zeb, he's a friend of Mick's. They did foundation together,' says Rob.

'Call him over, call him over,' says Bianca, tugging on Rob's sleeve.

'Hi, Zeb!' she calls out, but he doesn't hear.

Suzanne comes through the door. She starts talking to Zeb.

'That's his girlfriend!' says Rob.

'Oh, that is Suzanne's boyfriend!' says Bianca, looking disappointed.

The head of painting strolls into the canteen. He is a small man with hair that grows like moss. He stands with his feet apart and his hands on his hips inside his jacket, and surveys. He strides over and addresses us, and the tables nearby. 'Welcome to you, first years!' How are you settling in?' he says.

'When can we see your paintings, please?' says Bianca loudly.

I like the bell sound in her voice.

'Well! There are some in the library on slide, and quite a few catalogues of the shows I've had,' he says rather smugly, then takes a breath in to announce something else.

'No! the real ones! Can we see the real ones?'

His lips press together, slightly annoyed at the interruption, but he puts an easygoing face on things. 'One day I'm sure we can arrange a trip to my studio. Now then!' he rubs his hands together.

'When?'

He ignores her, and speaks up. 'I'd like you all to come to the lecture theatre in half an hour so we, the tutors, can introduce ourselves to you.' He bows a little, pointing his hands at himself.

'And you,' his hands go out to the side, 'can meet us! And then we can learn a *little* bit about what we expect from each other. Thanks very much!' He puts his palms up in the air and nods. 'See you later!' he says, and twirls round so his jacket twirls too.

'Creep,' says Bianca.

The next time I see Zeb is in the corridor when I've got lost on the abstract floor looking for film and photography, because we are doing animation. He is carrying a roll of chicken wire and some ping-pong balls. The balls are dropping and bouncing.

I start chasing them and pick one up; the other one drops down the stairwell and we both look over and can hear its musical bounce echoing as it falls through the floors.

'Well done!' he says, nodding at my eyebrow, and I just laugh.

And when I've finished drawing a hundred and seventy-two pictures of a small man doing a dance so his hips wiggle, and his arms wave, for one and a half seconds of film, I help him move the rest of his stuff down to his new work space. We talk about living in London, and the microbiology of the Thames.

Zeb is in the second year. He was put on the abstract floor until his paintings began to grow a dimension and they moved him down to sculpture. When he began to project film on to them they moved him back up to film. Then the pieces began to move so they put him next to the technician's office. Now they make sounds as well as moving, so they've put him on the mezzanine which used to be a storeroom.

'They don't know which box to put you in!' I say.

'I know,' he says.

4

The weeks begin to follow a routine.

On Tuesdays we have a class with Geoff. He teaches us how to make our own pastels with sieved earth and rice water, and lamp black pigment, by baking chicken bones in a biscuit tin until they are burnt; and how to size canvas and make primer with titanium white and rabbit-skin glue.

Wednesday life drawing class with Karl is compulsory for the first term. Thursday evenings is art history. Long lectures in the chilly lecture theatre, with Andrew Mackinley-Davis, who uses words like 'polemic', 'dialectic' and 'post-postmodern'. We come out of the lectures with glazed eyes.

On Friday afternoon it's 'museums and galleries'. We can choose what. It even includes an afternoon watching films if you want, at the NFT or ICA, as long as it's in a cinema with initials.

The rest of the time we spend in the studio, or drawing outside.

I'm sitting on the windowsill above the radiator, looking out the window at the far-away tower blocks on the horizon. They look blue.

'What do you vote, then?' I say.

'Museum of London,' says Rob.

'Sounds drab!' says Bianca, taking the coffee pot off the heat.

'Why not the V and A?'

'I don't want to look at *decorative* art,' says Rob.

'*Decorative art*,' mimics Bianca over the coffee pot.

Bianca has been moved up to the abstract floor, and it has become our habit to gather in her new space and drink real coffee that she percolates in her silver coffee pot on the ring she melts the wax on.

And after drawing in the cold wind all day, or struggling with a painting that won't work, or an afternoon stretching canvases till your thumbs are sore, it is a relief to gather in Bianca's space and sit on the windowsill above the radiators, looking out over the trees, and watch the weather changing in the sky.

'Tom says we should definitely go to the Hayward.'

'Who cares!'

'Paul says we should start with the National Gallery.'

'Which one's Paul?'

'Oh, I loathe them!' says Bianca.

'Tom's all right.'

'Who's got your goat now?' says Rob, crossing her legs and leaning against the wall.

'No one has my goat,' says Bianca indignantly. 'I have my own goat!'

'I don't like the small one, he's venomous,' says Cecile.

'Is that Paul?'

'What did he say to you?'

'That my work was twee.'

'That's very nice of him.'

'He's a bloody moron.'

'Have you seen *his* pictures?'

'No, what are they like?'

'Vertical stripes, that's all, vertical stripes of varying thickness.'

'You got to be careful what they tell you, they don't bloody know.'

'You know what Zeb calls them?'

'What?'

'Art officials!'

Bianca lies down on the battered chaise longue. She pulled it out of a skip. She wants it to lend some elegance to her painting space. It is faded orange-pink, worn through at the end, where the horsehair stuffing is coming out.

She puts her forearm over her eyes.

'Art officials,' she murmurs. 'Oh, I get it!' and laughs.

'You get tired easily,' says Roberta, sipping her coffee.

'It's because I have an illness,' says Bianca, still with her eyes closed.

'What illness?'

'Hepatitis.'

'Hepatitis?'

'Yes. Hepatitis D. I am very fashionable!' says Bianca languidly.

Rob finishes her coffee and gets up.

'Well, I'm going to the Museum of London. If you want to come, I'll meet you in our space.'

I follow her downstairs. We have been moved to a lovely space next to a big window. We've divided it with a butter muslin curtain that catches the light in its folds and glows white.

We pack our materials.

'I don't think Bianca will come, do you?'

But she is already at the studio door.

'I am coming!' she says. 'I have three sketchbooks, some charcoal, some coloured paper if we want to do collage.' She opens her bag. 'A box of oil pastels, three Conté sticks, some watercolours . . .'

'Hang on, hang on, Bianca, we're going to look at the museum.'

'I know, but I can't not take my things. Here, will you take some water?' She turns to me.

In the end we walk down the road with three canvas bags, two rolls of paper, seven sketchbooks and a vast assortment of media.

We take the bus along King's Road past the glittering shops, and the twiggy branches of the overhanging trees hit the window in the top deck so that we duck. We get off at Sloane Square and dive into the choking air of the Underground that shunts us to St Paul's, where we explode out of the darkness into the sunlight. We walk past St Botolph's, where there is a little garden and a fountain squeezed between the glass and concrete of the city like a slip of London from another time. We ride up an escalator in a glass tube and travel down a concrete walkway across a tangle of thundering roads and reach the Museum of London.

Bianca wants to go to the rooms that show Roman London. She's proud of her ancestors, and takes it personally when we call them invaders. Roberta and I wander into the Stone Age, where the sound of macaque monkeys squealing is played on a tape, and trilling birds, to mimic the sounds when London was a tropical jungle.

Rob unrolls her paper on the floor and begins a huge drawing in brown chalk of cave bears and rivers and crouching people, animal-headed women and large-leaved plants, and I have to walk away from her throbbing images in case I get pulled into her world, because me, I'm still looking for mine.

And underneath it all, under the shining glass and the old bones and the sounds of mammoths, and clay pots, behind the light-up displays and the touch-and-sniff, the lists of plants, the wall charts of climate change from the Palaeolithic to the Mesolithic, and the glass cases of rounded stones they brought to the river from Cornwall and Cumbria, Scotland and Ireland, maybe it's there, waiting for me to find it.

Rob has her paper spread out on the floor, sitting happily with her long dark curls falling on the page, her legs out at right angles, leaning over the drawing, with schoolchildren walking around her, stopping to glance at the mysterious animals and ancient landscape that flow out of her chalk and commenting to each other and whispering, two little boys in red V-neck jerseys pointing at the women with their breasts exposed, and giggling, until the teacher, with her clipboard, ushers them forward into the Bronze Age.

I look at the pots from 4000 BC marked with fingernails, and wonder, whose fingernail was it? who were you? and what did you think? It says here you thought the Thames was a deity and that's why you came from every end of the islands and beyond to throw your special stones into the water. When Pall Mall was a field of marigolds and mugwort, when artemisia was flowering in Mayfair and the ice had receded like a miracle, and the grass seeds had been blown on the warm wind, and the birch trees grew and the oak forests, and the red deer followed, and then along the river and through the trees you came and gathered round the hearth fires at night, that sent sparks upwards, the air filled with the smell of aromatic herbs and wet earth; and dawn, by the huge river, the reed warblers echoing off the water. A time of plenty, it says. I just like thinking of them all, sitting around in the woods, where Piccadilly is now, fashioning fine flint blades and listening to the birds.

I sigh. I don't like my little drawings of imaginary people sitting next to a river, dressed in skins.

I wander along the corridor following the timeline of Celts, Romans, Saxons, Danes and through a doorway into Londinium 47–550 AD.

Bianca is sitting by a replica of the Temple of Mithras, found beside the buried River Walbrook, listening to tape recordings of Roman soldiers shouting at each other in Latin.

In the large dark room the glass cases glow yellow and light up the faces of people as they wander through, like sleepwalkers, led by their headphones that are speaking them back through time.

We come out of the Museum and pass London Wall.

'Roman! says Bianca with triumph, and Rob looks cross.

Through the tall buildings of the city we can see the dome of St Paul's.

We step out into Ludgate Hill, and smartly dressed people are spilling out of doorways, rushing down the pavement and across the road and queuing at every sandwich shop. It is the city at lunchtime. We walk through the crowds and stand at a bus stop.

The big red bus opens sliding doors; we climb up the stairs and swerve down towards the glinting river.

5

I didn't know it when she said it, but it means something when Bianca says she'll ask around. She puts the word out into her enormous network of Italians, Venezuelans, Chileans and Portuguese, and within days you have a new sofa, a part-time job, a removal van, a free TV, or a new place to live.

The bedsit I move to is no palace, but even though the skylight is stuck open and the washing machine is broken and the kitchen as small as a cupboard, I prefer it to the double glazing, the blotchy linoleum, the striplighting and smell of institutions that I thought would gobble me up like that insect that lays its eggs in a frog and eats it from the inside.

I thought that would happen to me. I'd be sucked out somehow.

But thanks to Bianca, I have my own place now.

And every morning I cycle through the rowan trees, past the pyramids of cauliflowers and oranges, the stalls of red and brown handbags and different-coloured dresses, and climb up the stairs to the studio where Roberta paints her mysterious paintings.

I'm envious of Rob's paintings.

Downstairs in the basement, Cecile is painting huge flowers. Upstairs, Bianca is making work from glinting metallic paper, gold leaf and melted beeswax mixed with pigment; beautiful collages that glint in the light and glow in the half-light.

And I am painting London.

It is autumn and the city is lit by yellow trees. I walk around the streets, looking at paintings that haven't been painted yet, and I draw on the corner of streets at night, and by the river in the day, and from cafés high up above the road so I can see the distance is blue. And I take the drawings back to the studio and tape them on the wall to paint from. I paint Sloane Square from Peter Jones with a circle of trees and a red bus going up Sloane Street, and I draw Cambridge Circus from the Fruit of the Loom pub and paint the turquoise lamp-posts and orange brick buildings and a sky cut in half by the clouds.

In London the clouds have a habit of cutting the sky in half, so the sun shines from beneath and lights the buildings up yellow so they glow against the grey sky, and even the tower blocks look beautiful, lilac and grey with glowing pink windows reflecting the sunset shining against the dark evening sky.

And I learn about near, far and middle distance, and tone from dark to light, through all the in-betweens, and complementary colours that glow and shine together.

I look for them in the city streets and I see the sun shining through red leaves, next to green, and glistening on the wet grass.

I see a large yellow sun between dark lilac clouds, so it looks like a big eye with rays of lemon-yellow eyelashes.

I see an orange globe flashing at a zebra crossing when the sky is turning blue.

And Bianca calls it the yellow season except for the ash trees, their leaves flame-red, the tips purple so they glow from within like embers. I paint the dark street with brown madder, magenta and translucent Indian yellow painted over white, so it glows. The streetlight shining in the darkness, illuminating the trees.

I must have been invisible when I was doing the drawings for it, because a man raced past me with a bag in his hand. Not long after came a plump man, puffing, and then a lady with her hat askew, wheezing and clip-clopping on unsuitable heels. If they'd asked me I would have told them where he ran. But I didn't think to tell them, I was just watching the night.

And I paint the river. The beautiful river.

I go down to the river in the dark, and see the green lights reflected in the water, just after sunset when the sky is streaked with pink and the starlings gather and fly under and over the bridge with their startling precision.

I paint the river from Westminster Bridge, looking over St Paul's; from Albert Bridge when the leaves are turning, streaked with pink light at dusk; from Battersea Bridge, looking down towards the park and the serene gold Buddha.

I even persuade Rob to get up before sunrise to paint the dawn, and we sit on the police pier at Blackfriars and paint the sun rising over Tower Bridge. A grey green before dawn light that slowly turns to pink and lights the water, and then the streaks of yellow begin beyond the blue distant buildings, and we paint with watercolours, one, two, three pictures in as many minutes because the colours change so fast and the sky turns pink then yellow as the sun rises and shines down the river in a ribbon of light.

But Rob doesn't need the river, or the park, or the houses with the lights coming on, she doesn't need the street lights turning from pink to yellow or the turquoise shadows or the purple London night, or finding a place high enough to paint the bend in the river, or see the distance is blue. She doesn't even need the colours. She can make them in simple black and white, drawings and paintings endlessly pouring out of her, like dreams. Landscapes with paths and trees, and a man with a crown who holds his penis erect, and women who squat and give birth to other women, and horses, and people who she knows but has never seen; she knows how to make an unseen world into pictures and I want to know too.

6

'Will you come and help or just keep watch?' Rob says.

'Keep watch, why?'

'Well, they might not allow it.'

'You're only going to collect some earth.'

She shrugs. 'Well, you're not allowed to do lots of things that are perfectly reasonable.'

Ever since we went to the museum she's been obsessed with these ideas she won't talk about, only now they have to be made with mud, not just any mud, though, river mud. That's why we end up going to Battersea Park just before the gates close so that the twilight is beginning to fall and all the blackbirds and robins and song thrushes and blue tits in the park are singing their separate songs together in a big dusk chorus, and climb over the fence by the weeping willow with a trowel and a spade and four plastic bags, and dig up the mud from the river where it is low. But it's not the Thames, it's 'Tamesa', Rob says, which means 'the dark one', and she says a prayer to the river which embarrasses me slightly before we dig, which goes, 'Oh dark water, I am your daughter', but I am rather glad of the rhyme, and we spade the mud into the bags until they are full and ridiculously heavy, so we have to spade some of it out again, then realize that we can't climb up the walls that we've jumped down from, and

we have to call one of the joggers to get the park attend-
ant who we've tried so hard to avoid, so that he can fetch
a ladder from the gardens in the quadrangle where they
grow the bedding plants and get us out.

He says, 'What the hell are you doing down there?'

'Collecting mud for my painting,' says Rob.

'But she won't tell you the details,' I say. 'She's not telling any of us.'

'Oh, so you're the helper.'

'I am,' I say, as I climb back over the fence.

'Well, good luck to you. If you run outa mud just let
me know.'

'Thank you, we appreciate it,' says Rob, picking up the
bags.

'Tell us when the art exhibition's on so I can see what
you're up to,' he says, following us down the path.

'Certainly will,' says Rob.

'You sure you can manage with all them bags of mud?'

'Yes, we're fine, thanks,' says Rob, and we trudge out
the gates, the night turning blue, and the green lights
rippling over the dark water.

Zeb says that around every river is an invisible river. It
extends all around, down and to the side for 500 feet,
and it's full of micro-organisms, and the health of the
river depends on the health of the invisible river. And
I suppose that around every city is an invisible city also.

7

We walk into the dark courtyard, and through the glass wall we see Bianca and Cecile having tea in the lit-up canteen.

'They look like they're in an Edward Hopper painting,' says Rob.

Bianca sees us, and waves us in to join them.

We sit down in the canteen with the bags of mud.

'Where have you been?' says Bianca.

'Oh, don't ask!' says Rob.

'All right, I won't!' says Bianca, and turns back to Cecile. 'So anyway, what happened? She's telling me about the portrait commission. That awful woman's husband, and the photo of her smiling, with all her teeth showing?'

'Oh,' Cecile groans. 'He came to collect it, and said I'd made her look like a horse! I had to go to her gilt house with chintz everything and paint her lips again, this time closed, so the horse didn't show!'

'Oh my God, the horse!' Bianca squeals in a high-pitched voice.

'She wants a portrait that makes her look ten years younger!' says Cecile, who is so poised and demure-looking it is surprising when she swears. 'And fuck him! I changed it three times and he didn't offer me a penny more!'

Zeb walks past our table with his empty tray, and Bianca catches his arm.

'When are you going to show us your sculptures, Mister Zebedee?'

'When do you want to see them?' he says.

'Anytime!'

'Come on up, then!'

So we all troop up to the mezzanine, in a row, with Bianca making faces at us.

There are skylights in his space but no windows and the sink faces a wall. It is a big low sink with taps underneath it in the pipes. His space is crammed with bits of television sets, plugs and wires, old radios, their inner wiring exposed. There are projectors and canvases and cameras, some half taken apart. There are hammers and screws and rolls of steel wire, and copper tubing, and then there are his sculptures, which light up and tinkle. Strange otherworldly beings that have a logic of their own. Zeb's logic. Some ping rubber bands, some project light through bottles of different coloured water which quivers on the wall in a slow rotation.

'Wow! they are so fantastic,' says Bianca, touching them with her thin fingers, and looking them up and down.

Zeb stands in the corner, his hands in his back pockets and his head leaning over to one side.

He likes artists called Tinguely and Twombly and scientists who propose eleven dimensions.

He says he's seen his sculptures when he travels in dreams to other planets, but his don't work as well as those did.

'You like putting things together?' says Bianca, examining the constructions.

31

'And taking things apart,' he says, laughing.

'I wish you'd take apart my washing machine!' I say.

'I'll come and have a look if you like,' he says.

I didn't expect him to say that.

'That would be great!' I say.

Bianca looks at me out the side of her eyes. I glare at her. Bianca likes making up stories, even if she knows they aren't true.

'Well, I could come on Saturday morning,' he says, crouching down and looking through a box of tools.

'Thanks,' I say.

8

'Well, how late are you?'
  'Six weeks.'
  'Since it should have come, or since your last one?'
  'Since my last one.'
  'But that's not long, it's only two weeks.'
  'I'm never late.'
Rob looks down at the bags of mud, and puts her hands
on her head.
  'I suppose I better take them home.'
  'What are you going to do?'
  'Bake it, then sieve it.'
  'What?'
  'The earth. Make it into pigment!'
She looks at me and realizes, and we both laugh.
She shakes her head.
  'Oh, it'll be all right,' she says.
I nod. 'Course it will.'
  'I'll have a baby, I mean, why not?'
  'You'd be a great mum, Rob.'
  'Just didn't expect it quite so soon.'
  'You might not be, though. It's only two weeks.'

9

On Saturday morning I am sitting in my kitchen, and the doorbell rings.

I run down the stairs to let Zeb in.

'D'you want a cup of tea?' I say, showing him into the kitchen.

'No no,' he says. 'I'll get on with it,' and he has soon pulled the machine out from the wall and begun to undo it. I leave him to his deconstruction and sit next door, hearing all the little noises and clinks and thuds of the washing machine being taken apart. When I look through the curtain of plastic strips the washing machine is all over the floor, lined up in little rows, all the cogs and tubes and washers.

He looks up.

'I'm working out how it works,' he says.

'Don't you know?' I say.

'Well, no, I've never taken a washing machine apart before,' he says, moving the pieces slowly along the floor. His tall body is folded, and he is crouching on one knee. There is something graceful about his movements.

'Don't worry,' he says, looking up and smiling at me. 'It'll work fine!' and within an hour it is chugging away.

I watch him unfolding himself, standing up and stretching. He has to lay his hands flat on the ceiling.

'It's all right, isn't it, your little pad.'

'Yes, I like it. Look, you can see the river,' and I show him through the gap in the houses, and the rain pouring in slants.

'And you've got the market,' he says, pointing behind his head.

'Yes, I'm going there in a minute.'

'Well, I hope you've got your canoe!' he says, and I laugh.

'Look, Zeb, can I give you some money for this?'

'No-oh!' he says in a cascade of notes. 'It was fun!'

'Fun?' I say, thinking of my panic at all things mechanical.

'Yes, some people do crosswords,' he says, patting me on the shoulder affectionately. 'Anyway, it was my pleasure. Right! I'm on my way!'

'You're going to get soaked!'

'I will survive!' he sings as he walks down the stairs, and shouts 'See you!' when he slams the front door.

So I give him the magic shells instead. I leave them in his space wrapped up in a small drawing of a washing machine.

They open under water. I bought them in Chinatown when I was drawing pictures of Cambridge Circus.

I'd been lured down Gerard Street by the glowing lanterns and coloured paper decorations in the windows of the little shops, and out of the icy wind that was biting my face with cold rain, and making my fingers numb.

The lady in the shop couldn't speak English but she nodded at me and smiled and spoke Chinese and made delicate movements with her fingers and managed that way to explain what the little shells contained. I took them home and put one in a glass of water and waited. Nothing happened.

But next morning, I looked up and saw the shell had opened; the pink and yellow and blue paper flowers had unfurled, along with green fronds, and there in the glass was a miniature underwater garden.

10

Rob is preparing big pieces of paper seven feet tall, painting them with a wallpaper brush and PVA to coat the surface, and the smell of baked earth fills the studio, sweet and soft. Rob took the earth home, and baked it in her oven, while she waited for the line to turn blue. By the time she'd sieved the earth to a fine raw umber powder, and ruined the sieve, it was definitely dark blue. She said Mick was over the moon.

She is going to mix the earth, baked and sieved, with cold-pressed linseed oil.

'So you're sure?' I said.

'Yes,' she said.

'Well, well, well,' I said smiling, and I could tell by her face that she was glad too.

'But I want to keep it quiet for a bit,' she says, her eyes looking upwards to the ceiling, and I nod.

Behind the muslin curtain, on my table next to the window, I have a piece of smooth wood for mixing colours.

I notice a matchbox sitting there. I pick it up and push it open. A little yellow jack jumps out attached to a spring. It startles me and makes me smile. It must be from Zeb.

I make it ping out of the box a few times.

Then I leave it on the windowsill and pull a canvas out from under the table and get to work.

I rub the white surface of the canvas with rose doré, a translucent pink pigment made with gold. It is a delicate pigment; if you mix it with even the tiniest amount of another colour it disappears into it.

The colour prefers not to be mixed but to be laid over a white ground so the white shines through it and lights up its delicate pinky orange hue.

The surface is ready. It is a colour field.

I squeeze the tubes of oil paint on to the palette, one by one.

I love the colours and their secret singing.

Aureolin, a gentle golden yellow that is soft and hums, and high-pitched lemon yellow, sharp and startling, then the low velvet tone of alizarin crimson, and the seductive cobalt blue. It fills me with longing, if cobalt blue was a man I'd run away with him. He calls with a longing to far away. Blue is a calling-away colour and its sound is a sound so beautiful it makes you want to leave the earth. Not red though, red pipes up, especially cadmium scarlet. 'Do-do-doooo,' it says like a trumpet, it runs in your blood the same sound, 'yes, this is life!' It gets hot and passionate. If you put it in a painting it jumps forward, 'I am here!' it says, 'right here, ME!' and I love red for that. Then the beautiful violets, half red, half blue. Cobalt violet, singing in the range next to pink, but with more majesty, more mystery, and ultramarine violet, gentle, tender, like the shadows in twilight, but deep, with dignity and a hidden depth, like someone who walks among people but knows they are really a seraph.

Then translucent golden green that is like the sun shining through leaves, cinnabar green, spring leaves unfurling in the new light, chrome green, heavy like a green stone washed by the waves.

I couldn't work in the studios with music blaring because the ideas can't gather in the silence, and besides, you can't hear the colours.

I mix them on the palette.

The rose doré ground is ready. Orange pink. It is a small canvas, a foot square, but big enough for a world. I put some cinnabar green, some rose pink mixed with white, some royal blue. The colours sing together on the surface and already there is a space and a distance, a place for something to arrive.

I love the feeling in the studio, of the presence of the reality that we call into our pictures. It fills the empty space with invisible threads of light that touch that other realm. The ideas hang in the air, becoming more real with imagining, more robust and less wispy, until they are so real that they come and sit on the end of the paintbrush and get mixed in with the colours and appear on the canvas unexpectedly. An idea you might have had months ago will suddenly appear fully formed and look at you from the primed surface. The threads gather in the corners and on the ceiling like spiders' webs, but they aren't musty, they have a singing presence. You can feel them. They are halfway in, half out, between realities.

Roberta makes a quietness around her when she works. It is deep and palpable. I can feel it on the surface of my skin. She breathes and concentrates and the concentration makes a deep feeling that draws you into it; without her the ideas fly about untethered, with her in the room everything gathers and is brought down. We fall into deep concentration together, like a stone falling to the bottom of the sea, down and down, to the forest of coral, the flashes and flits of colour, the rippling underwater light.

I tell Rob her baby must be influencing us from his underwater world; half in and half out of this reality, his spirit still resident in the place where anything is possible. I think he must dart about among the ideas, spinning them around like toys.

11

'What happened? What happened?' says Bianca eagerly, when I walk into her space.

'What d'you mean, what happened?'

'On Saturday with Zeb!'

'He fixed my washing machine!'

'Nothing happened?'

'No. Nothing *happened*, Bianca'

'If you were Italian something would happen,' she says, looking dejected.

'Look, he's a friend. I like him,'

'Ah, how dull!' she says, waving me away.

I laugh and sit down on the windowsill, but I don't tell her about the jack-in-a-box.

There is a smell of resin. She is using egg yolk mixed with pigment. There are brown bags of pure cobalt blue, and ultramarine. The colours jump out at you when you open the bags.

The eggshells quiver as she walks across the floor, to place her pictures on the nails to look at them.

Her work has become more sturdy, on wood instead of paper.

As her collages have become more robust it seems she is getting fatter.

'Have you put on weight, Bianca?'

'Do you think so?' She turns round delighted. 'Have I? I hope so. I want a nice fat bottom.'

I love the smell of wax, it's like churches, and Bianca's paintings glint and glow like icons.

She goes out on Sunday mornings in Brixton with her dustpan to sweep up the hundreds of little green-tinted cubes of coloured glass from windscreens that have been smashed the night before, to use in her work.

'Are you religious, Bianca?'

'Don't be ridiculous! I want to sell my pictures to rich women in fur coats who wear too much perfume! They like things that glint!'

'You only pretend to be a cynic!' I say.

Cecile comes in with Rob, who has a big library book under her arm.

'Time for coffee!' says Bianca.

Cecile sits down next to me on the windowsill and Rob sits on the chaise longue, while Bianca unscrews the silver coffee pot and heaps in the coffee.

'Look!' says Roberta, opening the book and smoothing the photograph with her hand. 'They're amazing, don't you think they're just amazing!'

Bianca shrugs. 'You aren't interested in anything after 2000 BC.'

Roberta closes the library book of megalithic stones and puts her hands on her hips even though she's sitting down.

'Our history didn't start with ROME, you know!'

I start laughing. 'You two! Honestly!'

'All history books start with Rome!' says Roberta, turning to me. 'You should know, your dad's a historian.'

'Really, is he?' says Cecile, turning to me.

'Yes.' I nod, and think of the stacks of dusty books and the typewriter with its red and black ribbon, and the rubber bands he used to give me, that he kept in a box, lots of different-coloured rubber bands.

'There is a whole *history* of art!' says Bianca.

'Here we go! The Italian Renaissance!' says Rob.

'All over the world!' says Bianca, gesturing the whole of the world. 'You can't just ignore it!'

'I can do what I like!'

'There's a standing stone in London, did you know?' says Cecile, but Rob isn't listening.

'For you the only art is Italian art!'

'Actually, the period I like is Byzantium.'

She has postcards of the golden mosaics in Ravenna on the wall.

'Where is it?' I ask Cecile.

'It's opposite Cannon Street Tube station, under the Bank of China.

It used to be as tall as two grown men,' says Cecile, 'and it's been there for thousands of years. It's supposed to keep London safe. I'll lend you the book.'

'Thanks.'

'Maybe your dad knows about it. Did he tell you any stories about London?' she asks.

'Yes, he did, he told me stories all the time when I was little.'

I look out the window at the huge sky.

I remember a dragon dancing on a floating stage, and men pulling oars through water lilies in time to flutes. I remember the pigeons falling out of the sky with their wings on fire. I saw the city in the flames with the wind blowing outside after the twilight had turned the sea pink. I looked into the orange flames and saw it burning, and after that it was always there. I looked for it even if the story was from another time.

'All I'm saying is, open your mind. You only see one thing.'

'Well, same to you, Empress Theodora!'

'You can like whatever period you like!'

'And so can I!'

Roberta opens her book and turns the pages slowly. The coffee pot begins to hiss.

Cecile gestures with her eyes about the other two, and smiles.

'Has he published a book?' she says.

I look at the bottom of my empty cup.

'He hasn't finished it.'

And I remember the pages stuck together and the blurred writing where the whisky had spilt and the words had run into each other.

'Well, I'm sure he will,' she says kindly.

He's on his own now. On his own in that house. Alone with the wind blowing against the windows. And I don't want to think about my dad all alone in that house by the sea with the wind blowing against the windows.

'Can we change the subject now, please?' says Cecile.

'Of course!' says Bianca, who will have an argument about anything and forget it.

I look at Rob sitting under a brooding cloud of silence, and catch her eye.

'I'm in a bad mood,' she says.

'We don't mind,' says Bianca.

'I'm not in a bad mood actually, I'm pregnant!'

Bianca and Cecile open their mouths at the same time.

'How lovely!' says Cecile.

'Porca Madonna!' says Bianca.

'What are you going to do?'

Rob shrugs. 'I'm going to have a baby!'

'Wow!' says Cecile.

'Oh well,' says Bianca.

'It's not coming till the summer, I've got plenty of time.'

'How exciting!' says Cecile.

'Plenty of time!' says Bianca, shaking her head.

'What's the vote for this afternoon, then?' I say, before another argument starts.

'Giacometti,' says Roberta.

Bianca is walking about, pouring the coffee into our cups.

'See!' says Rob, holding out her cup. 'I like him and he's Italian!'

'Wow, a baby!' murmurs Cecile.

'Where's it on?'

'The Serpentine.'

'Let's walk,' says Cecile, looking out the window. 'It's a beautiful day.'

12

We walk down to the Fulham Road, Bianca and Rob behind. We have to persuade Bianca out of the second-hand clothes shop in South Kensington and drag her past the V and A up Exhibition Road, but none of us can walk past the Royal Academy Shop and we walk under the ornate stone gate and up the stairs. Bianca and I buy sketchbooks. Rob is wearing a big coat with holes in the pockets. The paint stand is hidden behind the palette knives. She buys a tube of titanium white, but when we come out into the street she produces handfuls of stolen tubes from the coat lining.

'You are a criminal!' shouts Bianca.

'Shut up, Bianca!' says Rob.

'O wow, Rob, carmine! £25 a tube.'

'You're terrible, you're terrible,' I say as I look with joy at the colours.

'Wait, look!' She hands me another tube.

'Oh, far out! Cobalt violet!' A colour as expensive as a jewel.

Rob and I have a locker where we keep our materials. Although we have our own, we also share. It gives us a chance to try new colours.

These tubes are for both of us.

'We've got umber, ultramarine, and here, look! Cadmium green.'

'Everyone does it!' says Rob.

'That is not a good rationale!' says Bianca.

'Yeah, like you're so squeaky clean!'

We walk into Kensington Gardens and the sunlight shines on the grass, the air is clear and the shadows are long because the sun is low.

We walk along under the tall plane trees, past the big dark Albert Memorial, to the Serpentine Gallery.

The tall thin sculptures make us quiet. We walk around them in silence. There is a room where the monumental figures are tiny.

'He spent ten years making small maquettes before he made them big!' Rob whispers, reading from the board. 'Ten years!'

'That's some gestation!' I say, smiling at her.

She laughs, and rubs her belly. 'Blimey, imagine having to carry it around for ten years!'

We walk out into the sunlight. The air is cold, but there is warmth in the light.

We walk under the trees and Rob takes her big coat off and we sit on it under a chestnut tree. She sits with her back to the huge trunk with her legs jutting out among the roots. I lean sideways and get out my sketchbook.

Bianca is doing qigong exercises. Cecile is copying her poses.

They both make an arc over their head with their arms, and stretch one leg out to the side, and bend the other. They move the arc from side to side, bending first one leg, then the other.

Their long shadows look like Giacometti figures slowly dancing. I am drawing them with pink chalk.

'This is called the rainbow!' Bianca calls out. I nod, looking up at them and down at my page. Kensington Gardens stretches behind them all the way to the Round Pond. People are walking along the paths in the grass from the Albert Memorial down to the Serpentine.

I close my book, now they are doing 'moving hands like clouds'.

They come over and lay themselves down on their coats. Cecile looks at my drawings.

'So why d'you think he wanted them so long and thin?' says Bianca, twirling a piece of grass.

'Maybe it's a pared-down thing, pared down to the core,' says Rob.

'It's the inner self, isn't it?' says Cecile in her cracked naked voice. 'The one everyone tries to hide.'

A dog leaps through the grass and sends a murder of crows flying up into the air, cawing. The dog is a poodle with ears that bounce, it is young and puppy-like. It bounces towards us and leaps on to Bianca and begins to lick her face.

'Get off, you horrible animal! Get off me, I loathe you! You are revolting!' She pushes it away and then kicks it. It yelps and its owner comes running after, calling, 'Fidelio, Fidelio.'

'Fucking Fidelio!' says Bianca, wiping her face with her sleeve.

We are laughing.

A large black crow swoops down and walks up and down before us. I open my sketchbook and paint with black ink, filling the whole page with the crow's head and shining beak.

It is hard to draw him as beautiful as he is. I follow the line of his head and his wings.

The crow caws. I paint his black eye. He walks slowly round in circles on the grass. His wings shine white in the sunlight.

13

When I walk my bike back home from college the sun has gone but the sky is still light; everything retains its colour, the grass is green, the pillar boxes still red, but the street lights have come on and glow in the gloaming. There is a tweet tweet beginning for the twilight chorus and the tall trees are black against the sky. The horizon is pale yellow, and shining pale blue, and the houses light up their coloured windows, and it is neither day nor night, and the dusk is alive with the colours of both.

Then Zeb is walking beside me. We are both surprised.

'Hey, how's the washing machine going?' he says.

'Singing a duet with the fridge,' I say, laughing. 'The sculpture going OK?' I ask.

'Yes, fine. How's the painting? You getting into it?'

'Sort of, bits and pieces.'

'That's good, bits and pieces is good.'

We pass by a garden behind railings. There is a gap in the railings covered by red and white striped tape. We walk past in silence. I've always wanted to sneak into one of those gardens in London squares. The kind that are locked, and look green and enticing.

'I've always wanted to sneak into one of those gardens,' he says. 'They look so enticing.'

'That's just what I was thinking!' I say, astonished. 'You spoke my thought!'

'Come on, let's!' he says.

'Oh, shall we? Someone might see!'

I chain up my bike and we look up and down the street.

'Go on,' he says, 'no one's coming, now!' and I dive under the tape into the rhododendrons. He follows. We are both giggling like naughty children.

'This is ridiculous!' I say in a loud whisper.

We climb through the rhododendrons and into a garden full of trees and low bushes and, in the centre, a lawn of grass, gently sloping to a fountain that is silent.

The trees have a presence that fill the garden.

By the fountain are three yew trees, and surrounding them are tall beech trees, and it is quiet, except for a crow calling from the corner of the square in a tree whose naked branches are reaching into the sky.

We make out a face in the foliage of the yew tree.

'Can you see it? Look there, see?'

'Oh, that's the nose, yes, I can.'

And we lie under the yew tree and look at the face in the dark branches and it looks and looks at us with intense eyes.

The crow caws again from a corner of the garden, we can see its black shape against the darkening sky, and Zeb says that crows see in two dimensions, and that's why they walk along like that, looking from one eye then the other, clocking two realities at once.

And I say it must be the great-great-grandson of the crows that have always lived in London, and imagine all the things they have seen if you could go back in time.

I begin to feel cold.

'I better go,' I say, standing up.

'Yes,' he says, 'me too.'

We sneak back through the rhododendrons under the striped tape.

He smiles and I notice he has asymmetrical dimples.

We go in different directions then, and as I bicycle through the night streets, the lit-up shops flashing past, I remember that he has one eye that looks at you with laughing in it, and the other one looks right into you.

Two-dimensional eyes.

I put my key in the lock and go through the green door; there are chips in the paint. Underneath, you can see it was once a mustard door, and before that it was pale blue. The stairs are narrow and the carpet is worn where the feet have walked. I walk up three flights, and let myself into my little flat.

I take my coat off and leave it on the bed, and go through into the kitchen.

The kitchen is very small, with enough room for a fold-out table and one chair.

I sit down in the dark and listen to the fridge. It has a language of its own, a repertoire of sounds that it chugs and hums and trembles through with dramatic pauses night and day. There are strips of plastic between the kitchen and the bedsittingroom which I have tied together and fastened to one side, so the doorway looks as if it has a hairstyle. I get up and put the kettle on. I make myself a cup of tea, put the light on, and take out my sketchbook. I look at the crow. I take out the drawings and put them next to each other.

I look through the window, up at the sky. There are pigeons flying in a flock over the buildings. The roofs are lit up by the moon's blue light. The street is in shadow or lit by yellow street lights. The pigeons are flying in a circle through the blue and yellow light.

The pigeons descend in a cascade and land on a roof.

And I look at the blue-black crow with a black eye and through the eye I see twin hills, I see the stillness and a wide river reflecting the sky. I see marshes and small islands and fires being lit and glowing in the dusk. I hear the sound of marsh birds and the zither-zing of swans in flight. I'll go down to the river and walk by the pale pink globes that light up the evening, and tomorrow I'll bike through the city to Cannon Street, and visit the London stone.

14

I cycle along the street, feeling wide open, colours splashing over me like waves in the sea. Clashing colours, honking noises, people with their different feelings trailing behind as they rush up the street. The air is cold but clear. The wind has blown the last of the leaves off the trees and turned autumn into winter. I ride along Knightsbridge and set out recklessly round Hyde Park Corner, sticking my hand out in front of buses and taxis, but I get pulled into the wrong stream and find myself sailing past Piccadilly and round the corner into Grosvenor Place. Sometimes you have to go with the flow on a bike in London or you might get squashed under the wheels. I dismount and take my bike down the steps into a tunnel that has colourful graffiti and someone playing the guitar.

Far away in my mind I think of dad and wonder if he's out walking along the cliffs in the wind.

I push my bike along the echoing corridor and into Green Park. I walk under the naked trees. I bike across the park to St James's Park, until I am told 'you're not allowed to bicycle in here', by a man in a maroon jacket, and I walk slowly round the lake and stop on the bridge to look at the water.

Has he built a fire in the study? Or is he wearing his thick blue jersey under his tweed jacket so his arms bulge?

I get out my sketchbook to draw the trees and the water and the tiny buildings in the distance that are just dashes and dots on the page. There is a stillness here after the traffic frenzy. It is a blue cold winter feeling.

Is he all right, d'you think?

I put my sketchbook away and then I remember the stone that has stood in the centre of the city for more than two thousand years.

It must have stood in stillness once. It has seen the cars pass, and before that the carriages, and before that the litters and the chariots. It has watched the people come and go, the Saxons, the Danes and before that the Romans and before that the Celts.

I walk over the bridge, and out a gateway down Horse Guards Parade to King Charles Street.

The stone was here before Charles walked under the ceiling painted with cherubs on his way to the block, before Elizabeth's dancing courtiers and dresses sewn with pearls, before Henry's madness and Eleanor's gentle hand.

I find myself in Whitehall and think I'd better look at the map.

I like wandering about the streets, it's like slipping in and out of different periods in history.

At last I come out on to Victoria Embankment and the Thames, bringing its blue river light, breathing its fresh river breath into the clogged city air. I ride on the pavement alongside the water, under Hungerford Bridge and past Cleopatra's Needle.

After Blackfriars I get tangled in a web of alleys and lanes; White Lion Hill and Knightrider Court. The air is dirty and sweat is pouring down my skin.

The stone was here before Alfred, the king with the

wisdom of an elf, before Canute told the waves to go back, before Arthur and Uther and Merlin's chilling prophecy, before Caesar and Boudicca, before Hengist and Horsa, before Estrildis and Brutus Greenshield.

I come to Walbrook where the buried river runs and at last, the Bank of China.

But when I squat down on the pavement opposite Cannon Street Underground station, and peer behind the bars and into the alcove, I see a small piece of whitish stone. It is shabby and the glass is covered with a layer of grime from the wind of passing traffic, and maybe there is nothing remarkable in this sorry piece of limestone, that has stood the test of time but that is all, and I walk away disappointed.

But when I navigate my bike through the jam on Ludgate Hill, and ride on the pavement along the Embankment so I can look at the river, when I chain my bike and walk across the footbridge to the Hayward Gallery on the South Bank so I can watch the water slipping under my feet, something in me stirs.

And as I reach the other side I know I can't walk up the steps to the gallery because something is rising through me like water bubbling up from an underground spring, and I see gold light behind my eyes.

And when I walk under the bridge and along the river, watching it glint and ripple, I feel a wide-open hope spread through me, that makes me stand still just to breathe the feeling of it.

And when I go back to college I draw pictures of the paintings I will paint; the forest and the beautiful river, the swans as big as horses and red wolves who roamed Cheapside when the Thames was a deity.

*   *   *

And I don't know if it is the spirit with his dark beauty trapped in the un-reverenced stone, or Zeb, who touches the edges of my dreams, and makes me wake up with a longing that is so intense, so deep, it feeds me with its mystery even while the emptiness of it could swallow me whole.

15

'Those bastard tutors!' says Bianca. 'It makes me bloody furious!'

'Pretentious! What about his stupid pictures!'

'Listen, he hasn't had a show for twenty years!' says Rob.

'Well, that tells you something!' I say.

Cecile had a crit this morning, and came up for coffee with red eyes. She doesn't tell you much but her eyes filled with tears when Rob asked her about it. She shook her head and swallowed and gave a little laugh, but the tears fell out anyway.

The tutors didn't think much of her big flowers.

'He just likes sticking the boot into other people's work.'

'It doesn't matter now,' says Cecile.

We are sitting outside in the quadrangle under the big tree. The day is mild and clear.

'Well, it does!' Rob says. 'They should allow us to take a friend in, to speak up for us,'

'That's a good idea.'

'So what exactly happens?' I ask.

'You have to take all your pictures into the assessment room along with all the sketchbooks', says Bianca, 'and the tutors . . .'

'. . . who are *all* men!' interrupts Rob, 'put the work all over the floor, line it up on tables, and against the walls, riffle through your sketchbooks, and then proceed to take the work apart, ask you the point of it, and tell you you're doing it wrong!'

'And when you're thoroughly devastated,' says Cecile, 'they pack you off with a set of instructions about how it *should* be done, how it *ought* to look, and what you're *really* trying to achieve.'

'Is it their habit to tear everyone apart?' I ask nervously. Cecile shrugs.

'Did they devastate you?' I ask Rob.

'I just told them I'm painting the "inner visions of my pregnancy",' she says in a wafty voice that makes us laugh, 'and they couldn't get me out the room quick enough!'

'Yes, tell them it's something menstrual,' says Bianca, 'that'll terrify them!'

'What do you do?' I ask Bianca.

'Oh, my English is really not very good, could you repeat the question?' she says, mimicking herself.

'What if you don't know what you're doing?'

'Exactly.'

'If only some of them didn't know what they were doing they'd be more sympathetic.'

The door to Sculpture opens across the quadrangle and Zeb and Suzanne come out arguing.

They both stop talking and she sits down with her arms folded. He squats down by her, then unfolds himself, his long legs make an upside-down W. I cannot hear what they are saying to each other but I can see that she is raising her eyes to heaven and hitting the air with the back of her hand. He is leaning sideways, reasoning with her.

He holds her forearm. She blinks her eyes, her lips press together and she looks away.

Zeb raises both his hands in a question.

'Those two are always arguing,' says Roberta.

'What do they argue about?' says Cecile.

'Oh, she wants him to behave when he meets her flash friends. Be different to what he is,' says Rob.

'Is that what Mick says?'

'What flash friends?

'TV people. She wants to work in TV.'

'Why's she doing sculpture?

'How should I know? She's got herself some job doing a commercial in Barbados.'

'Is Zeb going?'

'Doubt it.'

'It's probably very passionate,' says Bianca, 'very sexy to be so bad tempered.'

'Is it?' I say.

'And very addictive,' says Bianca.

'How d'you know?'

'I know all about boyfriends, I've had oh so many boyfriends,' says Bianca, lying down on the slab and looking up at the big plane tree, and stretching her hands out as if she wants to touch it. 'All about boyfriends, all about addiction.'

She draws the twiggy branches with her fingers up in the air, opening one eye and closing the other. Wherever she lounges she looks elegant. She wears a shirt from Guatemala with bright pink and green and blue squares and stripes, embroidered with red thread, and a pair of linen culottes with braces, both slung over one shoulder. No one else could wear the eccentric clothes Bianca wears.

'What were you addicted to?'

'Heroina! Now I have hepatitis as my protector. Without it I would go out and score right now!'

'Would you really?' says Roberta, rubbing her belly.

'Of course!'

I notice Zeb and Suzanne have stood up and she is gesticulating this way and that, shaking her head about so her long hair quivers.

I can hear the sound of her crossness from here but not the words.

'Everybody is addicted to something.' Bianca carries on tracing the twigs.

'Don't think I am,' says Roberta.

'Your baby! And your painting, and when it comes they will conflict!' says Bianca, who often makes pronouncements with great authority.

Roberta shrugs and smiles.

'What about me?' I ask. 'What d'you think I'm addicted to?'

'You are addicted to the pain of unrequited love!'

I put my hand up to my mouth. I want to say, 'We're friends, it's not like that!' but my mouth stays open behind my hand and I don't say anything.

'However, as we can see, he has his own addiction.' Bianca waves towards the arguing couple.

Roberta laughs.' Don't be silly, they're just friends.' She nods at me and Zeb.

'Hmm-hmm-hmm,' sings Bianca with her eyes closed.

The door to the sculpture department slams and Suzanne has stormed off in a huff.

'I didn't say they didn't love each other,' Bianca says with her eyes still closed.

'Yes, I think they do,' says Roberta, looking at the door. But Bianca didn't mean them.

I watch her as she lies there, the twig shadows trembling on her face. Sometimes she has to lie very still and be quiet. Her illness makes her suddenly tired.

'Does it make you tired being pregnant?' Cecile asks Rob.

'Nope!' says Rob.

'Are you looking forward to it?'

Roberta shrugs. 'Think so.'

'I loathe babies, they are so disgusting!' says Bianca.

'How can you say that!' says Cecile.

'No really!' Bianca says, getting up on her elbow. 'I was in a restaurant. A woman took out her tit and began to feed her baby, milk everywhere, all over the baby's face, all over the tit! Porca miseria! I stopped eating! I couldn't eat! It was too disgusting.' She lies back down and closes her eyes. 'They should hide them away! Roberta, when you have your baby, hide it! Put it away in a cupboard or something!'

I look at Rob to see if she's offended but she gives me a laughing exasperated look.

'Lucky your mother didn't think like that, Bianca!' she says.

'She did! She was a totally unnatural mother! Why do you think I am so fucked up! She telephones me with her anxiety: "Bianca, what are you going to do about this? What are you going to do about that?" When I leave the telephone I'm a nervous wreck! Listen, she could win a PRIZE for anxiety! She worries about EVERY THING! She's thinner than me!'

'FIRST-YEAR CRITICAL ASSESSMENTS' it says on the door.

I don't like waiting out here with all my work, I don't want to spread it all around the room and have them riffle through my sketchbooks asking the reasons for things and entering my private world as though they have special privileges. I have left the new drawings upstairs, in case the ideas get frightened off by the scrutiny.

Sinéad comes out the door and makes a face at me. Her eyes slide diagonally down to stare at the floor, as if to say 'You have no idea how horrible that was!'

Tutors follow her out with stretchers and stacks of sketchbooks, and pile them outside the room.

Inside, three of the tutors stand with their arms folded, talking to each other by the window. The door swings back and forth as the other two bring work through, back and forth, till all her work is outside the door.

There are five altogether. Terry, who's always drunk, Paul, the head of painting, Sergei, who made Cecile cry, Tom, who has a streak of kindness in him, and one with an orange beard who speaks to you as if he suspects you of something. I glimpse them all as the door swings back and forth.

'Would you like to bring your work through?'

I follow them in with a pile of sketchbooks. It is a big square empty room with splashes of paint on the floor and windows down one side. There are some grey tables near the wall and a stack of red chairs. They put the sketchbooks on the grey tables and the rest of the paintings round the room, propped up, or scattered on the floor.

There is the painting of Cambridge Circus, with turquoise lamp-posts and orange buildings, with a black and white sky and wet pavements. There is the purple sky and yellow light the night the robber ran past. There is the river in the dawn, and the river at dusk, and a portrait of Roberta painted with a carmine background. There are sketches of Sloane Square made with black ink, and watercolours of dawn from the police pier.

They flick through the sketchbooks and breathe in, slightly bored, as they look. They stand around looking at the pictures.

I am so glad I didn't bring my new drawings. The sketchbook is hidden upstairs.

Except one has slipped through.

Sergei picks it up and looks at it.

'Keep away from this kind of thing, you're better at drawing what you see,' he says, holding it in front of him with a finger and thumb for me and the others to see.

It is a blue figure with the head and wings of a swan.

Paul turns the corners of his mouth down and moves his head from side to side, assessing.

'I don't mind it.'

The red-haired man with the beard doesn't say anything but looks at me suspiciously. He flicks through a sketchbook.

Then he says, 'What are you trying to achieve here?'

'You mean at art school?'

'No, on the planet. Yes! At art school!'

'Umm . . . to learn to paint.'

'But what for?'

I wish I was Italian or pregnant, I'm sure it would make it easier to answer these questions.

'How do you justify being an artist?'

'I don't know.'

'I mean this is very nice . . . soufflé! but what about MEAT AND POTATOES! I'd like to see some MEAT AND POTATOES in your work instead of this . . . soufflé!'

I'm confused by the soufflé.

'Why don't you make more LARGE sketches?'

'She needs to make bigger paintings.'

'Yes, use less colour'

'And bigger brushes. Make a breakthrough!'

Paul nods. 'Yes, you need to make a breakthrough. This is all very well, but it's . . . very *pretty*.'

'Yes, you need to think outside the box.'

'As it is, you could even call it . . . illustrative.'

'Maybe go into monochrome. Try a seven-foot canvas!'

'Paint with a wallpaper brush. Expand your ideas!'

'Stay away from this imaginary . . . stuff,' says Sergei, nodding and putting the offensive drawing back in the pile.

I leave the assessment room in a state of shock, and carry my canvases and sketchbooks up the stairs.

'What was it like?'

Bianca is standing over the red ring with the coffee in her hand. 'I have just made a pot for you.'

Roberta is sitting on the sofa with her hands wrapped round a mug.

'Yes, how did it go?'

Cecile is on the mattress. She looks up.

I sit down next to Roberta. I just shake my head and can't find words. 'Oh, something about meat and potatoes.'

'What?'

'And soufflé. Oh, I'm just glad that's over, I don't know what I'm going to do next term, though.'

'Why?'

'Well, when they expect to see a seven-foot canvas in monochrome painted with a wallpaper brush!'

'Is that what they want?'

'Why do they always want everything to be enormous?'

'What do you want to paint?' asks Cecile.

'Small paintings, with more colour, from my imagination.'

She nods. 'Well, you do that then.'

I take my coffee from Bianca. 'Just as long as I don't end up with that bloody Sergei as my tutor next term.'

17

The next day when I go upstairs, Bianca is packing up her studio.

'Will this still be your space after Christmas?'

'Yes, thank God!'

'Oh, I'm glad. Me and Rob are keeping ours.'

'Are you going home for Christmas?' asks Bianca.

'Don't want to much,' I say.

'No? Not to see your mother and father? The family?'

'My mum's dead, Bianca.'

'What happened to her?'

'She died.'

'Yes. But how?'

'She drowned.'

'What happened?'

'No one knows really, she went swimming.'

'How old were you?'

'Five.'

'Can you remember?'

'No. I can't remember a thing about it.'

'Nothing?'

'The funeral, vaguely.'

'You blanked out the rest?'

I shrug. 'I suppose so. But I don't remember her very well, anyway, she wasn't around much.'

'What about your father? Did he remarry?'

'Nope.'

'Why do you say it like that?'

'Because I wish he had.'

'Do you?' says Bianca. 'A stepmother?'

'Someone to bloody look after him!'

'Is he old?'

'No, but he drinks too much.'

'Oh.'

'I think he's been holding it together for me . . .'

'. . . and now you've left, there's a big hole. Well, you have to live your life.'

'I just don't feel like . . . I mean, I feel I should . . .'

'Take care of him? Of course. In Italy you would. There was an old lady in Rome that looked after her father until she died. She was seventy-nine, and the father was still alive. He'd worn her out! Her whole life devoted to him.'

'Yes. I suppose they do that in Italy. Anyway, my dad's not a tyrant.'

'But he drinks too much.'

'Yes.'

'That's not easy.'

'No, it's a bloody nightmare.'

I sigh and look out the window.

'I don't know what to do.'

'Natale con i suoi, pasqua con chi vuoi!'

'What does that mean?'

'It means *I* should be going home for Christmas instead of staying here.'

'Are your family making a fuss?'

'You are telling me.'

I like it when Bianca uses phrases like that. It makes me smile.

'What are you going to do?'

'Stay here!' And her hands go out either side, palm upwards, as if to say 'obviously!'

'Oh, but Bianca!' I shake my head and look out the window. 'Am I supposed to go back there to look after him? Am I? Because mum's gone? Because he doesn't have a wife? Because he's all alone? Well, I don't want to!' I say, hitting the table. 'I don't want to sit in that house with him making clinking noises in the Weetabix cupboard, when it's bloody breakfast time, and slurring his words by lunch, and sitting slumped in that armchair next to the fire by teatime, and then making some big song and dance of opening a bottle of wine at exactly six o'clock as though that's the first drink he's had, and starting all over again. And there he is in that bloody armchair, his eyes all bleary, having revolting sentimental conversations about "Oh darling, do you love me?" when all I want to say is "No, I don't, you self-indulgent bastard. How dare you ask me that!" But that's not what I'm supposed to say, is it. I'm supposed to go home for Christmas and be a good daughter.'

'Who says you're supposed to? Just out of interest.' says Bianca, not in the least perturbed by my outburst.

'Everyone.'

'Everyone like who?'

'Magda probably.'

'Who is Magda?'

'Just a neighbour,' I say, and I look out the window for a moment, because she isn't just a neighbour. And I remember the smell of the woodstove and the steam rising off the wet clothes in the kitchen when we came back from the cowshed, and holding on to her trousers when we walked through the forest of cows.

'A neighbour?'

'No. More than that. She used to look after me a lot when I was small.'

'So he has someone nearby?'

'Well, they argued. They don't talk now.'

'That's up to him,' says Bianca, lifting up her hands. 'But you think you should go home?'

'Yes.'

'Because?'

'Because I feel so bloody sorry for him!' And then I put my head into my hands and cry great monster sobs, and Bianca doesn't say 'there there,' or put her arms round me and try to make me stop, she just lets me cry.

'He didn't use to be like this, you know, Bianca, he didn't, even after mum died. He was strong and big and lovely, and noble. Now he's, oh, he's ... he CRIES! He cries all drunk and sentimental and I want to hit him. That makes me horrible, doesn't it?'

'No.'

'I don't want to go home for Christmas.'

'Then don't.'

So I don't.

18

I sit on the radiator and look out on London in January. It looks naked and drab. The clouds are grey and weigh down the sky.

'Stop moping! I can't stand you moping, if you mope you must go downstairs!' says Bianca.

'I'm not moping! Wasn't it nice, our studio?'

'There was no light!' says Bianca.

No. The studio didn't have much light, that was the only thing; just a little frosted-glass window that opened about six inches, because it was on a metal hinge that squeaked when you opened it, so it only let in the sawdust-smelling air, and the sound of the saws, and the men shouting at each other as they stacked the wood on the lorries. But I got used to the darkness in a way. I had to make the colours glow.

'You see! You are being nostalgic. I can't stand it.'

'I'm not, it's just January, and I've got bloody Sergei as a tutor.'

'Well, you have lots of work to show him! You used that studio twice as much as I did.'

The idea of showing Sergei the new paintings fills me with horror.

'They might put some life into him!' says Bianca, smiling.

I laugh. Bianca's name for Sergei is 'the zombie'.

'What he needs is a few minutes in the corridor! *"AMEN! Praise be the Lord!"* '

We both laugh. Next door to the studio we borrowed over the holiday the Church of the Cherubim and Seraphim also had their premises, and we could hear them doing exorcisms in the corridor. Bianca and I would listen with our eyes wide open and hands over our mouths, as the strange wobbly voice cried out: 'Don't marry her! she is a baaaad person!'

'Praise be the Lord!'

'She will take your money!'

'Amen!'

'Find another woman!'

'Praise be the Lord!'

They had about five thousand candles burning every time they did a ceremony, and wore long white robes and pork-pie hats like bath-caps. The children wore the same in miniature and sang songs which rocked the studio.

We liked them being next door with all their incense and songs, speaking in tongues and spirit voices, and one day a big woman came to the door and asked me what I did, and I showed her my paintings, and she said in a beautiful low Nigerian voice, 'Ah! Your pictures are full of spirits.' I must have looked alarmed because she said, 'Good spirits, good spirits' and we both laughed.

I was thrilled she liked them.

'It just feels weird being back in an institution, that's all. No freedom.'

'Yes, with a technician upstairs to cut your stretchers,' says Bianca, 'and a shop in the canteen you can get everything half-price. Freedom is not free! It's expensive! We didn't pay for the studio, don't forget.'

We'd borrowed it from Bianca's cousin's ex-boyfriend, who went back to Italy for Christmas. It was behind the timber-merchant in Acre Lane so the air smelt of wood.

'Well, we made some money! I liked those jobs!' I say.

Through Bianca's network we'd found a studio *and* part-time work.

That's how we ended up spending a dark afternoon on a sunny day in a dungeon under the Coliseum, burning our fingers glue-gunning pearls on to Elizabethan dresses that the chorus complained about because their voices got lost in the ruffs.

The next time, it was a tiny room up in a tower, stitching hooks and eyes on to pink-embroidered pale green tutus with lots of netting. That was at Covent Garden. I had to explain to Bianca that someone was playing a joke on the receptionist when her high voice came over the tannoy, 'Could Mike Hunt come to reception, please.'

'Oh God, you are so romantic! Life as an artist out there is tough! TOUGH! It's not all pale green tutus!'

I laugh. 'No, I know that. But at least there's no Sergei.'

'Ha!' she says, pointing at me with a wagging finger. 'I know exactly what is wrong with you!'

I blush and look out the window.

Suzanne is making a sculpture in the courtyard down below. She has a welding mask on and her overalls undone and tied round her waist, so she is standing in the cold in her vest with her brown arms exposed. The sparks are flying.

She is back from Barbados.

'It's so vulgar to have a tan in January!' says Bianca, looking over my shoulder.

I can't help laughing at Bianca sometimes.

Of course I wish I hadn't told her, but I had to tell someone, and it's obvious I can't tell Rob.

It happened in a moment in the canteen, and it's annoying that Bianca was right all along.

'Hey! What about you and Geoff?' she says.

'Oh, Bianca, please. Just forget it.'

But one moment can change everything. One moment in the canteen.

I could hear the saucers being laid out in fours, then the cups being unstacked and placed in the saucer, and the tinkle of the little spoon; clink clop tinkle, clink clop tinkle, and Zeb was telling me about white: titanium white is a blue white, but it can turn yellow if you get the cheap kind; zinc white is a purple white, it has a metallic tinge; lead is yellow white; and I picked up the teaspoon to look at the white sugar crystals and the teaspoon flipped over and the sugar went on the table. I leaned over to wipe up the sugar and I looked at him.

I looked into his eyes.

And the moment opened like a flower and stood still. And I saw what a lie time is, because it all stands still. And eternity is right there.

For ever, I've known you for ever.

So I looked away. And now I can't stand next to him, or come into the room or pass him in the canteen without blushing or blurting out some rubbish, and we used to be friends, and it was easy. And anyway, Suzanne is Zeb's girlfriend.

19

Maybe I should tell him! I stand up quickly, woken by the idea and the terror of it. Quick! before I lose my nerve.

'See you later!' I say

'I didn't mean it, you can stay and mope!' says Bianca, following me to the door.

'No, it's OK, it's not that. I'll see you later.'

I run down the stairs to the mezzanine with my heart beating. The door to his studio is open.

Zeb is standing with his back to me. He is reaching up to a high place on his peculiar tinkling sculpture that looks as though it's come from another world. It lights up with coloured light, it twirls things and it tinkles. The sleeves of his dark blue paint-spattered shirt are rolled up above his elbows so his upper arms show. I can see his shoulders under his shirt and the curve of his biceps. He screws something high up above his head, so his arms reach up and make a diamond. His long fingers twiddle something and the structure shivers and tinkles. His head is tilted a little. I follow his black hair falling down his long back and his dark blue shirt is only half tucked in, and his long legs in jeans; one leg straight with the weight on it, the other sometimes a little off the floor like a dancer, as he reaches upwards.

On Wednesdays Karl sometimes makes us do drawings for three or four seconds and the model changes her pose.

I could do a drawing now with diluted ink: his beautiful shape, and the shirt half tucked in, that I want to put my hand inside, want to travel up the spine, under his shirt all the way to the back of his neck, touching the curves of his body, the smooth skin. I want to touch him. I want to touch him.

I run back up to the studio, clatter clatter up the glossy stairs.

I stand in the studio, breathing. I put my hands on my cheeks and look out the window at the white sky.

'Rob, let's go to the RA.'

'It's not Friday,' she says from behind the muslin curtain.

'Let's go anyway. We can draw.'

'But it's a collection. I don't like collections, I prefer one artist at a time.'

'Oh, but Rob,' I say, going through the muslin, to stand in her space, 'they've got the dancers, we might not see them again, and the Red Room, and Cézanne, and Kandinsky. Let's go. Come on.'

She puts down her paintbrush.

'Oh all right,' she says.

We get off the bus and walk along Piccadilly.

Pigeons are cooing and bowing, in sunlit corners of the pavement, making gentle burbling sounds as they circle one another, then flutter together on high-up ledges as though they are cliffs, with a sea of people below them, to-ing and fro-ing in tides.

We walk into the Royal Academy across the courtyard and up the wide steps.

When we enter the tall rooms, we separate. I walk slowly and look at Cézanne's pale blue mountain, hot light and cool green trees breathing the air, and Monet's pond, the light slipping over the ripples on the surface of reflected trees. I see how he paints a poppy field with cobalt violet and salmon pink, so it looks like sunlit red poppies growing as far as the eye can see, and how he paints the stalks of grass that glow in the shadow under a haystack, which is made of colours you can't describe, only they are the colours of hay in shadow: pink-grey, blue-grey, green-grey, yellow-grey, if you look close.

The red dancers blaze in the centre of the next room; bigger than life-size, moving all the time since they were painted, the red bodies vibrant against the blue, and singing with the green.

The dancers turn pink in a blue studio, and a pink chair stands in front, the white dashes on the blue cushion pulling the chair into the foreground.

I move through the big doors and see Chagall flying his wife like a kite in a purple dress, over green houses and a pale pink church, and friendly Kandinsky celebrating in rainbows and spillikins.

And then I find the one I like the best and need the most. It is a lonely curved path, in winter, with spindly black trees. But the snow, how he sees the snow! It is pink and yellow and many different pale blues reflecting the sky. The mountains are covered in blue fingerprints. The picture glows in constant twilight.

I look and look at it, till Rob pulls me by the sleeve and says, 'It's time to go,' and we walk out into the Piccadilly evening.

20

'What have you done, Bianca?' I walk into her studio space and it's orange.

She is lying on the chaise longue with one leg up, the other down and a piece of Paisley-pattern material over her eyes.

'I am suffering!'

'What's wrong?'

She sits up and takes the material away from her eyes.

'Oh, no, I can't bear it!' And puts the material back and lies down.

'What is it?'

'Oh, it's PMT. Why else does anyone paint their space orange!'

'You can repaint it! I quite like it.'

'No! No! Don't mention it! Don't look at it! I don't even want to imagine you looking at it!'

I look out over the city and into the far distance. I am restless too. Every dot of air has Zeb in it.

And I've got a tutorial with Sergei in one hour.

'Oh, you are in one of your far-away moods, go away! I can't bear you when you're like that!' she says.

I sit down on the end of the chaise longue.

'I can't work today.'

'But listen!' she says, sitting up, the Paisley pattern flying. 'I have a plan for you!'

She starts busily piling up pieces of wood.

'Oh, not me and Geoff!' I sigh and go over to the window

'Oh, yes, yes, yes, I have all these stretchers that need their ends cutting.'

I look into the courtyard, the sparks are flying from the welding gun.

There's Suzanne. I mean, it's not surprising, is it? Standing out there with her overalls half undone, the arms tied round her waist, with her long blonde curls tied up in a fetching cascade, welding that *thing*.

I passed by it with Rob and tried to get her to criticize it with me.

'I mean, look at it, what is that?'

'Well, she's just experimenting.'

'Yeah, but come on, it's pointless!'

'Well, it's quite a skill, welding.'

'Oh please. She just does it because she looks good in the gear. The welding mask, stripped down to the waist. You know, to weld a bloody pointless monstrosity that just gets bigger and bigger and tips over if you so much as touch it, loads of skill in that! Yeah, right!'

But Rob just looked at me then, and I thought I ought to shut up.

'Are you listening to me?' says Bianca, close to my ear.

She looks out the window at the welding.

'Ah! Like her sculpture, she is a spider!'

'No, I don't want a date with Geoff,' I say, walking away from the window.

'He really likes you and you like him, he's patient, you admire patience!' she says with a scoff.

It's true that he is patient. He bends over the ruler and cuts the wood to the right millimetre, when all the panic-stricken third-years are lining up to get their frames cut in time.

'Listen,' says Bianca, slowly putting the stretchers into my hands and talking in a kind of sing-song way. 'Just listen to me. You aren't going on a date, you are asking him to Silvia's party. Say it after me: "Would you like to come to Silvia's party?" See? Easy peezy lemon squeezy.'

I laugh. The phrase sounds funny in her Italian mouth.

'Up the stairs . . . up one floor,' she says as she steers my shoulders from behind out the door of the studio.

'Look, I've got a tutorial with Sergei!'

'There's time!' she says.

I walk upstairs and into the workshop with my pile of wood. The sky shines through slanted skylights. The room smells of wood. There is a circular saw in the table, and freshly planed wood shavings on the floor. Geoff is leaning over the ruler marking a notch with his pencil, which he puts back behind his ear. He looks up and smiles. He has short brown hair but the fringe goes in his eyes.

'You want to cut those corners?'

'Yes,' I say.

'What d'you want to do? Knock them together with corrugated nails?'

'Yep, that's what I'll be doing.' I nod.

'OK, here, use this vice.' And he sets up the saw so I can saw them through at the right angle.

I set to sawing away at the wood and think, what on earth am I doing this for? And can't think how I ended up cutting all these stretchers for Bianca. Then I remember a vague plan about Silvia's party and I look up at Geoff and watch him as he bends over the measuring and his hair falls in his eyes. He turns his lips inside as he measures. He looks up and catches me looking at him and smiles.

He looks down again and says from behind his hair: 'There's something really good happening this Saturday, want to come?'

'I . . . oh, what's that?' I say, trying to remember if that was the way round the plan was meant to go.

'Have you heard of Billy Graham?'

'Oh . . . yeah . . . the preacher,' I say, my heart sinking.

'He's a really wonderful speaker, he knows what life's about and he fills you with this kind of warmth . . .'

But I'm picking up my wood, saying 'Thanks so much for . . . you know . . .' trying to walk backwards out the door with a handful of planks.

I clamber down the stairs and into Bianca's space.

'What happened?' she says, 'Did you ask him out?'

'Of course he's a patient carpenter!' I say, throwing the stretchers on the floor, 'he thinks he's bloody Jesus!'

21

'Line them up so I can see them!'

Sergei is in my space. He is leaning against my table with his legs sticking out and his arms crossed. His glasses are on the end of his nose and the sneer is on his mouth, curling back his lips to reveal brown teeth. Eyes like nails look at things with a cold sharp pricking look.

I feel as if I am lining up my pictures so they can be shot.

I turn them to face him, some I hang on the nails and the others are lined up on the floor against the wall.

They have tender colours. None of them are finished.

He takes his glasses off and puts the end of the arm in his mouth, eyeing along the row and sniffing out, as though he's laughing at something.

They are my new pictures, explorations into another world that is hidden.

Sergei is shaking his head

'What are you trying to do with these, what is that?'

He points to a painting of two figures.

Phthalo turquoise, and alizarin crimson mixed with cadmium red, create a dancing vibrance, and as I tried to make the colours sing together, a winged man appeared in the paint and spoke to the figure sitting next to the river. It whispered in her ear and it stood on its toes, as one leg reached behind, its wings outstretched as though it had just landed. She listens.

Sometimes the images come by themselves.

I wanted the two colours to sing.

'What is that supposed to be?'

'It's not supposed to be anything. I wanted to make the colours harmonize, and the figures came along.'

'You're really better painting what you can see instead of this mumbo-jumbo. You're going way off track here, who are you trying to be?'

I wasn't supposed to answer that question.

He shakes his head. 'There's far too much colour in it anyway.'

'Well, I'm just experimenting.'

'Just experimenting! You've got no tone in it! It's all one tone. Don't you know anything about tone? You have to work out what it is exactly that you're trying to achieve, and then follow a plan to achieve it. You're all over the place. It's a mess! And what's that?'

He points to the painting with the blue figure.

She has a body made of water. She feels everything. She stands on the bridge with the water flowing beneath her and it is telling her its history in visions that flow through her like memories.

'That's a figure made of water.'

'Another cliché,' he says under his breath, 'angels and bloody mermaids. This isn't the eighteenth century, you know, things have moved on! Don't you look at what is going on around you?'

'I want to paint my own things,' I say, too quietly for my liking, suddenly transformed into a too-small person with this ugly smelly pale-skinned man with eyes like nails, and words like hammers.

'You don't know *what* you want.'

There is a tall painting at the end, standing upright. It is the largest and only just begun. I want to paint the spirit in the stone. The London stone. The first time I imagined him he was flying above the blue river over Albert Bridge and Battersea Bridge, and down to Blackfriars past Lambeth Palace and the Houses of Parliament. He flies over Tower Bridge to the Tower of London and his finger is pointing. He is making the sky orange and the air pulse and throb.

'What is this, an attempt at Chagall?'

'I was trying to paint the spirit in the London stone.'

'Ah, so we've gone from the eighteenth century to what, the New Age? Is this a New Age fad?'

'No,' I say, offended on behalf of the ancient spirit. 'No, that stone has been there since before the Romans! It was probably erected by the druids.'

'Druids!' He puts his forehead in his hands and shakes his head. 'Oh God give me strength!'

He looks up and his face is suddenly yellow, the rims of his eyes are red. He opens his mouth and I see his brown teeth.

'Are you an idiot?' he blares at me.

'What's wrong with that?' I say.

'What world are you living in? Airy fairy land? Escaping into some world of your own!' He bangs the table to give emphasis to his words. 'Live in the real world!'

He sighs and looks down. 'Here you are, tra-la-la-ing through your degree, painting fairies and fauns. I'm just trying to bring you into the real world,' he says in another tone.

'But is there any point,' he says under his breath, standing up and brushing his coat and walking out of my space without a backward glance.

I stare at the table he's been leaning against.

Roberta pokes her head through the curtain.

'Wasn't too bad, was it?' she says.

'Are you joking?'

I look at her with my mouth open, and all my joints go limp.

She laughs.

'Come on,' she says, putting her arm round my shoulder and guiding me out of the studio. 'Don't worry about the zombie! He hasn't painted a picture in twenty years!'

'I know. That's what makes him lethal!'

22

'I think you should wear this one!' says Bianca, putting a red velvet dress over the side of the bath.

She flicks through the dresses in the wardrobe.

I'm sitting in the armchair between the chipped stained-glass window and the communal dressing table, which has a row of twenty lipsticks under the mirror. One of Silvia's copper-coloured bras is lying in the doorway.

'Or this one?' She holds up a green Indian dress with gold thread and sequins around the neck.

I shake my head.

She looks at it with her head tilted.

'No? OK,' and puts it back. Clip clip through the hangers.

'Here is one of Silvia's.' She holds it up. It is a communal wardrobe for the overflow of clothes. The dress is gold, ruched, 1940s-looking.

I shrug. 'I'll try it.'

I pull off my T-shirt and pull the gold dress on.

'Take off your trousers!' shrieks Bianca. She gets up and pulls the dress down and zips it up, then steps back and looks at me sideways.

Silvia steps in the doorway and picks up her bra.

'What do you think?'

I find it touching the way Bianca speaks to her Italian flatmates in English if I am there.

'Yes, you look very nice, I like it, I like it,' she says. and crouches a little, to see in the mirror and put dark purple lipstick on her lips.

She doesn't seem to mind that it's her dress. Silvia has long dark auburn hair, and a curvy body.

'Well, I think you should try the red one,' says Bianca

I feel constricted by the structure in the seams, and breathe out with relief when she undoes the zip.

The girls Bianca lives with do textiles at Goldsmiths, and the flat is hung with velvet curtains printed with spirals, and quilted spreads sewn with appliquéd animals are thrown over the sofa and chairs. A piece of pink silk is tied around the shade, which tints the light in the sitting room.

I walk in, wearing the red dress. Bianca nods, and points her finger at me.

'This one! Yes, this one! What do you think?' She turns to Silvia.

A huge cauldron of minestrone is bubbling on the stove in the kitchen. Silvia stands in the yellow-lit doorway, holding a huge chunk of Parmesan cheese wrapped in silver foil.

'Yes, I like too,' says Silvia.

'Now shoes,' and Bianca gets up, takes my hand and leads me into the corridor, where there is a long row of shoes.

'Try these!' She calls through to Carlotta, 'Porti quelle rosse sta notte?'

'No.'

'Allora, try these.'

I slip my feet into shoes that are far too high.

Bianca kneels back on her heels and looks me up and down with satisfaction.

'Ha! ha! now you can steal him!'

'Are you sure this is the best way in, Bianca?'

We have climbed in the end of the garden, which is more of a waste land, two gardens knocked together behind houses that are mostly squats. I am walking in the dark on high-heeled shoes, through piles of rubble and old tyres and a forest of sycamore saplings, my heels sinking into the mud.

Bianca is giggling. 'Maybe not!'

As we near the party we hear the dooff dooff dooff of reggae beats thumping under the grass. A bonfire is crackling and sending sparks into the air. Some home-made torches have been stuck in the ground and light up flickering patches of the garden, and smell of paraffin. The sky above the sparks is a clear indigo night and the red moon looks strangely afflicted. There is a dark bite in the bottom corner. The moon is being swallowed.

Many people are piling out of doorways on to the grass, and the smell of chicken and rice and minestrone flavours the air. Silvia has brought the cauldron of soup, and bowls of food are spread out on a table that has been hauled outside, along with bottles and glasses and paper cups. Inside, the people are thick, bodies are sweaty and pulsing together with the music.

The thumping rhythms fill the air and the drums pulsate in the ground and the bass pounds in our ears.

There is the smell of marijuana mixing with the chicken.

I feel suddenly nervous and the air has become strange. The moon is half swallowed by the black shape. The flickering torches leave their imprint on my eyes so my vision is dotted with purple and blue flashes over the dark garden. Bianca is surrounded by people. They chatter away like geese in Italian and Spanish. She has a big piece of Parmesan in her hands, wrapped in silver foil, which she is undoing and grating into the huge pot of minestrone. I can smell the cheese from here through the clouds of aromatic marijuana that two tall men with long dreadlocks are smoking with their backs to the bonfire. The flames fly up behind them, making them into black silhouettes.

The moon has been swallowed. It feels cold without loss of temperature and quiet although the music still plays. A glimmering, eerie feeling.

Zeb walks up the steps from the basement. He must have slid through the bodies. He stands still, looking. He can't see into the dark.

He could be an Apache, with his long dark hair. But I think he's a Crow man.

He sees me and nods. He walks towards me and the quiet intensifies. Time stops passing. His eyes look at me out of the dark and I can see the fire reflected in them. He stands over me like a tree.

He opens his mouth, but doesn't say anything.

'Look at the moon,' I say. 'It's just been swallowed.'

Everything feels wrong. Disjointed. Jangling.

My voice doesn't seem to synchronise with my mouth. I speak, and hear it echoing.

A thin sliver of red moon appears out the other side.

He looks up at the moon and back at me.

His eyes are strange.

Bianca is suddenly there beside us. 'Zeh-Beh-Deeee!' she calls up at him, holding his hand and reaching up to kiss his cheek. She winks at me.

'Look, you must have some wine! Where is your cup?'

'I'll get some,' says Zeb, going over to the trestle table.

I watch his back walking away and stooping over the table.

'Here! I have a bottle!' she calls to a knot of people next to the tree, and walks over to them, holding her bottle up in the air.

I look across at Zeb but now Suzanne is at the table too and she is talking. She wears a yellow dress and it shows off her tan from Barbados.

'Blondes should never wear yellow!' says Bianca, coming back with her bottle. 'It clashes with their hair! I will break up the fight.'

She walks across to the table, and smiles to one and then the other. Suzanne doesn't smile. Zeb glances over at me and hands Bianca a cup. She comes back.

'Here you are.' She pours it as she walks towards me.

'Thanks.'

I take my wine under the tree where Rob and Mick are lying on his coat with their backs leaning against the trunk, gobbling chicken and rice from paper plates.

'How are you?'

'Did you see the eclipse?'

'We're not going to stay that late but you can get a lift back with us if you like.'

I nod and wander round the garden to look at the shadows and the purple flashes. I can see Zeb and Suzanne having an argument in silhouette in front of the bonfire. I'm sick of him and his love life.

I wander past them into the seething mass of bodies in the basement. Silvia is dancing with her boyfriend. He is a muscular black man in a white T-shirt, he has a bald head and it shines. Silvia gyrates her hips slowly, looking at him all the time. Her hips move but her head stays in the same place.

I close my eyes and dance. The music fills the darkness, pulses through me in colours, and sweat runs over the surface of my skin.

The music becomes slow and people are pressing up against one another. I slide through the writhing bodies to the doorway and the garden. On the edge of the crowd Zeb and Suzanne are dancing. She has her arms in a circle round his neck.

Bianca is at the top of the stairs. She nods over at them and shrugs.

I walk past the embers of the bonfire. The torches are spent and the garden is dark. Rob and Mick are cuddled up under the tree. Mick has big arms and he squeezes her to him.

'Are you ready to go?'

I nod.

'Come on, then.'

We drive up Acre Lane, past two people fighting, with a crowd shouting around them. I feel dark, closed in by the buildings, and deep down within me is a crying sound. We drive round a corner to Clapham Common and the sky is purple with orange clouds.

The trees are dark against the sky. We flew the kite here. Zeb brought fishing line and attached it to the string, it just kept going higher and higher, until it was a tiny speck. When the fishing line ran out he let it go, and Bianca said, 'I didn't realize your intention was liberation!' and we all laughed.

Suzanne wasn't there. She wasn't there for the whole Christmas holiday, when we'd met up in the Portuguese café and had crispy custard cakes and fish-balls with the Italians every Sunday.

I have to put Zeb out of my mind. Not feel these feelings. Fold them up, put them away somewhere, then take them out and paint them secretly.

We drive past Battersea Park gates and I look into the dark trees, and then out on to the bridge. I love the river at night, reflecting the coloured lights. We cross the river and I feel the water flowing beneath us. Rob and Mick are talking to each other, but I can't hear. There is a crying sound. Far away. It is the sound of the moon. It hangs over the river, eclipsed. But there is another moon; to find it I have to follow the sound to within my own world. I know it. I have painted it. There is a forest there. It is still. Sometimes the moon disguises itself and looks at me with intense eyes. When I find it, and paint it, the crying will stop.

We drive along past the barges with glimmering lights outside, and up Edith Grove. Litter is being blown about the street by the wind, and a huddle of men in dirty clothes sit drinking on a traffic island lit by yellow light. They are calling out, their arms flailing, and I don't know if they are sad or singing. The city has a peculiar atmosphere, as though it has slipped through time to another century, or the veil between time is thin and other centuries are showing through. Zeb knows about those things.

We drive up and along the streets and stop outside the peeling porch of my house. A drunk man is curled up outside my door.

'Oh dear!' says Rob. 'You've got an alkie on your doorstep.'

'D'you want me to help you shift him?' says Mick, as he pulls the handbrake.

Something hits my chest. I breathe in quickly.

'Oh my God!'

Roberta looks at me.

The breath is knocked out my body.

'It's dad!'

Part Two

1

'We'll help you get him up the stairs,' says Rob, making a decisive move that wakes me from my shock.

He is a dead weight when Mick and I try to lift him, and smells of sour alcohol. He mumbles and groans as we lift him. I open the door and he falls on to the mat. My one room, with a small kitchen at the back, is too small for his presence. It fills the air with his weight. I open the windows. I have a sofa and a bed, a table and a chair. In my kitchen there is a small table covered in formica with bananas and apples on the shiny white surface.

Rob has made tea.

We have laid dad on the sofa and he has fallen to the side and now his head is on the arm so his face is pulled sideways and his mouth is open.

Mick is standing up, looking out the kitchen window, through the gap between the houses where you can see the dark river under the purple sky.

I look at Rob, bewildered.

'He didn't say he was coming.'

'Is he always like this?'

'You mean drunk?'

She shrugs with one shoulder.

'Yes, I mean, it's been getting worse.' I sigh. 'He's all

alone in the house now and . . . Oh, I don't know, I don't know.'

I get up and look round the door at him lying squint and uncomfortable on the sofa. The sour alcohol smell fills the room. I don't want him to be there.

'I don't want him here, I don't want this.'

'Well, he's here,' says Rob, 'and he'll sober up.'

'And then what? What's he come here for?'

'To be with you, I expect.'

'I don't want him here. I can't look after him.'

There's such a horrible combination of disgust and tenderness and anger and panic in me that I begin to tremble and I put my shaking hand on the door lintel to steady myself.

'Sit down,' says Rob. 'Just sit down a minute and drink your tea.'

And I think of Bianca still at the party and Zeb dancing with Suzanne. Then I look over at the sink and start thinking odd things, like Mick's back pocket is torn and maybe he should sew it up and will Rob do it, and then I imagine her sitting under the light, sewing up his pocket.

The surrealness of the night continues. The apples, pears and bananas are too bright, divided by their bamboo squares. The flat feels overcrowded with energies that do not belong here.

'You must go home,' I say, looking up. Even Rob looks strange. Her lips are purple.

I blink my eyes. 'God, I feel as if I've taken acid or something. D'you think someone spiked the drinks?'

She looks at me. 'No, I don't think it's that.'

I shrug.

She gets up and Mick turns round. He puts his arm round her.

'You'll just have to send him home when he wakes up.'

'I can't imagine him, I mean, getting on the train, oh well.' I give a half smile. 'I'll be OK. Off you go.'

They close the door. My flat is too full. His presence is heavy.

I sit on my bed and look at him. My eyes are too wide. Something in me is trembling.

'Dad? Dad?'

He moans.

'Dad?' I lean across to shake him. His head falls off the arm. I move to catch him, and tug him back on to the sofa.

'What are you doing here, dad?' I know he won't answer. 'What d'you expect me to do?'

He suddenly opens his eyes and clutches my hand with both of his.

'I'm frightened, Eve. I'm frightened of dying.'

'But, dad, you're not going to die.'

He holds my hand so tight that it hurts. And squeezes his eyes shut, but his mouth is open, his teeth clenched together in a look of acute pain.

'Oh, dad!'

I sit back on the bed.

He suddenly, violently, rolls off on to the floor and lies on the mat between the bed and the sofa. From the acrid smell and a trickling sound I realize that he is pissing on the floor.

'Oh, for fuck's sake, dad!'

I get a bucket of water and a cloth.

'For God's sake, dad!'

I pull off his trousers. I wrap him up in a towel, and ease the mat from underneath him. I mop up the piss and take the mat between my thumb and finger and rinse it in the sink. Then I shove it out the window, weighted down by a packet of washing powder and a pan filled with cutlery.

When I go back through to mop the floorboards he is lying in a foetal position with the towel wrapped round him. He looks like a big tiny baby.

I take the blanket off my bed and throw it over him.

'For goodness sake, dad!'

I lie under my duvet and look at the yellow window on the ceiling. I don't want to close the curtain, so the yellow streetlight shines into the room making the shadows brown and the light lurid.

I can feel a presence in the room that isn't just dad. As though he has brought something else with him. I'm afraid it will get into me when I'm asleep. I lie with my eyes wide open. A blue window is flicked around the room by the headlights of a passing car.

2

All morning, at college, I've been listening for sounds: someone clattering along the corridor, bumping against the thin partitions, slumping down somewhere. Like he might turn up any moment in my painting space and piss on the floor, then fall over and lie with his chin resting on his breastbone, and his legs splayed out at right angles.

I am scared he's going to come in to the college and show me up! That's what they used to say at school: 'Oh, my dad, did you see what he was wearing? He really shows me up!' That's when you're thirteen, it's all right to be ashamed of your parents, afraid they'll make you conspicuous, make you ashamed of them. That horrible feeling squirming inside your belly that makes your toes curl. They really do. They curl sideways so you stand on the outer edges of your feet. It makes you hold your breath but the cringing is the worst part. Everything seems to turn inside out; all the intestines and the stomach. You clench it but it does it anyway.

Rob puts her head through the curtain.

'D'you want that?' she says, handing me a cup. 'I don't want it.'

'Why not? It's still hot!' I say, taking the coffee.

'Dunno, it's making me queasy,' says Rob, sitting on the stool and getting out her tobacco to roll a cigarette.

'So what about your dad? Where did you leave him?' She licks the paper closed and puts the fag in her mouth.

'Should you be doing that?'

'Listen, I'm down to three a day so shut up.'

'OK, OK.'

'Well?'

'He was still sleeping when I left this morning,' I say, looking out the window.

'So he's usually like that?'

'Mostly, I suppose.'

'What's he doing here?'

'I have no idea.'

'Maybe he wants to come and stay with you.'

'Oh my God.'

'You'll have to kick him out, it's your life.'

'Rob!'

'Well, you have to be like that, alcoholics are hard work!'

'Is that what my dad is?'

'Obviously.'

'Oh Rob, I just hope he doesn't come in here drunk!'

'Why should he?' says Rob.

'To see me, I suppose.'

'Well, he might find a friend!' Rob laughs and gives me a nudge.

I know she means Terry and I laugh half-heartedly.

Rob picks up her bag. 'I'm going down the Housing Benefit,' she says along with a puff of smoke and stomps off with the fag in her mouth.

There is a feeling of drama in my body. A trembling that I cannot quieten. I feel shocked. Something in me is shaky and unsteady. And all my ideas, which usually congregate in a humming throng of colours, are scattered about in a disconnected distance from each other.

There is an emptiness around me where the ideas usually are, and all I see is the dream that I woke from with sweat on my face, trying to cry out that it wasn't my dream.

I'd been pulled down a tunnel with wet walls. The ragged people had despair in their faces. My dad was there and they were clutching at him. There were broken bottles among the filth. The dark river in the tunnel was full of rubbish. They saw me, and began coming towards me.

'Let's get her,' one said.

I tried to run on the slippery stones, and woke up shouting, 'This isn't my dream!'

I want to paint the dream to get their pale bony faces outside of me and on to the canvas. I can still feel their groping fingers and smell the stench of the river.

I mix the colours on the palette: chrome green, raw umber, Naples yellow.

I paint their greenish faces on the canvas, in dark filthy clothes.

The painting has grown ugly. I don't like looking at it. The colours have turned to sludge. Sometimes all you can do is make a mess. When I try drawing with charcoal and spill the turps over the drawing so the charcoal smudges I decide it's time to stop for lunch.

I walk into the clatter of the canteen, and the smell of beans and chips. The dinner ladies stand behind the chrome counter chatting to one another, holding long silver spoons. I buy my sandwich and coffee. The wall down the side of the canteen is made of glass so that when you come into college at lunchtime you walk past a row of chewing faces. Suzanne is sitting with her friends next to the glass window. They are talking loudly together and laughing. I sit down in the corner by the wall. Suzanne has her chair tilted back. They are looking out the window.

'What the hell's he doing?' one says.

Then they are all quiet, their faces sideways.

'Oops, no! Didn't make it!'

I look, but cannot see what they are looking at.

'Someone should tell Stan or there'll be a whole crowd of them here in a minute.'

'Oh-oh steady! Nope! Down again!' and they all laugh.

'Oh God, I think he's puked!'

'Here's Stan!' They all look out the window and are silent for a minute.

My arms and fingers have gone limp so I have to put down my sandwich. I know who they are looking at out in the courtyard.

Stan, the caretaker, has white hair and black eyebrows and a name so unpronounceable he's called Stan.

'What's he saying?'

'Asking him something.'

He's a bear from an Eastern European country with huge hands, and even before I see him walk back across the courtyard and through the glass door I know he will be coming to find me.

He walks through the double doors of the canteen. He looks about the room and sees me. He motions to me with his finger, just quickly; a little twiddle in the air.

I get up from the table and leave my coffee and sandwich. I follow Stan out the door.

The eyes in the glass wall follow me. I feel as if my body has turned into thousands of little slithery balls that all slide up against one another and slither.

Slimey slithery sliding balls. I am glad big Stan is with me. I want to hold his hand.

He puts his big body between me and the wall of eyes as he bends to talk to dad, who is slumped down next to the Henry Moore sculpture with his legs splayed out at right angles and his chin resting on his breastbone.

'Here is your daughter.'

Dad looks up. Tries to sit straight.

'Evie, there you are! Evie.'

'Oh dad!'

'Oh there you are, Evie. Evie, there you are.'

I try and lift him and Stan helps and together we hoist him up to sit on the edge of the wall.

'Dad, let's go home'

I try and hitch him up by putting his arm round my shoulders. He stands and staggers. He's a dead weight. Stan hitches him up the other side.

'Home later, now bench,' says Stan, and we stagger with him to the bench on the other side of the road.

I look up at Stan, who nods to me and walks back over the road. I sit with dad on the bench out of sight of the wall of eyes.

'Evie, oh Evie.' He holds on to my shoulder.

'Dad, for God's sake, what are you doing here?'

He is sitting bent over, feeling the raised blotches on his forehead. The drink has poisoned his blood.

'I wasn't like this,' he says pointing at the pavement.

He looks up at me with watery eyes. 'Evie, I wasn't always like this!'

'I know, dad, I know.'

'I wasn't . . .' and he tries to stand and falls back down. He tries again to pull himself upwards but he crumples down with a wobbling movement, puts his head in his hands and sobs out a dark painful cry.

I sit on the bench with him, not knowing what to do.

Zeb comes through the door, and walks quickly across the courtyard and over the road to us. I can see Suzanne in the darkness behind the glass door with her hands on her hips. He comes over to the bench.

'It's my dad,' I say out of awkwardness.

'Had a few too many? Done it myself,' he says.

Dad looks up at him and growls.

Zeb wants me to feel better, but there are too many feelings in me with him there as well, and I can't bear his presence.

'Can I get you something, Eve? Some coffee?'

'Go away,' I say, my voice cracked, 'please just go away.'

'OK,' he says, and goes back over the road.

Then I feel I've been sawn in two, but not across like the woman in the box. Lengthwise, like a fish when they pull the guts out.

3

The stairwell of the house my bedsit is in always smells of damp. The carpet in the hall is thin and worn and olive green. Under a chipped mirror is a table where the post piles up and every day I flick through it to see if there is anything there for me. But there isn't.

How did we get back? Somehow. After I'd left him to sleep under my coat, after plastic cups of black coffee from the machine outside the lift, after hauling him up, weighted down by his heavy arm and steering him along the King's Road and clambering and nearly falling into the bus, and pushing him out at the stop, when he fell against the wall and banged his head, and all the people going home with shopping or coming back from work didn't really pay attention to us at all, we finally climbed the stairs, and this morning I'd left him lying on the sofa, still sleeping.

Not all of the strip of olive green carpet is nailed down to the yellowed wooden stairs. You have to be careful the carpet doesn't slide underneath you. The landlord doesn't like to fix things. Dad had slid on the stair carpet when the three of us were trying to haul him up the stairs.

I wonder if he is sober, and I roll the piece of paper in my pocket as I walk up the dark stairs.

When Bianca saw the painting of the nightmare, and heard about dad, she had marched me up to Miss Pym's office and looked through the telephone directory to find out the time and the place of a meeting for alcoholics nearby. I have the piece of paper rolled up in my pocket to give to dad.

'Darling,' she said, 'he is an addict like me!'

There's a skylight at the top of the stairs. The glass is crusted with something brown and translucent, but I prefer the dingy light to the bare light bulb that hangs down on a long wire and reminds me of a horror film.

I put my key in the lock and open the door.

Dad is sitting on the sofa. He is dressed and everything is neat, his hair combed to the side. He stands up. He is sober.

'Evie,' he says.

'Hello, dad. I'm going to make some tea.'

I throw my canvas bag on the bed and go through to the kitchen. I feel awkward and so does he. I put the kettle on.

'Listen, dad,' I say, unfolding the piece of paper.

He stands in the doorway of the kitchen.

'Darling, there's a letter for you,' he says.

'Where is it?' I say, looking round the door.

He is putting his shaky hands in one pocket then another.

'Oh, I must have put it down somewhere,' he says glancing up at me apologetically and looking about him. 'Where *did* I put it?'

'Oh dad, couldn't you have just left it downstairs?' I say impatiently. 'That's where I always collect my post.'

'Sorry, darling,' he says, looking about the room, 'so sorry, I know I had it.'

I sigh and go back into the kitchen. I light the gas and put the kettle down on the stove, and then I see that on the table next to the biscuit tin, standing against the empty teapot, is the letter. It is from him.

I take it out of the white envelope and unfold it. I read the letter, in his beautiful handwriting. It is a gentle letter. It tells me how sorry he is for being this way. That he loves me, that I am a good person, that he is ashamed. The letter makes me cry, because I feel so sorry for him. Cry for his shame, for the way he makes himself loathe himself. He is a good noble person, and that noble nature is horrified by the drunk. I know that he is, and so am I. When you love one and see it being destroyed by the other, what can you do? All you can do is go into the next room where he's standing with his head bowed and pull his big arms round you and cry into his jacket, and say, 'But I love you, dad, don't worry about any of that, so what, it doesn't matter, dad, it doesn't matter.'

And he strokes my hair and whispers into it about how sorry he is.

'I know,' I say. 'It doesn't matter.'

'But, darling, it does.'

And he's right. It does. It does matter. It tears you apart, that's why it matters. And forgiveness has nothing to do with it, because it still tears you apart.

The kettle whistles and I make the tea and blow my nose on his big handkerchief and we sit squashed together round the kitchen table, and I unfold the crumpled piece of paper with the address and the time, and he takes it and nods. 'Yes, darling', he says, 'tomorrow.' And I squeeze his hand and nod at him. 'Yes, dad, please.'

4

'How's it going?' says Rob, coming into the studio with a new roll of paper.

'Oh, it's OK.'

I tell her about the letter, and the meeting. 'It's at the church, practically opposite.'

'That would be good.'

'Oh, it would be such a relief.'

Rob puts down her shopping and goes to fetch tea, and I go back to my work.

I have been painting a strange picture all morning, I know it is horrible but I have to paint it; a girl with many slithery arms and legs like an octopus walking past a wall of eyes. I am painting the feeling I had. It has many tentacles and the face of a frightened child.

I smell him before I even hear him but he is already in my painting space. He is looking over my shoulder, breathing down my neck. I am startled and look round with a jerky breath.

'Oh my God, Sergei! You scared me, please don't do that.'

'I am walking round the studios, it's my job.'

'Well, you could knock on the wall or something.'

He ignores me

'What is this? Art therapy?'

'I don't know what you call it, if you want to call it that,' I say, confused, wanting to hide it away.

'This isn't an art therapy course.'

I don't answer.

'Surrealism is one thing but there has to be a reason for it. It comes from the imagination, but it isn't *self-indulgence.*'

'I'm painting what I feel,' I interrupt him.

'What you feel!' His eyes look at the ceiling and he nods with his usual sneer.

But last night dad left me his letter; the sad beautiful letter from the man he once was, and Sergei's quivering wet lip, his cold eyes looking at me with their closed blue gaze, repel me.

'Fuck off, Sergei!' I say in a tired voice and I turn away from him.

'I beg your pardon?'

'You heard,' I say, turning back to face him, and raising my voice. 'And I'll tell you why! I'm fed up! Fed up of you coming into my space and criticizing everything I do, fed up of your useless advice. So just go away!'

He pats the air with his yellow hands as though smoothing it down.

'There is no need to become over-emotional.'

I just stare at him. He swallows like a lizard, with unblinking eyes, and turns to leave, saying 'Women!' under his breath.

'Far out!' says Rob, putting her head round the curtain. 'It's about time someone told that old bully!' She is laughing.

I take the tea from her and shrug. 'Oh Rob, to be honest I don't care about Sergei. I just hope dad goes to the meeting. I just hope he goes.'

5

But he didn't go. He looked at me with bleary eyes, lifting his eyebrows and blinking slowly, unable to shape the words 'Sorry, darling'. He was slumped in the chair, an empty vodka bottle at his feet when I got back from college.

'But dad, you said you would!'

It was no good talking about it because he just made gestures to the window, his eyes looking lost then returning to mine, his head shaking slightly, and trying again to shape the words, until his eyes looked at nothing and he didn't even try to speak. And I kicked the door with tears in my eyes.

'Oh dad, for fuck's sake!'

And in the morning, with his hands trembling, he made tea, and he was present in his eyes, and once again he said, 'Yes, I will today, I promise.' But when I came back he hadn't gone anywhere except the off-licence and his watery eyes looked at me sadly and he put his hands up in a helpless gesture, until finally one morning I took the kettle from his shaking hands, when he was trying to fill it under the tap, and I pushed past him to light the blue flame, and said, 'Dad, just GO! I don't care where!' And when I came back the flat was empty.

That was three nights ago, and I don't know where he went.

I didn't mean it, dad, and now I don't know where you are. You didn't take your keys. You're somewhere on the street, and where did you sleep last night?

I open the front door, half expecting to find him on the doorstep. The sky has a threatening look. It's going to rain.

I walk past the church and look through the railings to see if he's asleep on one of the benches.

I run across the road to take the short cut down the alley. There aren't many cars yet; I woke up so early that the market is only just being set up. A man in an apron, and a fag in his mouth, is joining two poles together. 'It's gonna piss down in a minute!' he says, jerking his head at the sky.

I walk by the skeleton of the market, the bare metal stalls with no awnings; boxes piled on the pavement and bits of wrapping blowing about on the road.

I thought he'd go to the address on the slip of paper. I thought it would all be solved. He'd find out what to do. Find people to help him.

And I imagine him curled up on a damp piece of cardboard.

A black and white dog comes up to me and sniffs me and goes trotting off down the street.

Roberta came with me to the police station, but that didn't do much good.

The sergeant said, 'Do you know how many people there are in this city, young lady?' in a tired voice. His colleague must have taken pity on me because he pushed him aside and said, 'How long has he been missing, love?' and took out some forms. I said three days. He gave a little smile and didn't look at the sergeant, who was pushing his chin back into his chin and nodding with his lips.

'That's no time at all!' he said, patting my hand. 'He'll be back, don't you worry,' but he wrote down the details anyway.

Rob was waiting outside on a low wall, smoking one of her three roll-ups of the day.

'Well?'

I shrugged. 'They say he's not officially missing after three days.'

I walk along by the closed shops and people are unlocking the roll-up metal sheets with loud grating sounds. Suddenly the sky darkens and the light turns greenish. It starts to pelt.

I keep remembering the night before I left home in Cornwall; and dad looking up the stairs with those eyes.

I run for shelter and stand under the awning of the Turkish cake shop.

That 'you're leaving me' look that he'd tried to hide.

I stick my hands in my pockets and look at the rain falling outside the awning. The road shines and trembles with busy drops.

But I'd seen it in his shoulders too. His jacket had that weighed-down look, even when he took it off and hung it on the back of the chair there was that round weighed-down look on it, and when I picked it up once, to try it on, the jacket weighed my shoulders down too, so it looked as if I carried something, and it made it hard to breathe, and I took it off quickly and felt frightened.

Now the rain comes in sheets, slanting and bouncing off the pavement. I feel the wind of it on my ankles.

Where is he going to go in this rain?

I'd been upstairs packing up my paintbrushes in an old dishcloth, sorting out the tubes of paint, when I heard him on the stairs.

'Would you like a cup of tea?' he said.

It was a little white room that looked over the moor and the blue hills. I liked looking on to the land. I used to set my easel up and paint out the window, watching the light change the colour of the hills from deep green to glowing orange when the sun shone. Then I painted out of the window that faced the sea; the Mount in the far distance changing colour every day, sometimes obscured by the mist, sometimes dazzling yellow, lit up by the sun, sometimes like a mysterious green isle.

The sea changed all the time; rippled like a snake-skin on a cold grey day, with a sky dark and brooding; then pale blue that glowed so gently it made your heart limp; then in the morning when the sun rose and the sky was flushed and rosy the sea would turn pink. The whole bay between the distant Lizard and Land's End would be pink. I loved painting the bay. I loved watching the sea.

I still loved it, but he didn't. He hated the sea now.

The drops drip from the awning to a slower rhythm. The air is filled with raindrops, water slants all landing on the pavement so it is a sheet of bouncing drops, making puddles in the dips, and rivers in the gutter, the traffic whooshing through it.

He'd looked up the stairs with the tea in his hand and said, 'We've been all right together, you and I, haven't we, Evie?' and I looked down the stairs and his face was at the bottom looking up, with my shadow falling over it.

'Haven't we, Evie?'

'Yes, dad, of course we have.'

He'd nodded 'I'm so glad,' he said. 'Something good came out of it.'

I'd followed him downstairs.

'Dad, you'll be all right, won't you?'

I knew he'd say, 'Yes, be off with you, get on with your packing, you've a train to catch tomorrow.'

But he didn't.

He looked at me and he breathed hard with his mouth open, and closed his eyes for a few minutes with a frown on his forehead.

'Dad? What is it?'

'Oh, it's all right, Evie,' he'd said.

'Will you be all right, dad?'

He'd looked away, out the window, and said, 'Oh, there's a storm coming in.'

He wouldn't be.

I'd known he wouldn't be and so had he. He couldn't lie about it and it was stupid to ask him to. But he also didn't want me not to go.

He just didn't have enough to live for on his own.

A slender boy walks through the rain, smiling, with his hands out, doing a strutting bouncy walk. It lessens. Only a few drops come through the air now.

I walk out along the wet streets.

That white breathing face.

The gaping mouth, looking out of the window at the grey sea.

When I reach the turning to college I meet Rob coming the other way, pushing her bike.

'Any news?' she says.

I shrug, and shake my head.

'Come on,' she says, putting her hand on my shoulder. 'Let's get a tea and sit by the river a bit.'

We go to the newsagent that sells takeaway tea, along with newspapers in every language, and boxes of exotic vegetables.

'It's all right, Eve, he'll turn up,' she says, as we walk down the street towards Albert Bridge, past a man lying on a bench, his coat tied up with string, and I double-check to see if it's dad. His face is old and grey. He has white bristles. He is asleep on a rolled-up sleeping bag.

We cross the beeping road and lean over the wall to look into the olive-green water. On the other side are the calm trees of Battersea Park.

'It said in the letter he didn't want to burden me. What does that mean?'

She shrugs and blows on her tea, then sips it in little slurps.

I watch the river water slipping over itself. It runs fast and full after the rain.

'He's not going to throw himself over the bridge or something. He won't do that will he, Rob?'

'No, I'm sure he won't.'

We sit down on the bench held up by Egyptian figures with the faces of people and the wings of birds. Grimy daffodils tremble in the traffic wind. The sky is low and heavy. We sit in silence for a long time until our tea is finished.

'Think it's going to rain again, Rob.'

'Listen, things work out in the end,' she says, and squeezes my arm, as we get up from the bench and leave the river behind.

As we walk fast in the spitting rain along Oakley Street, Rob tries to tell me not to worry, and dad has to live his own life. I just nod, and stick my hands in my pockets, while all the time planning the places I will go and look: the railway stations and Underground stations where there are waiting rooms; tunnels and passages where there is shelter and warmth.

Then suddenly, as we reach the King's Road, a car drives through a puddle, just missing Rob, and I see blue glass smashing into small splinters and pink water splashing on a wall, and then an almighty crash, and I wonder why I am seeing Zeb's sculpture splintering to pieces in my mind.

'Can't you just leave him to it?' says Rob, after we've got back to the studio and hung up our coats and unpacked our bags.

'How d'you know I'm not going to?'

I am sitting at my small table and Rob is taping a huge piece of paper to the wall.

'Because you've got the *A to Z* out, and you're planning where to look,' says Rob, who must have eyes in the back of her head.

I shake my head at her intuition, and put the book away.

'Well?' she says, standing in the doorway, holding the muslin curtain aside. 'Why not? Why can't you let him go, and find his own way? It's his life.'

'I don't know,' I say, undoing the cloth full of tubes of paint.

The reason is too deep for me to reach, yet I know that part of me is inextricably linked with his dark journey, and it fills me with dread.

'He's a grown man, Eve,' she says, and lets go the curtain.

I look at her figure moving about behind the see-through muslin that absorbs the light from the white sky. Rob's huge pictures of women painted out of river mud glow from the walls. They are seven feet tall and smell of baked earth.

'Anyway, how d'you know he's on the street, there are places he can go,' she says with her back to me, as she sizes the huge piece of paper with long strokes.

'I just know,' I say, looking down at the colours I am mixing. Cadmium yellow, cobalt green and blue, lamp black. I have left out any form of red so nothing can go brown.

The cobalt blues and greens are making gentle combinations that calm me. The picture is by the river. The road is green because of the light.

Why can't I just leave him to it? I say to the green painting.

'Better that he's gone!' says Rob matter-of-factly as she bends to size the base of the paper.

I look at her as she kneels and swishes the size with a wallpaper brush, then look down at my colours. Lamp black has got in with the cadmium yellow and turned it a rotting green. The colour of the slime in the river when the water is low, I think to myself, and from deep down in my imagination comes an image; the slime they find the bodies in when they are pale and cold, and I shake my head to dispel it.

6

I wait among a crowd of people outside a lift. We push together as it arrives with a ping, and troop through the silver doors. We squash inside, breathing each other's breath, and with a clanking grinding sound we lurch upwards, trembling beneath the arhythmic flicker of a zinc-white striplight.

The cool air of the night hits my face. I walk beside a looming building and through tall trees. I am glad to be out in the air.

I've been looking in bus and train terminals, in Underground tunnels, under bridges, on park benches.

I've been to Paddington to look in the alcoves of the echoing station, to bleak and windy King's Cross and the nooks and crannies of St Pancras, looking at the grimy faces to see if I can see dad's. I've been along brown tunnels lit by yellow light, up escalators and down tiled stairwells, going to as many places as I can with my one-day travelcard.

I walk under the bridge. The streetlights reflect off the river and throw glimmering shadows on to the underside of the steel girders and gently stroke the dignified faces of the bearded refugees with trembling water light as they sit, pale and proud, on their makeshift cardboard beds, each bowing slightly when I look at him. They have lost their home and their possessions but they have their souls still with them. They do not belong among the people who crowded my nightmare when I woke and knew I had followed dad into his dream. The place his soul had slipped. I walk up the dark stone stairs.

I stand on the bridge and look into the black water and see the green lights reflected in rippling lines until they crash and splinter apart, broken into by the wake of a night-time police boat. At the same time a siren makes a frantic eee-aw eee-aw along the road and a blue light flits between the trees and fades away. He must be somewhere in this huge pulsing noisy city; lying on a piece of cardboard or a bench along the river, under a bridge or up a dark dirty alley where the restaurants put their rubbish, out of the cold wind. It is blowing in my face from the river, and the black water flows under my feet.

I have a feeling in me, clogged and heavy like red mud, and it has a sound, a moaning sound.

I don't know if it belongs to me or dad, and I walk into the middle of the bridge where the traffic is loud. I lean over the edge and make the long red moaning sound into the wind, and the feeling uncoils and flows out my mouth and is carried away by the river; and the sound has memories in it. They dig into me and pull up more memories from the mud. They flow through me and unfurl in the windy air; and I remember being held in his arms next to the fire, in the warm green room, and walking with him along the cliffs, he shielding his eyes to look at the far-away islands, and along the shore, the sun shining on the belly of the waves so it seemed they were lit from within. I remember the bonfire in the woods at night when all the trees came in close, and we baked potatoes, and I remember him walking with his big stick in the long grass, me collecting things to show him, snail-shells, twigs and feathers. And I remember his eyes at night, 'Bless you, darling!' 'But I didn't sneeze, dad,' and the light from his eyes when he smiled. And I remember him walking by the graveyard on the anniversary, and not even looking over the wall.

I walk back across the bridge and away from the river and the indigo night.

Poor dad. He couldn't bear the pain of losing her.

I duck beneath the scaffolding and walk between striped poles past the skips. I peer into the dark brown shadows of a tall doorway at the bodies swaddled in sleeping bags that are tied with string. Dad doesn't have a sleeping bag. The yellow streetlights bounce up and turn the sky orange.

I walk across Trafalgar Square past the huge lions, and climb on to a bus that zooms along the Haymarket and drives so fast round Piccadilly Circus that a woman falls over and shouts 'We all want to get home, love, but have a heart' at the driver, and I sit on the lower deck and look out at dark and bright Piccadilly flashing past, too tired to shield my screwed-up eyes and see if I can spot dad in a dark doorway.

I remember picking petals out of the grass when the wreaths had tumbled over each other in the wind as though they were racing. The men chased them, their hair blowing sideways, and the women held their black hats on to their heads so they wouldn't be blown down the oblong hole that was surrounded by planks of wood holding down tarpaulin; you could only just see the red mud cut clean and plummeting down into the dark. Dad threw a handful of earth in and handed me some earth to throw in, and I threw but it landed on the tarpaulin. I thought it was a kind of game. And above our heads the sky was moving, and through the salty blowing air I could smell the earth.

After dad let go my hand, and I looked up and saw his face contorted and felt a tear-drop on my face that had been blown on to my cheek from his eye, so I knew that he was crying, the wind blew a crowd of dark clouds over the cemetery and it began to rain sideways so even the people under the umbrellas got soaked down one side. And I got pulled next to someone's legs, but dad stood in the rain with his hair being plastered down straggly over his eyebrows, his mouth open and his teeth showing, but not his tears, and the raindrops splashed on the planks of wood and poured into the oblong dark and made a drumming sound, and the piles of earth on either side began to move in red muddy rivulets down the grey flag-stoned path. And someone put a mackintosh round my shoulders, but dad stood on his own, getting wet to the bone.

The driver speeds so fast around Hyde Park Corner that we all lean sideways and hold on to the poles. He doesn't even stop at the bus stop at the top of Knightsbridge, and cross shouting voices are left behind in the night as we career along the road, while frantic people pull the cord, ringing the bell to stop him so they can get off.

I climb off the bus and walk along my road, and up the stairs to my bedsit. I take off my clothes and get into bed without putting the lights on. I don't want to remember any more.

I lie in bed, listening to the girl upstairs practising the violin and hitting the wrong notes. But the musical notes in the wide black night are beautiful and comforting, coming from her body movements I can see in my mind's eye, and her longing and her hope. The big wide night, lit by a pale half moon, embraces the sound and me in bed, and her longing, and the nearby river, and the street-lights and the person clipping along the street outside. It is holding it all, and the sound of the violin accompanies it, colouring the night with its warm sound, and gives the night a heart.

7

Today the studio is cold. Rob hasn't arrived yet and I miss her presence.

I am mixing the colours on my palette but they are making horrible combinations. I put down the palette knife, and look out the window at the trees and the grey buildings.

Sometimes I am afraid of the white canvas, afraid of what can happen on the smooth sized ground, the mistake that can turn all the colours to mud. It's always the same mess. It must wait somewhere for its chance; and then it slips down the brush and on to the surface. It gets itself in all the colours and gobbles them up with its deadness. It gobbles up the clear bright colours and regurgitates them so they are ugly next to each other. It turns it all to mud, but not the mud we scooped out of the river that has been baked in the oven so it fills the studio air with a warm sweet smell, not that kind of mud; and I look through the muslin curtain at Rob's paintings and wish she would arrive.

At coffee time the door opens and Rob and Cecile and Bianca all come through the door, talking at once.

Rob plonks her bag down.

'Eve, you forgot Karl's class.'

'Oh, it's Wednesday!' I say, putting my hand up to my forehead.

'We were doing three-second poses,' says Bianca, mimicking the poses and changing them every second to show me.

'It's all right,' says Cecile, 'he didn't take the register.'

'That's the second time, Eve,' says Rob.

Bianca comes through the curtain to look at my picture.

'Oh Evie, your paintings are getting uglier and uglier.'

'I know,' I say. 'It's awful!'

'Well, it isn't just about making pretty pictures!' says Rob through the curtain.

'It's because you have a worry,' says Bianca.

'I think it's interesting', says Cecile, leaning over to look.

'Interesting is always an insult,' says Bianca, laughing. 'What happened to all your beautiful colours?'

'Are we going up to the abstract floor for coffee?' says Cecile.

'Well, I'm not staying here for Rob's instant!' says Bianca, making a face.

'Are you all right?' says Cecile as we follow the other two out of the door.

'I suppose,' I say.

'You think everything should be beautiful,' says Rob to Bianca as we walk up the stairs.

'Well, who wants something ugly on the wall?'

'You aren't really, are you?' says Cecile to me.

'No,' I say, shaking my head. 'I suppose not.'

'Then you should only express nice things, should you?' says Rob.

'No! Look at Goya. I'm not saying that!' says Bianca.

'Sounds like it.'

'But why paint in those ugly colours? Eve has a sense of colour!'

'You have to paint what you feel sometimes.'

We walk into Bianca's space, filled with light from the huge windows, and glinting gold and crimson.

It is a dark and light day, with sunlight through rain, and lit-up buildings against black clouds. The racing rain-drops have rainbows in them. Bianca's collages catch the light and also the dark, reflecting the weather that shines and glints and glowers over the city.

'Not everything can be pink and gold!' says Rob, with disdain in the 'p' of 'pink'.

'Well, not everyone wants *mud* on their walls!' says Bianca.

Cecile makes an exasperated face at me.

'Who cares what they want on their walls!' says Rob. 'What about Francis Bacon, he's not pretty.'

'I didn't say that anything had to be pretty! That's what you said.'

The conversation continues and includes Frida Kahlo and Brueghel and though I want to join in, something in me is listening to a far-away sound, as though dad has taken part of me away with him.

Bianca goes to fill the coffee pot for another cup and returns with her face animated and a little flushed.

'Oh my God, I just heard some gossip on the landing.'

'What?' we all say, looking round.

'It's not good. Not good at all.'

'Well, tell us!' says Rob impatiently.

'She smashed his sculpture!'

'Whose?'

'Zeb's.'

'When?'

'Who did?'

'Suzanne, of course.'

'How could she?'

'Poor Zeb.' I turn to the huge window looking out over London.

I'd seen it in the puddle when the car tyre split the water to smithereens.

'Why, though?'

'Were they having an argument?'

'He's split up from her, that's what I think.'

I look across the buildings at the far-away distance as they talk about who heard it from who, and who said what, and I think of Zeb walking down the road, looking forlorn.

Rob stands up, rubs her back and says that whatever's happening in anybody's love life it's time she got back to work. Cecile nods, and Bianca gets out a sheaf of gold leaf and sits down. But I don't want to go back downstairs to my mess of a picture. I just want to sit up here above London and watch Bianca glueing gold leaf to a piece of wood. When she leans close to it the outbreath from her nose makes the gold leaf flutter.

'Why don't you go and see him?' says Bianca, after the other two have gone downstairs.

'Who?'

'You know who! He likes you, you like each other. You told him to go away, remember.'

'I can't, right now. I just can't.'

'I know your father is missing, Eve. I know that it's hard for you, but . . .'

'I just can't deal with all the feelings. I feel stretched taut like a drum with too much in me. One more feeling and it would all split apart.'

'What would split apart?'

'Whatever it is that's holding me together! I'm just somewhere horrible at the moment.'

'And Zeb isn't?'

'Well, he's not in the horrible place my dad's in.'

Bianca looks up at me. 'And I don't think you should be either!'

The sun comes out and floods the studio through the raindrops, and the gold glitters and flutters to the floor as Bianca stands up and says, 'I know! I'm going to take you somewhere!' And begins to pack up her sketchbook and collage materials. 'He's the patron saint of Londoners!' she says, pulling on her coat, 'and we are Londoners!'

'Bianca, what are you talking about?'

'Come on, downstairs! Get your stuff! I'm taking you on a pilgrimage!'

'But you're not religious.'

'No, but I am superstitious,' says Bianca. 'And I think you are losing it.'

'Losing what?'

She just looks at me.

'D'you think so?' I say.

'It's in the eyes!' she says, pointing at me with two index fingers.

So I let myself be led downstairs to get my coat and sketchbook and out the door into the sunlight and the rain.

8

On the top deck of the bus Bianca gets out her guide-book and translates from Italian about Rahere who went to Italy and saw a vision of a six-winged animal with lion's feet who took him up to the top of a mountain to meet St Bartholomew who told him to build a church in Smithfield, because it was a holy place.

'The meat market? Really?' I say.

We climb out the bus and walk down Smithfield, past men in blue and white striped aprons, carrying dead pigs and cows from refrigerated lorries down metal ramps and through the gates of the meat market.

We walk away from the road and the iron smell of blood down Rising Sun Court and come upon a grey church and a grass garden dappled with sunlight from an overhanging tree, hidden behind buildings, with a feeling of stillness. We walk into the garden. The quietness encloses us. From the branches a dove calls roo-coo, roo-coo.

Sometimes you walk through an invisible curtain that divides one atmosphere from another. It is a gentle thing, but within the gentleness is something that could completely rearrange you. Your whole being might turn into dots and become part of the air.

The garden feels separated from time.

Bianca and I go down the steps into the church, which envelops us in flickering darkness and the smell of frankincense.

And I feel as if we have fallen beneath ordinary reality where the air is thicker.

We walk past a statue of Bartholomew carrying his own skin.

'Poor thing, is that what happened to him?'

I light a candle for dad.

Bianca is turning the pages of an enormous red leather book with gilt-edged pages.

'Rahere built it in 1123 with the help of children and beggars,' she whispers, and the whispering fills the air with 's's' that linger and echo, as she tells me stories from the Book of the Foundations.

'So many people were healed that he's only going to tell us about the ones he's seen with his own eyes! the writer says,' she whispers.

'Maybe he can heal your hepatitis,' I say.

'Oh no,' she says, 'if I didn't have hepatitis I'd go and score heroin straight away. It is my protector!'

While Bianca sits at the back of the church in a tall wooden pew, making collages with metallic sweetie wrappers nailed smooth, I wander up the dark corridors and wonder what it was like being alive then, shuffling up the aisle with your legs in a basket, pushing yourself along on sticks, so you could get to the altar among the songs and the glimmering candles and be healed by a saint you can't see. And far away I hear a church bell and I feel the reverberation of the sound in my cells.

We sit outside the church for a while. The rain has stopped. The little garden glistens. Bianca has bits of coloured paper all over the bench. I draw a picture of St Bartholomew by a wide blue river and a church built by children from the time when people were healed by invisible hope.

A wind blows through the plane tree and Bianca's pieces of paper flutter. She chases them across the grass.

Then the bells start ringing, dong-dong ding-ding-dong, in different rhythms. Once they must have rung all over the city, telling about times to pray, and the hermits who guarded the gates of the city and the holy wells, with their long matted hair and ragged clothes, would have closed their eyes.

We walk away from the sound, out of the old gateway and past St Bartholomew's Hospital and into the city streets to catch the bus home.

9

It is Saturday, and the college is closed. I bike along the river with my paintbox, a jar of water and a tube of white. I chain up my bike in Victoria Gardens and walk between the plane trees that eat up the traffic fumes and keep London clean, and up the steps to Lambeth Bridge. The dark clouds have gone and the river shines with light.

I stand on the bridge, looking towards Westminster, and paint the curve in the river. I follow the wall with my paintbrush all the way up to Westminster Bridge, which is distant from me, but little on the page. I follow the arches with the tip of the brush, making sure they are small enough, and behind the bridge, the dome of St Paul's, a curve and a dash of blue. My brush follows the line of the water's surface. I put in the trees in Victoria Gardens, then a frenzied tumult of dashes and spires, and among them a circle; the face of Big Ben.

The brush follows my eye. I paint the surface of the water. Little dashes far away, ripples nearby; a small boat in the far distance, a large passenger barge on the bottom of the page.

I wait for the paint to dry and look into the river and watch the water slipping over itself, brown and deep. Down there among the stones, something is lodged. I see dark orange rust spots behind the silty water, and the rippled blue surface that reflects the sky.

The sun slips out and the Houses of Parliament light up, all spiky.

I turn the page and draw with my pen.

A barge moves over the water and under Westminster Bridge. A yellow lorry crosses over the bridge at the same time, and an aeroplane moves slowly across the sky and disappears behind a blue and grey striped tower block. I keep up with my pen. They describe the near, the far and the middle distance, and help me make the small page into a big space.

Tied-up boats slide gently over the up-and-down of the water in the ribbon of reflected sun, sending tiny ripples and dots of light over the surface. Then the clouds come from behind me and little spots of rain begin to smudge the ink.

The castellations of Lambeth Palace begin to drip downwards into the trees.

The bridge vibrates with the weight of a bus.

I walk towards the café on the river, opposite Lambeth Palace, in the rain. It sits over the water and the windows look down the river to Westminster.

The window-pane is covered in raindrops. I can see Westminster Bridge in the misty distance.

I draw the frowning sea serpents coiled around the globes of light, and the green lions holding circles in their mouths along the curved wall.

I turn the page. I am learning the scene. I draw quickly in black ink, the spiky towers, the distant bridge, the curve of the water, the lions and dolphins in squiggles and the pavement under the trees, with the castellations of the palace behind. On the bench is a man. I am making him up. He is hunched on the bench. The trees are holding the sky in twiggy branches.

I turn the page. I draw just the man on the bench, I can see the trees and the bench and I copy the shapes, but I am making up the man. He is surrounded by dark shapes. They are crying out somehow.

I turn the page. I can't go there.

I take out my paintbox. I think I am painting the olive-green water, and the verdigris lion, but the paint coagulates on the page and there is the figure stooped over on the bench, surrounded by other figures. I draw them in the paint. They are the people of his despair. I'd felt their presence in the flat and entered their city in my dreams. Their eyes were hollow, their mouths chewing nothing, fingering me with greedy hunger, and I'd fled from them along a dark underground tunnel, knee-deep in water, and woke myself trying to scream.

I close the book and don't care if the pages get stuck together. I am comforted by the sounds of the coffee machine and the smell of coffee, and the man in a knitted yellow hat that keeps his hair in a bundle. I look out the window. The other side of the river is more and more hidden by white mist; the spiky Westminster towers poking up in ghostly silhouette, Big Ben's face still visible, but the river beyond the bridge is obscured behind white, and raindrops rush down and make the surface of the river shiver with hundreds of droplets.

When the rain stops I walk out into the white day. The air is clear, washed clean of dust, and the wet pavements reflect the sky. I feel heavy. As if weighed down by a memory that is living in my chest. I stand still. It is living under my breath. If I stop and close my eyes and stop breathing maybe I will see it. It is far away.

Then I see his crumpled face.

When the wind had come along with the rain, and the black sky had broken and lashed his hair, his face crumpled into a strange shape; while everyone stood under the umbrellas, he stood by the gaping hole with streams of water running into it, and clenched his hands together instead of holding mine.

I walk along by the benches that are placed up on little plinths so you can see the water.

A smartly dressed man in a hat and a brown raincoat, with a crease in his pinstriped trousers, lays a newspaper on the wet bench and sits down on it. He looks like he belongs in a 1950s film when everything was dark red and pale green.

I wonder if the gold and silver statue people will be standing still beyond Hungerford Bridge or maybe they're worried the rain will wash them clean.

I look into the water. It is swollen with the rain.

I am remembering the cold church with the wind outside and an old lady saying 'Poor child' as if I wasn't there, while I touched the face of a mermaid carved into a chair. I looked round at her while my hand felt the contours, to tell her that I knew she meant me, because my mother was dead, but she looked away, and I looked back at the mermaid who had strange eyes.

I breathe in the river wind. The mist is lifting. I copy the smart man and climb up the steps and put my sketchbook down on the rain-spattered bench.

Big Ben booms out his dong that colours the air. I take

my book from under me and draw his portrait. He started life as a drawing, and before that he was just an idea in Pugin's mind. He is difficult to draw. It is easier to draw quickly.

But suddenly I put my sketchbook down and leave it on the bench to go down the steps and lean over the side and look into the flowing water.

I had new goggles. I wanted to swim in the seaweed forest, deep down where the waving fronds grew high, and the sun made shivering underwater ripples on the sea floor.

I saw it floating upside down with its mouth open; it slowly bounced towards me and touched me, a dead dogfish, with white stuff, omelette-like, coming out of its mouth. I screamed all the breath out of my body, and heard the scream fill the water. I fought my way back to the surface, heavy without air, and spluttered into the above-water daylight, coughing out the water I'd gulped instead of breath, until I was hauled out, laid flat on the rock, and she'd blown breath into my body through my mouth, until the gurgling water in my lungs spewed out of my mouth in a long stream.

The sun comes out from behind the clouds and lights up the river.

The water glitters and I close my eyes and feel rippling light on my eyelids.

But I am still seeing memories.

I remember Mrs Tregenza held me against her white apron, and I didn't like it because it smelt of fish, and I didn't like her fishy hands, that sliced the long silver mackerel bellies so the red guts tumbled out in bloody coils, fingering their way through my curls.

'He'll be back in a minute, darling, don't cry,' and she'd jigged me up and down against the scaly oily apron until I'd seen dad outside and run into the drizzle to be with him. His hands had made tense starfish and clenched together in a jerky rhythm but in time with each other, I couldn't hold those hands, while Bob was murmuring to him and making my dad's face go strange. And the pavement was slippy and the sea came into my Wellingtons, as I hurried after him between the boxes of fish with their red eyes staring. They didn't frighten me. It was the rhythmic pulse of the starfish hands.

I open my eyes. The sun has gone again and the water is brownish green. I turn back to the bench and sit down next to my sketchbook. I open it and draw a little girl underwater, swimming next to a dead dogfish.

Then I remember it. The image that was conjured in the slant of light, by the words that came through from the kitchen along with the cooking smell: 'They've found the body by Lamorna, the eyes wide open,' and I'd imagined my mother wrapped in seaweed, the kind like hair, her eyes staring, with a frill of egg-white floating from her mouth.

It must have all happened within a few days.

I nearly drowned and then she did.

I bicycle slowly back. The memory has opened a shaking space within me. I bike past Millbank and the wide stairs of the Tate, through Pimlico and the red houses of Chelsea, and by the silver river all the way home.

I climb the stairs and lie down in bed although it's not even time for the streetlights to come on, and lie looking at the ceiling until my eyes close on their own.

10

I wake up with a start. It is dark outside. I can still hear dad's voice calling to me out of my dream. It is so real I think it's in the room. There is a car alarm going off in the street. I switch on the light. It's only 11:30. I get up, put my clothes on without thinking, and pick up my keys. Surely if I follow the feeling I will find him.

I go down the stairs and out into the street. There is a wind blowing. The sky is dark blue, with stars. I walk down the dark streets, looking up the alleys and along the King's Road, lit up with coloured light, people coming out the pub in crowds. I pass three men, their arms round each other's shoulders, singing 'Here we go here we go' and laughing.

'All right, love?'

'Hello, lady of the night.'

I walk up to Sloane Square. Two figures are lolling in the centre of the square, under the trees. I feel like I've walked into one of my paintings. One of the men gets up and falls over.

I walk up Sloane Avenue towards Knightsbridge. The wind is blowing through the leaves. A police car whizzes past me, its siren blaring, the blue lights flashing. I feel the wind of it, it drives so close to the pavement.

The sky has gone brown with orange clouds. I walk along Knightsbridge beneath the tall buildings, imagining

I am following his footsteps, sure I'm being led to him, if I just follow my feet.

Under the hotel in Knightsbridge some old men are sitting by the big-leaved plants, and chatting to the doorman in his top hat and gold buttons, but dad is not with them. I trudge on up to Hyde Park Corner. I keep thinking I'll just go on a bit further. I'll find him if I carry on.

By the time I've walked up Green Park and Piccadilly to the Circus I feel as if my body doesn't fit together. People sit around the fountain under Eros, dressed in ragged clothes, with lurid faces which change colour in ripples under the advertising lights. The lights make rhythmic circles and zigzags and wave patterns and flash out Coca-Cola and Fuji film.

Cars are zooming, more sirens flash past, and the sounds begin to echo.

Maybe I will find him if I carry on down the Haymarket, maybe he's sitting on the steps of the National Gallery or among the lions made out of melted-down guns. That's the sort of thing Zeb tells you; and the cross on St Paul's weighs the same as seven cars, and reality is 80 per cent invisible.

Someone by the fountain is screaming. Two men are fighting on the pavement. I see the man's head wobble as it is pounded by the other man's big fist. I run away from them, down a dark street, past whistling scaffolding pipes. A man gets up from the bench on a ledge, and bursts into tears.

A night bus slides past and opens its doors. I recognise the number and clamber in. I sit down and close my eyes.

11

'You look fucking terrible!' Rob says as she comes through the muslin curtain into my space.

'I feel it, Rob!' I say, sitting down on the stool.

'No, really, shit! You look bad. You're a state! Your eyes have got rings under them. Look at yourself!' she says, getting up and fetching the mirror she uses to paint self-portraits.

'Oh don't, Rob, I don't want to look.'

'Listen! He's missing, he'll turn up, you can't spend your nights and days tramping the streets!'

'Yeah, but what if he turns up dead, Rob? What if he turns up in the river, or frozen to death on a piece of cardboard?'

'It's spring, it's getting warmer.'

'It was freezing last night! And that wind.'

'Yes, and you were out in it, listen to me! It's not your responsibility! Are you listening? He's NOT your responsibility.'

'That's just words, Rob. What if your dad was out in the street? Probably drunk in a gutter?'

'I think you should go and see Safi.'

'Who's Safi?'

'The college counsellor.'

'Oh and she'll help me find him, will she? The police were fucking useless!'

She shakes her head at me, and puts the mirror down in my space.

'Look in the mirror,' she says as she goes through the curtain, 'and see Safi.'

I look at myself. My eyes are wide open and scared-looking, with dark rings. My face is shockingly pale with a yellow tinge, and I have a squint look.

I stand outside the red door. And look at the label. Mrs Safi Irfan.

'Oh, bugger this.'

I walk down the stairs halfway to the canteen, then turn around and go upstairs again, and stand outside the door. I breathe in and knock.

'Come in,' says a voice from within.

I open the door.

She sits behind a desk, and looks round to me.

'Come in, dear,' she says.

She has a soft Indian accent, her hair is grey at the roots and dyed dark chestnut. She has high cheekbones and dark eyes.

'Sit down, do you want to sit down?' she says, standing up. 'I can make you a cup of tea if you want to talk for a little bit.'

I want to walk out the door but I am touched by the pretty way the words sound in her mouth.

I sit down.

'Would you like a biscuit?'

All the consonants are softened, and there is a melody in the sentences.

I just nod to everything she asks, that way ending up with a biscuit, a cup of tea with two sugars, none of which I really want.

I would like to sit in here and listen to her saying ordinary things all day.

'My dear,' she says kindly, 'you are here to talk to me?'

'Well I . . . yes,' I say.

'What would you like to talk about?'

I look out the window at the white sky.

'It's my . . . well it's about my . . .' I swallow and look at her, and her look is so deep that it reaches into me where my tears are; the look says, 'It's all right, you know,' and the tears begin to silently pour out my eyes.

She sits nodding slightly until the tears stop.

'My dad,' I say in a whisper.

'Yes.' She nods. 'It is difficult for you.'

I feel as if she knows it all already.

She has seen him on my front steps, slumped against the railings, and us dragging him up the stairs. She knows that he pissed on the floor and I had to change his trousers, and about the beautiful letter he wrote.

'He said he was sorry, you see,' I say, and she nods. 'Sorry because of all of it, that he didn't want to be that way.'

She nods.

'And I remember . . .' I say, shaking my head slowly at her while the words are stuck, and the memories are in the air round her head, so I'm sure she sees them too, 'I remember how he was.'

She nods. She can see how he was; so noble and tall.

'He doesn't like what he's become, you see.'

She nods. 'And its hard for you, too,' she says, and something cracks in me and and I begin to sob.

'You see, he left because he's ashamed, I made him ashamed, that's the thing, and now he's out on the street in the cold. On some park bench,' and the tears pour down my cheeks.

'My dear,' she says gently, 'you didn't make him ashamed.'

'I did!' and my voice has a screech in it, 'I did! I told him I didn't want him in my flat, that I couldn't put him up, I couldn't cope with him. TO GET OUT. To get out.'

'And what if I were to tell you that you did the right thing?' says Safi.

'The right thing' sounds beautiful in Safi's mouth. The trill of the 'r' is soft. It opens some kind of doorway in the air that reveals many possibilities. The doorway closes abruptly.

'But what if he DIES on the street? He might DIE!'

Safi stays perfectly still.

'That is his choice.'

The melody in her voice makes the word 'choice' end on a high note. And I hear that his choice comes from a place within him that I cannot reach.

'You cannot make that choice for him.'

I nod, she has made me see it.

'And you cannot protect him from it.'

I look at the many-armed deity Sellotaped to her diary. She turns the book round for me to look at, the colours are pink and green and gold.

I talk with Safi until the sky darkens and she switches on the light. I tell her about the far-away memories; the day mum went missing, and Bob telling dad, and her funeral, and dad crying in the rain. I tell her about nearly drowning and the dead dogfish, and my mum's kiss of life. I tell her about Magda and the farm, and escaping from dad's despair to come to London. When I stand up to leave she comes round the desk and takes my hand. Her eyes look into mine.

'You don't have to be in there with him,' she says. 'Despair is a lie. There is always hope.'

And I see the spirits of his despair whispering their lies, and I see hope as a bright place brimming with possibilities. Safi's words contain reality in them. They are not empty.

'Come and see me again. Ring me any time,' she says, giving me a telephone number, and I take it and thank her and walk upstairs to the abstract studios to see if Bianca is still working.

But the studio is empty and I look out over London as the streetlights come on, and sit among Bianca's pictures in the glinting dark.

12

I go and see Safi again and tell her things I've never said before.

I tell her about dad, and how he used to tell me stories on the green sofa while I looked into the flames, how we went walking together on the cliffs and the moors and fishing sometimes when he had the time. I tell her about finding all the empty bottles in one go and noticing the bleary look in his eyes, and the scared feeling as it happened more and more, and the horrible fear it turned into, watching him slowly fall apart.

Safi asks me about mum, and I remember how I longed for her when I was small, but never really knew her. She was on the stage, and I imagined it as a huge platform on stilts. She used to walk out of the station in high-heeled shoes and lean over to kiss me, and then she'd be gone again, waving out the window; and the longing in me that was attached to the train and the waving hand would stretch out long and thin as the train moved away, and after the train disappeared I would cry into dad's jersey.

I remember all the feelings because of Safi's eyes. She has eyes that overturn places in you, that turn over pages in your mind you haven't seen for years and look at them with you.

I tell Safi that I missed mum when she died but not like dad did. I felt dad's howling grief in the depths of me and saw it every day in his eyes. And when I got older her absence sang through our lives like a sad song you hear in the distance.

Safi says an absence can have a powerful presence in people's lives and I see a person-shaped emptiness behind dad, and feel its magnetic force, and realize that's why I had to get away.

'Your mother is not an absence, Eve,' says Safi, 'that is your father's pain. Your mother is a presence,' and I close my eyes and feel light feelings pass through me in whispers. And even if it's faint and far away, I can feel her presence, and I wish I could find dad so I could tell him that.

'But you must let him go,' says Safi, 'and set yourself free.'

And even though I don't understand, I can feel what Safi means, and I breathe in and look out the window at the sky, so it fills up my lungs with sky light.

And she asks if Magda is my aunt. I say no, she was a neighbour, but I used to call her auntie. 'Did she look after you?' And I remember the smell of the slurry in the farmyard and the sound of the cows breathing, and the warm kitchen with the wind outside and the coats steaming in front of the stove. 'Yes,' I say, 'she was like a mother to me.' Safi nods, and I tell her how I used to hold on to Magda's legs when my mother came back because they were safe legs. Safer than my mum's in her high heels, that wobbled and clipped and clopped. And besides, she might say, 'No don't, you'll ladder my stockings.' And I didn't like the nylon skin that could break into ladders if you touched it.

I tell her about the argument Magda had with dad. How I didn't even know what it was about, but I was a teenager and took my dad's side. She says, 'Why don't you ring her?' I say, 'She doesn't have a telephone.' 'Then write to her,' she says.

So I do.

13

I am sitting next to the window in my studio so the light shines on to the palette. The colours I am mixing are neutral and quiet.

I told Cecile I was tired of the ugly colours.

She said the ugly colours make the other colours look more beautiful, but I said I was tired of those colours of despair. She said, 'What colours are those?' and I said, 'Like Indian red mixed with Prussian blue,' and she mixed it to see what colour it made. She said she thought that was rage, maybe rage gone stagnant. I said, 'Yes, it could be that.'

We were sitting downstairs in her space after her tutorial, and she was fed up because of what the tutors had said. It was an insult, after all.

That space down on the ground floor isn't like the other studios; less cosy, people do huge pictures and there are ramps and pulleys and loud music, and I looked at her pale delicate face as she considered the colour she had mixed. She has naturally red lips and orange eyelashes, and was frowning slightly as she put her head on one side. Its true that her pictures are huge, and stretched above us in flower shapes and spirals so you could be looking at undergrowth or outer space; but I never feel that Cecile really belongs on the ground floor.

Then I mixed the scary green from cadmium yellow and lamp black, just to show her, and told her it was like the rotting seaweed at low tide, that when you walk through you have to keep your mouth shut because of the flies. 'But it could be despair, couldn't it? Wouldn't that black-green weigh you down? I mean it wasn't one to lift your spirits, was it?'

She said, 'No, you're right, you'd have to be careful of a colour like that, it might murder someone!'

I laughed and said, 'Especially if a bunch of tutors had just told it to "get a job painting window displays!"'

And we laughed at the idea of the colour having a tutorial.

'If anyone ought to paint window displays, it should be the head of painting and his endless vertical stripes,' said Cecile, and I nodded in agreement.

But even so, she looked at the green and said, 'I can imagine painting with that colour, it all depends what colours you put it next to.'

I said, 'I'm sure you're right but I'm not taking any chances. I'm going to make my paintings out of grey from now on.'

So I'm mixing neutral colours now; browns and greys and dirty whites. Colours that speak like stones and bricks, scaffolding pipes and cement. Unnoticeable colours. The blue-grey of the paving slabs after the rain, and mud stuck in the grip of tyres, the colours of rags and dirty string, and sacking and wet cardboard and paper blowing across the street, and the bone colours of discarded bus tickets pressed into the road by lots of feet.

These colours and their tiny shift towards blue, hint of purple, or tinge of pink, I like them. They comfort me.

14

'No, I'm not saying I don't like them,' says Bianca, balancing on one spindly leg of the chair and trying to do a pirouette holding on to the table edge. We are sitting in the canteen next to the glass window.

'It's just they're not those beautiful colours you used to use. I mean, people go through phases, don't they? This is your drab phase.'

I laugh.

Rob shakes her head.

'What?' says Bianca. 'It's my opinion. Come to the Rothko! That'll cure you!'

'Oh, let's go,' says Cecile. 'I really want to see those paintings.'

'The colours are fantastic!'

'Yes, and the real thing is completely different from the reproductions.'

'Yeah, some just don't, do they.'

'Don't what?'

'Reproduce.'

'Cézanne doesn't, either. You don't get what he looks like in the flesh, until you see him.'

'The flesh?'

'Stop being so annoying, you know what I mean. In the paint, then.'

Bianca's chair skids sideways and she ends up sliding down the glass wall, so Rob has to catch her and the chair and pull her straight, while Bianca is squealing and Roberta is laughing.

Suzanne walks into college arm in arm with a man with hair so short he looks bald, and sunglasses on the top of his head although it is not sunny.

'Is that her new boyfriend?' says Bianca, looking round.

They walk through the door into Sculpture on the other side of the quadrangle.

'Is it?' She turns to Rob.

'How should I know?'

'Because of Mick. They're friends, aren't they?'

Rob shrugs. 'Doesn't mean he tells me everything that's going on in his friend's ex-girlfriend's love life!'

'Have they really split up?'

'Who knows with those two!'

Bianca looks at me. But I look away at the grey paving stones. So what if I like drab colours.

Bianca puts her elbows on the table and cups her face in her hands. She slides across the table so she's looking up at me, her mouth stretched wide, and lifts her eyebrows up and down.

I laugh at her.

Rob and Cecile get up and take their plates away.

She slides back again and sits up and cricks her neck from side to side.

'I'm glad you're back,' she says. 'It's like you've been walking in the realm of the dead. I didn't like you being a zombie!'

'Is that what I seemed like?'

'Yes! You got lost.'

'Was I lost?'

'Yes, of course! Junkies do it! They go off. You look in their eyes and they're gone. I have done it myself!'

'Where did you go?'

'Oh, I don't know, into oblivion.'

'I wonder where I went.'

'Maybe your soul was out looking for your dad.'

'I'm glad it's back, then,' I say, looking out at the quadrangle through the glass, and the pigeons pecking under the statue.

'Listen, come back with me for the weekend. Come to Brixton. Get away from your little place and stay with us. You need some good food. You need some normal life. OK? Then you will be able to do the most normal thing in the world, and go and see,' and she inclines her head upwards to the mezzanine, 'that friend of yours.'

'Thanks, Bianca, I'd like to.'

'We can go for a walk, we can make a nice dinner,' she nods. 'It's a good plan.'

15

It is a grey London day. It looks like it might rain.

The air is damp. I am on the bike following Bianca's pink and green Guatemalan shirt. She gets off her bike at the embankment and we cross over the thundering road. We stop to look over the wall into the water reflecting the white sky.

'Let's bike through the park,' she says.

So we cross Albert Bridge by foot, just to see the river flowing under us, and lean out over the water and shout each other's names into the wind. It begins to spit and we hurry through the park gates and ride our bikes with our heads down against the drizzle, to the shelter by the fountains. We stand in the shelter to wait until the drizzle stops. There is a man in there. He has a low voice and his voice booms round the shelter when he says, 'It's wet, isn't it.'

Bianca says, 'You must be an opera singer.' He says that he is, and he's from New York and here to sing Mozart. Bianca says, 'Oh could you sing something for us, please.'

He booms out 'Don Giovanni,' and it makes the hairs on the back of my neck stand up and my mouth fall open, the sound is so big.

But Bianca glances at me, and says to him, 'Oh, not that, please' so he sings 'Moon River' and the sound reverberates around the shelter, and I look outside and the trees are glistening in the evening light, and the river turns into something sorrowful.

'Oh, it's beautiful!' says Bianca. 'It's heavenly.' And he laughs and his laugh also fills the shelter.

We cycle away when the rain stops and realize we didn't ask his name.

We ride between the glowing green playing fields and into the trees and bushes that line the lakeside paths, past the blue boathouse, and the café and the ducks on the rippling lake, and the peacocks and peahens who strut about behind wire mesh calling their plaintive call, and through the gates into the rush-hour traffic. Bianca winds her scarf round her nose so she looks like a bandit, and we dodge and weave between the cars following the 137 round the corner and up Queenstown Road. We dismount and push our bikes up the hill. Then Clapham Common spreads out before us large and flat, where we flew Zeb's kite. He attached it to a fishing line so it reeled out and out, and up into the sky, until it was a tiny speck and there was no more fishing line and Zeb let it go, so it floated off into space. It must be up there at the edge of the ozone by now. And we cycle along the tree-lined road and round the corner into Acre Lane. We pass the timber merchant where we had our studio and the air smells of newly sawn wood. Past the café where we had our bacon sandwiches and mugs of tea, past Reggae Records and the sari shop, and the Ritzy Cinema, where I automatically check the old men gathered on the steps drinking Special Brew, and into Bianca's road.

When we've chained our bikes to the banisters we walk up the stairs. On each landing there is a different-coloured strip of stained glass, and as I follow Bianca up the stairs the strip of coloured light passes over her, changing the colour of her clothes. Red, green, yellow, pink. When she stops at her front door and takes out her keys she has a strip of turquoise light across her face.

'Why did you tell him not to?' I ask.

'Not to what?'

'Sing that song.'

'Never mind why.'

'Why?'

'Because it's the father's ghost singing and I thought it would be bad luck.'

And I stand still, on the doorstep, while the strange feeling passes through me.

We have fennel tea made from what looks like dried grass stalks, from a flat black teapot that Bianca bought in the market. The tea smells of liquorice and tastes of aniseed, and Bianca tells me a story Silvia has written, about a woman whose body is a landscape: her breasts are hills, her thighs are valleys.

Later, Bianca's sitting room flickers with candlelight, and there is a smell of garlic and herbs. She is standing at the table with three grey squid on a newspaper, attempting to cut out the ink sack. The ink is spurting out onto the newspaper.

Giacomo has brought two pots of sturdy basil, and a jar of damson jam he made himself. There is Eduardo from Venezuela, and his wife Anna, and Cesar from Chile, who is cooking the tomatoes in the kitchen ready for the squid, and looks through the door every now and then, to join in the conversation, in his apron and holding a wooden spoon.

His wife Maria Ines is bringing the pudding.

'Here, help me,' says Bianca and hands me a knife, and I cut into the strange quivering flesh.

When Maria Ines arrives we cram round the table in the sitting room and everyone is talking a mixture of Italian and English about which shop sells fresh food, and what the food was like in Egypt, where Giacomo just went. The coloured velvets glow and flicker, and Eduardo touches my foot under the table, and I frown at him because he's sitting next to his wife Anna. We drink wine and eat, and the wine warms me along with the laughter and the red velvet curtains printed with spirals, and the coloured throws on the sofa, and the cushions glinting like gold in the candlelight.

Bianca gives me an embroidered nightdress and I sleep in her big bed, listening to the sirens outside and the crowds of people coming down the road shouting, after the pubs have closed.

In the morning we lie in bed and Bianca tells me another story Silvia has written, about a woman who has a fold-up forest that she unfolds around her when she feels like it.

We get out of bed to make coffee.

We pass Silvia's open door. She is lying diagonally across the bed with one arm flung above and her auburn hair cascading sideways.

She opens her eyes and looks at us.

'Allora?' says Bianca. 'Last night?'

Silvia stretches and smiles. 'I was dancing till three.' 'Make me a coffee!' she says, and folds back the covers, 'and come in with me.'

'Get in,' says Bianca. 'I'll bring it.'

A piece of lace covers the armchair and a copper-coloured bra is slung over the arm.

I climb into the bed next to her.

'Did you sleep well?' She has a kind of lisp.

I lie beside her. Her skin smells of milk. I ask her about the story. She says, 'I will read it to you.'

I close my eyes. I can smell the forest that she unfolds around her. The flowers exude a thick scent. I smell the forest floor in her hair: the leaf mould, the moss, and the tiny orange chanterelles with earth still clinging to their roots.

Bianca brings in the coffee.

There are animals in the forest too. I smell their fur and their nut-flavoured breath.

'Move over!' says Bianca, so I am squashed between them.

Siliva laughs. She has freckles on her face. Her lips are stained dark purple.

'Oh, but I like me,' she says, and lies back. Her arm behind her head slowly stretches up through her hair. 'Everybody likes me.'

Her long silky auburn hair exudes a fragrance.

She turns over and flings her arm round the dip between my ribs and my hip.

'You smell nice,' she says. She has a low soft velvet voice. She squeezes me and her hand moves over my breast.

'Oh, you have enormous breasts!' she says, laughing. 'How did you keep them hidden so long?'

I start laughing, her laugh is infectious.

'Did you know her breasts were so big, Bianca?'

'Yes, I have noticed!' says Bianca, sipping her coffee.

'Remember it took half an hour to get the gold dress off!' says Bianca, and starts to laugh, so she spurts coffee and has to put the cup down, and I am sandwiched between their giggling bodies.

'Shut up!' I say.

'No, listen!' she whispers, putting her finger up.

'What?'

The door opens down the corridor.

'It's Carlotta's boyfriend. Call out to him, Silvia! He's so English, let's pretend we've had a night of passion.'

'Oh Tony! Tony!' says Silvia in a low seductive voice.

Bianca and I listen. He passes the open door.

'Would you like to join us?' says Silvia.

He clears his throat like a caricature of an Englishman, and walks past the open door with a startled face, and Bianca puts her hands over her mouth as though she is ashamed, but Silvia is laughing, and the sun shines through the thick lace curtains and lights up our faces in intricate patterns.

16

The sun shone all weekend. But now the raindrops are
dripping down the window of the studio. They even drip
in shadows over the cotton duck I have stretched over the
frames. Sometimes the sun comes through and lights up
the drops in glinting colours then disappears again, and
all the coloured lights go out.

I have knocked the frames together with corrugated
nails and stretched the canvas till my thumbs are sore,
and now I'm waiting for the soaked rabbit-skin glue to
melt into gloopy liquid so I can size the surface.

We went with Silvia to her African dance class after we
got up. Partly because Bianca had told me, and I wanted
to witness, the cascade of love talk that hurtles towards
Silvia from every corner when she walks along Railton
Road.

'Oh please, darlin', talk to me. I want the whole street
to see me talking to you.'

'Beautiful queen!'

'Oh sugar!'

'Woman sweet honey!'

Bianca and I stood at the back of the class in T-shirts
and leggings, and watched the leopard-skin leotards
and gyrating-in-time bodies moving in breathtaking
synchrony with each other and the djembe players; while

we jumped too soon, kicked a beat after, moved our hips in the wrong direction, and ended up getting the giggles because we couldn't keep time at all.

The studio is filled with the animal scent of the melting rabbit-skin glue. It gets up your nostrils and stays there for days so you think you smell it everywhere.

In the evening we went to the crypt in Lambeth to listen to jazz, and the drummer couldn't keep his eyes off Bianca. It was a dark little place under an old church and I wondered if it was old enough to have been there when William Blake lived in Lambeth. My ears were ringing because I stood too near the saxophone.

I stir the glue round and round. It is melting into a smooth honey-coloured liquid. The texture is just right. I take it off the heat and let it cool.

On Sunday morning we biked along Brixton High Street and up the road, past the paper factory to the Portuguese café in Stockwell. Bianca sang 'Sunday Morning' into the wind with her own words. Everyone who came to dinner was there, as well as Giacomo's boyfriend, and Mikhail, the refugee from Serbia. We sat outside in the courtyard and ate fishcakes and drank galão, and they talked about politics and the war; then Bianca told them about dad. I was embarrassed at first. In a minute, everyone was talking about my father. About alcoholics and people going missing, about where he could be, and who they might ask to help look for him, and when did you last see him? and what was he wearing and how old is he? and where did you look? and how are you feeling? and did you go to the police? no, they're never any help, and how long has he been drinking? and what! He has no wife, ah well, he drinks because he's lonely, and so you have no mother, poveretta! and the plates piled up and they ordered more coffee and custard pastries with burnt tops, and I told them about the dark tunnels, and the railway stations, and the benches looking over the river. And by the time the conversation moved to Giacomo's cousin who went missing in Mexico, to Mexican food, and Steve Hatt in Essex Road, the best fish shop in London, I felt as if everything I went through all alone and full of terror, had been somehow warmed by the light of their attention, been taken from a dank ashamed place and aired along with sunlight and coffee and turned into stories that people share on Sunday morning, and even though dad is still out there, missing, I feel less strange in the world, and less alone.

We walked round Brockwell Park after all that coffee, and ended up in the little garden among the lavender and green hedges, watching the blue tits sipping water out of the fountain.

It was all to make me normal, Bianca said, normal enough to do a normal thing like go downstairs to the mezzanine and knock on the door.

When I've sized the last canvas and they are standing in a row against the wall, stinking out the studio, I get up and look out the window at the sun trying to come out and decide it's time to go and see Zeb.

17

I walk downstairs into Zeb's space. He is sitting mending his sculpture.

The light is streaming in and shining through the bottles of coloured water so they shimmer and tremble on the wall in sunlit reflections. Each time he twiddles a screw the water light twirls and trembles on the wall.

He looks up.

And looks down again.

'Howsit going?' he says to the screwdriver.

'Fine,' I say to my fingers.

'Could you pass me that screw,' he says to the back wall. I look behind him and pass him the box, and one of us drops the box, so I say, 'Sorry' and we both bend to pick them up and bump heads, and both say, 'Sorry,' and I sit back down and he takes a screw and the rest lie scattered between us, twirling across the floor till they come to rest.

He screws the screw into the metal frame, biting his lip.

I breathe in and look at the door

'Looks like it'll be all right, then, the sculpture,' I say to the door.

'Mm-hmm,' he says, another screw in his mouth.

'Better go now,' I say, getting up and rolling across the screws.

'No, don't go yet,' he says. 'I'm nearly finished it.'

There is a tiny squeaking noise as he screws in the last screw.

'There! Look, it stands again,' and he wobbles it to show it's steady and all the glass tinkles, and the coloured light shivers on the wall.

'Yep,' I say. 'Looks good!' I nod. 'Steady, anyway.'

We both nod at the sculpture for a few minutes.

'D'you think . . .'

'D'you want . . .' we say together.

'What?'

'No, what were you going to say?'

'Just thought we could go and get a coffee.'

'Yeah.'

We clank downstairs but our awkwardness can't fit through the door of the canteen, and we stand in the hall looking out the window until the sunlight pulls us outside.

We cross the courtyard and sit on the bench on the other side of the road, out of sight of the wall of eyes. And I remember sitting here with dad. But now it's Zeb I'm sitting next to.

'Are you . . .'

'Is your . . .'

'What?'

'No, you.'

We look at each other.

'Honestly, what are we like,' he says.

I smile.

'Your dad?' he says gently.

'He's still missing,' I say and look at the tall building of the art school; the layers of glass and concrete, stretching up into the sky to catch as much light as it can.

'Somewhere,' I say, and lift my chin at London. 'Somewhere out there.'

A silence falls. With Bianca I can leave my worries for a while, but with Zeb I feel all the way down to the deep places.

'Are you still looking for him?' he says.

I glance up. His eyes are looking at me. His look says, 'It's all right, you can say what's true.'

I close my eyes. In the dark part of my mind I can see my dad's journey; by the river, down alleys, on benches, in tunnels. I can see the empty buildings, the littered paths along dark canals, the bridges by gasworks and steps that lead nowhere, and tears are in my closed eyes.

'Oh, Zeb, I can't find him.'

'No. I know you can't,' he says, putting his hand on my shoulder. 'I don't think you're meant to.'

'I never know about "meant" to.'

'I don't think he wants you to.'

'Find him?'

'Look for him, even. I don't think he wants to be found, do you?'

He looks at me and his eyes are so deep they reach into me. I look down at my hands and my voice comes out cracked.

'Oh, Zeb, I know everyone says so, and sometimes I think it's true.'

And suddenly the lovely time I had with Bianca breaks apart and something comes up from underneath. And I hear a voice crying, 'Help me, don't leave me to this. I'm ashamed of how much I need you.' It is calling into the dark to be found, to be found, to be found.

'My poor dad,' I say, and Zeb puts his arm round me.

'Oh Zeb, my poor dad,' and Zeb holds on to me and says, 'It's OK, it's OK.'

We sit on the bench and the breeze blows through the branches of the big plane tree. It blows through the weight that sits between us made of feelings about dad.

When the feeling eases I see the weight between us is not just dad. And when I ask Zeb about Suzanne, he draws his arm away from my shoulders, leans forward, presses his long fingers together, and breathes out slowly in a big sigh.

'I mean I've got my own things to sort out,' he says, looking off down the street at the cars zooming along the King's Road.

In my mind's eye I see a slender shard that must have leaped out of one of the bottles, and pierced him when the sculpture smashed. She'd meant it to, it was made of an intention, not of glass, and it has wounded him.

'The school is taking the second-years to Barcelona next week,' he says. 'Just for a few days.'

'Yes, I know,' I say. 'It'll be good.'

'There's a chance a couple of us could do an exchange.'

'Exchange?'

'With the art school in Barcelona.'

'Oh Zeb, are you going away?'

My voice is quiet because I don't want him to.

'It would just be for a couple of months next term,' he says. 'I think I need to get away for a bit.'

He turns back to me. 'Eve, I'm so glad you came to see me. Look, even if I go, I'll be back!'

I put my hand on his arm and nod, and his eyes look at me like sunlight.

18

'What did he say?' says Bianca. 'Did he talk about Suzanne?'

We're on the Tube going to the Rothko show, sitting in two twos. Rob is sitting at the other end of the carriage with Cecile. The Tube is full of bodies pressed together, breathing the same breath in and out.

'Not really,' I say, but we are going through a noisy juddering and she can't hear a thing anyway.

'What?' she shouts.

'I said not really.'

Two Japanese girls sit opposite us in orange and purple platform shoes. Bianca keeps looking at them.

The train slows down and Rob and Cecile are making signs at us from the other end of the carriage.

'We know! We know! We're not morons!' says Bianca.

We come out the station at Embankment and walk up the steps and across the footbridge beside the thundering trains. People are playing drums. Cecile is excited about the colours she is going to see.

We stand on the footbridge and a passenger barge passes underneath us and we look down the river to St Paul's.

'Let's get a move on,' says Rob.

Bianca slips her hand through my arm.

'You could have asked him to come and see the show. Ask him round to dinner at my house next week.'

'The second-years are going to Barcelona next week.'

'So he's going to Barcelona?'

'Yes,' I nod.

'And you don't care?'

I look at her but I can't say anything.

Cecile looks stricken when we pass a man in a wheelchair with no legs because everyone has given their change to the smiling djembe players.

She stops on the bridge, trying to find change in her handbag.

'Come ON!' says Rob.

Cecile finds a coin and slips it into his cup, looking relieved.

We walk across paving stones, up a concrete stairwell, through a glass door, and into the galleries of the Hayward.

In the beginning there are pictures of houses and landscapes. But then he sets the colours free; and the canvases emanate colours like notes of music that go right through you in harmonies of pink and red, yellow and blue, blue and crimson. They bathe us in coloured light. The combined colours sing together. As I walk through the galleries my whole body hears the colour harmonies as though it is a big ear. When I reach the last room I feel as if I've swallowed the colours and they are singing within me.

He paints the colours of sunlight and the colours of earth, and the in-between colours of twilight. And then he paints the dark.

In the last room the paintings are black; huge spaces of many-layered black.

They make me hold my breath. Oh my God, I know where he went, from all that light, to no light at all.

'They were the last paintings he did before he killed himself,' says Bianca, subdued. And we look and look at the colours of his despair.

'Poor Rothko,' says Bianca.

I nod but I am thinking about dad.

We gather outside the gallery, jumping and shivering to keep warm. Rob's going to Waterloo to take the Tube, she only lives by London Bridge, and Bianca says she'll walk down with her and get the 59 to Brixton. Cecile is meeting her husband at the Royal Festival Hall to hear a concert by a famous Japanese violinist.

'You all right?' she says, looking at me, concerned, her hair blowing about her in the wind.

'Course!' I say. But I feel overcome by an agony of leaving them.

'OK, see you then.'

I turn away, embarrassed by the intensity of my feeling, and wave at them without looking round, then almost run along the concrete walkways of the Hayward.

I just thought we would all walk across the footbridge together, by the thundering trains and see the river, in the dark, gliding beneath us towards St Paul's.

When I walk across the footbridge alone I feel desolate. I lean on the railing and look into the dark water. It looks like black oil. I can hear a far-away sound. It is beyond reach. I hear it with my ear that hears the colours. He is walking in the cold wet wind. He needs the cold and the wet to distract him from the scream within him.

Because the abyss has no edges.

He doesn't want to be alone with the moaning wind. There are others like him. I see them in the tunnels, their coats tied with string, and I speak into the dark river, 'It's not hopeless, dad, there's always hope. I love you, dad. Don't let it go black!'

But even when I've got home and cooked spaghetti and hung the washing on the squeaky pulley, and washed my hair in the basin, I can hear the voice of his despair, speaking in my blood.

19

And when I sleep it calls me in my dream.

It is an ugly light, the yellow light that lights up the black night and turns it brown. He is in the doorway of a filthy tunnel that smells of urine.

'This is where I belong,' he says. 'This is dark enough for me.'

'Help me!' he says to the dark bricks. 'Help me!' he cries out in a cracked voice, collapsing on to the wet pavement that reflects the lurid light.

It is not a cry but an animal that moans in him. The tunnel is still echoing his moan.

'I can't get free. I am trapped here, and I can't get free. Find me!' he cries, 'because I cannot find you. Find me!' he cries, in the voice of a child. 'I'm afraid!' And the night swoops around him, dripping, and he shuffles himself into the corner away from the water reflecting the yellow light. His feet are wet from the puddle, and he clutches his knees under his chin. Folded up, waiting, while he quivers and trembles from cold. He has reached a place of darkness. He has gone down a tunnel with wet walls and found the wind.

There is a feeling weighing down his shoulders and clenching his breath.

'Where is hope?' he cries out, but no sound comes out of his mouth because of the wind. First he hears it in his ears, like a roaring, and the roaring separates him from sound, and he is in a world of silence. The wind comes once more and he no longer feels the hard, the cold, the wet. It separates him from his senses and the world disappears. There is no smell of traffic wind that blew down the tunnel, or urine that stank from the walls. There is no lurid yellow light and no sound at all, except the wind receding into the distance. And he takes a long breath till all the air is gone.

Then, from far away, lying curled up like a baby, his hands between his legs, from above, looking down, he sees himself. 'Was that me?' he says, in a clear voice.

I wake up with a start and vaguely remember the dream.

'Dad?' I say to the bedroom. I want to go back to sleep to find him. I feel that he is free, like the sun breaking through cloud in rays of light, and something in me responds and shivers, shaking off its own darkness.

'Are you all right, dad?' I feel something light pass through my atoms in waves. It is strange.

20

'There was a bad frost last night!' says Bianca, pointing at the white camellias, their petals tipped with brown.

'It's confused all the flowers!' says Cecile.

Karl has sent us out to draw in the cemetery, the space under the trees. First we had to draw each other upside down in the studio, and Rob said, 'For fuck's sake, this is doing my head in!' and Bianca said, 'It's meant to.'

'Oh, why's that?'

'Because you don't need your head, you need your instinct!' said Bianca, mimicking Karl. That's when he sent us out to find a cemetery to make a space on the page.

'Why it has to be a cemetery, I don't know,' says Cecile. It was Bianca who chose Putney and we all clambered on to the number 11 and took it all the way to Putney Bridge.

The river is silver. The sky is pewter, and we go through the gates of the cemetery past the camellias and walk through the cemetery and between the yew trees that spread their branches over the gravestones and drop their needles over the graves. Crows fly about among the tall beech trees, cawing at each other and dancing from one branch to another. We sit down under the metallic sky.

For some reason I feel happy, touched by an inexplicable hope. Maybe dad is all right. Maybe, after all, dad is OK.

'It's gonna bloody rain,' says Rob.

'No, it won't, it won't,' says Bianca. 'Just sit like that. I want to draw a Madonna next to the tombstones.'

'Look, he just wants us to make a space, not a bloody icon!'

'No, but wait, like that! I like it, it's good, please, Rob.'

Rob huffs and puffs, and sits down on the bench and gives in with a shrug, and takes out her own sketchbook to draw the big yew tree, and the path emerging underneath it, and the church beyond it and the graveyard all around it, and I draw both of them; one sitting on a bench, one standing under the tree, looking up and down, intent on their drawings. We stay absorbed until Bianca closes her book, cricks her neck from side to side, and looks about her.

'What did you draw, Eve?' she says, coming under the birch trees to where I am standing in the flowerbed.

'I drew the two of you.'

'Oh, did you? Let me look!'

I open the page and show her the smudged charcoal figures and the trees and the black and white sky.

'Oh yes, I like it!'

'I don't think I better show mine to Rob,' says Bianca, laughing at the same time as speaking. She takes it out. 'It doesn't quite work,' she says, laughing again.

I look at the picture, at the short legs and big belly,

'Well, the proportions are a bit . . .'

'I know, I know,' Bianca interrupts, 'but I wasn't measuring and you know I'm crap at drawing!'

'You always say that!'

Rob comes over, cautiously picking her way through the twigs.

'Time we were getting back,' says Bianca.

'No, wait! I want to see,' says Rob. 'Show me what you've done.'

But she doesn't like the picture.

'Never mind Madonna!' scowls Rob. 'Looks more like the hunchback of Notre bloody Dame.'

'Don't be offended!'

'I'm not offended!' says Rob, sounding more offended than usual.

We walk through the yew trees and between the stones to find Cecile, pale as a ghost, and chilled to the bone, who has been drawing bark.

'Trust you!' says Rob, looking at her drawings, while Cecile does a bouncing dance to keep warm.

We take the bus back in a hurry because Bianca has a tutorial with Terry.

21

'Why don't you just go and tell Miss Pym you want to change tutors?' says Rob when we're back in the studio.

'Can you? I mean, would she?' I say.

'Well, you can ask, can't you?' says Rob, mixing the sieved earth with an acrylic medium and setting to work on a new picture. 'Go on, she liked your blue painting, remember.'

Miss Pym likes turquoise. She always wears it, sometimes with white and black, sometimes with pink, but always there is turquoise, and when she passed our space one day and the blue painting was hanging on a nail, with the muslin curtain pulled back so I could see it from afar, she opened her arms wide at the blue river. 'Oh, I like that painting!' she said, and asked for the names of the colours. 'Phthalo turquoise and manganese blue, not cerulean, no, that's too opaque, but, yes, if I could afford it I'd try cobalt turquoise.'

I like Miss Pym. She has two selves. The top one is the efficient secretary that most people are quite scared of, including Paul, the head of painting. Everyone knows that Miss Pym runs the school. But the one she speaks under her breath is quite different; naughty and mischevious. To some she only shows her officious face, but the other one glimmers underneath. I like seeing it.

I knock on the door. She's sitting straight-backed at her desk with her arms leaning on either side of the open diary. She adjusts her spectacles.

'Yes, dear?'

She's in her efficient mood.

I clear my throat.

'Well, I was just enquiring if it was possible . . .'

'Yes, dear?' She looks up at me over her glasses.

'Can I change tutors?'

She looks down at the big diary and flicks to the back page. She puts it to one side and looks at her rota.

'Who do you have?'

'Sergei.'

She follows the names down.

'Yes, Sergei.' She is looking at the sheet.

'So . . .' she says, still looking at the rota. 'You don't like him . . .'

'Well,' I begin. 'It's just . . .'

'. . . either,' she says and gives a tiny laugh, then returns to her efficient look.

She purses her lips, following the list with her index finger.

'Andrew!' she says, and looks up and lifts her eyebrows up at me in a question.

'Fine!' I blurt. 'Absolutely! I mean is that it? Just that easy?' I say.

'Yes, dear . . . if I want it to be!' she says, breathing in, and looking at me. 'Now I've got work to do.'

So an hour later, when I'm called back, 'Hey, the secretary wants to see you!' I think it's because of Sergei, or maybe Andrew, and I wonder why she has arranged a chair for me sideways and placed the phone across her desk, so I can speak into it easily and not have to lean across, and I wonder why she hasn't got her efficient face, or even her mischevious face on, but instead a truly concerned look, and I ask, 'What is it?'

'The police, dear, they want to talk to you. they said you left them this number if there was any news.'

My heart starts to thump.

'Yes,' I say, and look out the window at the sky, breathing heavily and swallowing back my fear of the voice on the other end.

'We don't know,' the voice is saying, 'three older men. dead. may not be your father. identify. if possible. soon as possible.' May not be, may not be.

'It may not be,' I say to Miss Pym, handing the receiver over the desk, though the phone is near me.

'It may not be,' I say and smile weakly as I go out the door, then down the corridor to the studio where Rob is cleaning mud off her brushes.

'What is it?' she says, alarmed, and I wonder how she knows.

'It may not be,' I say, 'want me to identify . . .'

'I'll come with you,' she says, pulling her coat off the hook and throwing the rest of the brushes into the bucket so they plop into the water. I look at the surface of the water and the splashes on the floor

'Hadn't you better clean them? It'll ruin them, you know.'

So we slowly and carefully clean the brushes one by one.

When they are stacked together in the paint tin, Roberta says, 'All right then, are you ready?'

I must look scared because she says, 'It's all right, it's all right, I'll be with you,' and rubs my arm.

'Thank you, Rob, thank you.'

22

We are led into a room that smells of strange chemical smells like formaldehyde. There are white tiles on the wall, and silver edges. The floor is white, there is a trolley, and a white sheet covers a body. I know it is not my father from the shape under the sheet. It is too squat.

I am relieved, but there is another body under a sheet and she leads me towards the trolley. It was a cold night, cold that kills people.

Oh, dad. But it is not him; I can see from the belly that sticks up under the sheet, and the hair that is long and grey.

I turn away from the pale dead face, and then something strange happens: time slows down, it slows down so slowly that I can look carefully at every little crease and hair in the policewoman's face. I look at her mouth as it slowly forms the words, but I don't seem to be able to comprehend the meaning, because she slowly puts her hand in the small of my back to guide me, while her other hand gestures forwards, and opens the way.

I am filled with a strange sense of awe at the beauty of the world, and the humming sound of the air conditioning has many voices in it, singing in a low harmony, and when I look at the body under the white sheet on the third trolley, I know at once from the shape that it is dad.

I look at the white sheet, and in the long moment time seems to have wound down to a standstill, long enough for me to see clearly memories flowing past.

I see him holding up the crab, and bringing me my first yellow fishing net, I remember the rockpools like gardens of beautiful flowers, I remember the walks through the gorse when he held my hand, and lifted me up on his shoulders so that I saw, not only over the gorse that smelt of coconuts, but over the trees below, down over the rolling grass to the bay stretching out, with St Michael's Mount and the line of silver along the horizon. And tying ribbons to the twigs, and in his study that had a green light in the summer because of the plants that grew over the window and the sunlight shone through the leaves. And in winter with him in the big chair by the fire, and the orange flames that contained the mysterious city.

And then to my surprise part of me is clawing at the sheet, shouting, 'Dad, my dad!', wailing like an animal wails, tears pouring out my eyes, wrenching up from my belly, and I am collapsing forward on to the trolley, touching dad's cold body, and the policewoman is holding me, and pulling me away from the trolley, saying, 'It's all right,' and giving me something to hold, and I am sobbing over the body, and at the same time part of me is perfectly still in a gentle feeling, being held by my father's memory, not memory, his being, his invisible self. He is there, he is there, and it's all right. I can feel him, and at the very same time as this strange convulsion is racking my body, I am being held in the arms of my father's beautiful ghost; as though a door is open and two worlds are existing together that are quite different. And the world my father wraps me in has a singing light, and yet there is the hard floor reflecting the striplights and the metal tubes and the animal that is wailing a grief-stricken wail, but the two realities exist at once. And then the policewoman guides me into Roberta's arms, who is standing there. I want to tell her that it's all right, because she has tears in her eyes and strokes my hair. I want to say, 'It's all right, he's here! You can't believe how beautiful it is, how lovely it is to feel him here, and know he's all right, that he's with me. Can you hear the sound of the music in the air conditioning? Can you feel the ribbons of light that are flowing through this room? He's here, my father is here, and I can see memories,' but I can also see that the way I am behaving would make it hard for her to see that, because I am distraught.

Then another strange wave of reality comes. It is quiet; a kind of numbness. It is as though I can see it all, but I'm not really feeling it, and I am calm and it's different. I dry my eyes. I say, 'I'm all right, Rob, thank you for being here.' I turn to the policewoman and ask her what needs to be done, what is the procedure, I even use that word 'procedure', and she says 'this way,' and we all file out of the humming room, and along a corridor with yellowed peeling paint and through a door, and there is a table and file trays and plastic chairs and my mind is lucid but only for the black print on the forms. I remember every detail that I need to: postcodes and dates of birth, names and addresses and doctors. It's amazing. They all pop up in my mind, and

I am going through these strange motions with absolute efficiency.

When it's all done Roberta says, 'I'll take you home,' and she puts her arm round me and walks with me out of the building.

Part Three

1

I am relieved after the clamour of Paddington, the echoing voices, the rushing people and flicking stations, to lean my head against the cool window and surrender myself to the rhythm of the train. I don't have to do anything but sit here for six hours. I can just breathe and be held in the rocking motion and let the jittering strangeness of the last few days move through me. It is dark outside, and the people around me look quivering and pallid in the electric light that reflects us in the windows. I close my eyes.

I think of Zeb in Barcelona, sitting at a café in a narrow street with orange walls among a crowd of smiling people, and think maybe he will forget all about me.

I walked up the stairs to his studio when I came back with Rob from the police station. She said to stay with her and Mick that night but I had to get my things. I don't even know what things. I felt like my body was made of lots of bits and pieces that didn't fit together. When I walked up the stairs I'd gone straight to the mezzanine because I wanted Zeb. I wanted Zeb so badly but he wasn't there. I wanted to hold on to his big body, I wanted him to stand there like a tree. But the door was locked, so I couldn't even roll up his old paint-spattered shirt and hold on to it, I could only lean my head against the door and smell the inky smell of the keyhole then lift one foot after the other up the stairs. I'd known fine well he wouldn't be there. The second-years had been gone days. But I still went there imagining he might be. Just shows how daft you can get.

I open my eyes. A little girl is crying. She reaches up to her mother, who lifts her on to her lap and strokes her hair. The little girl is flushed and tired and her mother soothes her. She curls up and puts her thumb in her mouth and her eyes flicker up and down, up and down.

I look out the window into the dark. We are in the countryside now, passing fields and hedges. The trees are black against the dark blue sky.

I'm so glad they came with me. I don't think I could have done it alone.

They must have met outside the lift where Rob was waiting for me, because when I came back downstairs Cecile was there too, and had been to fetch the jam jar for the flowers. She even brought candles.

It was Roberta who had asked in the police station where exactly it was they found him. That was one thing I didn't have the presence of mind to ask. I think Rob is right about the river; because I closed my eyes when I threw the flowers in, and my mind saw a river of light, even though it was raining.

We caught the bus there, and bought the flowers from the woman at the top of the Tube steps. I picked the freesias out of the bucket. And we'd walked along the street by the river. It was a cold misty damp day and everything was dripping. There was no one there. It seemed like a miserable little alcove; a stone corridor leading to some steps. There was a piece of red and white tape lying on the paving stones, maybe the police had left it behind and I thought of dad there all curled up, and held him in my mind. We put the flowers in the jam jar and lit the candles and Cecile told us a Buddhist chant and the sound echoed off the walls. She said it would make it peaceful for him, and with the songs and the flowers and the flickering candles, I think it did. Rob said it was good it was by the river, because it was a holy river and it would take him home. We walked down to the riverside and I threw in some of the flowers and they floated along on the surface of the water to St Paul's.

And I was certain I could feel him with me; that feeling of being enfolded in something warm. He must have known we were trying to help the part of him that might get left behind, confused.

But I don't have that feeling now. I feel alone. Oh dad, I whisper to the cold window, now it's me who's left behind, confused.

When the train pulls into Penzance I step out on to the chilly platform and smell the sea air. I walk into the cold wind outside the station.

Magda is there, waiting.

She takes my bags, wraps me in a blanket, and puts me in the car. The red and black tartan blanket smells of cows. Straw and cows. We drive up the lanes and through the trees to her farmhouse on the hill.

Some people might say it was a coincidence she phoned when she did. I think it was a miracle.

She was so glad to get the letter from me, she said, and she was so sad to hear what I had to tell her. I could hear her sigh down the telephone, a long sad sigh.

When I get out of the car into the wind it's pitch black and I smell the slurry.

'There now,' says Magda. 'In you come.'

She sits me down in front of the woodstove, and it reminds me of being little, when I'd come into Magda's kitchen with my teeth chattering and she'd wrap me in a blanket so my arms were trapped and put me in front of the woodstove with the door open, and by the time she brought me hot chocolate I'd be warm enough to unwrap my arms. And that's what she does. She goes over to the stove and makes me hot chocolate.

'Thanks, Magda!' I say, taking the steaming cup from her.

'There now!' she says, and sits down beside me and pokes the fire so the flames flare up and sparks fly up the flue.

2

The day of the funeral is quiet and still. One of those days when you can hear the sea lapping at the bottom of the cliffs, and the sky is clear and the hills are lit up with sunlight.

I sit by the coffin in the cold dark and look at the twisted ropes that loop around the brass handles while the vicar, with his eyes closed, murmurs prayers.

I think of my dad lying inside it. I was surprised when I touched his forehead. Surprised by the cold. Magda waited outside the undertaker's when I walked up the long narrow room with dad laid out at the end next to an urn of false flowers, and when I leaned to kiss his forehead it was cold. Cold as marble.

The vicar is saying, 'He's at peace now,' and everyone is standing up. The sound of the organ fills the stone church. Magda looks awkward in her black dress, and we sing a hymn with words about finding rest, and peace at last, and I walk behind the coffin in a kind of trance and out the door into the light. I breathe in the scent of the flowers and feel like dad is holding me, as though I'm swathed in something soft. My mother's grave has been opened up for dad's coffin to be lowered into, and I realize his pain is over, the longing he always felt for her is finished, and I throw in a handful of earth that drums on the lid. I close my eyes and hear the skylarks and see the river of light.

Some people shake my hand and look solemn but I can't seem to focus my eyes properly. Magda says, 'Sit down on the wall.' I tell her, 'No, I'm all right, really, Magda, I'm OK.' But I can't get in the car, and have to walk along the cliffs with the waves crashing below and listen to the seagulls crying over the sea.

And as I walk along the narrow path through the tall yellow gorse I think, 'I'm glad it's over for you, dad.'

3

But for me, it isn't over.

In the next few weeks my thoughts don't fit together, and I walk around Magda's kitchen and the farmyard, trying to piece together my broken mind.

I felt it splinter apart when I walked into dad's cottage and saw the chaos of broken plates, empty bottles, piles of dirty clothes mixed up with books and letters and unpaid bills; and in the study, the stacks of paper that would never become a book.

I sit at the kitchen table feeling dislocated and unreal and no matter where I look I can't seem to find myself. There is an empty place where the colours used to be, and I look at the white page of my drawing book and the blankness says, 'There's no point to anything.'

I see puddles in the muddy farmyard that turn into faces and their eyes have the sky in them.

I go for a walk in the woods and put every feather I find in my hair so when I get back to the farm, my hair is so tangled and twisted into fifteen feathers that Magda has to cut them out.

I can't sleep at night and every morning I hear Magda crunch across the gravel under the window before it's light, on her way to milk the cows.

'Am I going mad, d'you think, Magda?'

'No, you're just exhausted. It'll work itself out,' she says, and sure enough I fall ill with a fever and feel like I am fighting a battle in my dreams.

I open my eyes a tiny crack and see a piece of light.

Where am I? I open them and see the window. Or is it a picture?

There is St Michael's Mount a long way away.

I reach out my hand to touch it. Maybe it's a picture. I lean back on the pillows and close my eyes.

I see dad's face under the sheet and the trellis of stories he wove across the room.

'There's his study to clear,' I say with a shock, 'and his face is so cold and so are his hands.'

Images keep swimming away from me like fish.

'Have a spoonful of soup,' says Magda's voice.

I feel sweat, clammy over my body and dripping down my neck, and a liquid heat behind my eyes.

'Did we bury him, Magda?'

'Yes, love.'

'Why's my hair short?'

'I had to cut the feathers out . . . Just a spoonful. It'll do you good.'

'I have to clear the cottage, Magda.'

I see the mess of broken crockery and the empty bottles on the floor.

'We've nearly finished it, Eve. I'll give you another pillow, then you can sit up.'

But I push her hand away. The sea of images crashes over me like waves; buildings that implode inwards, splintering bottles, dirty clothes, dark tunnels lit by yellow light. I am pressed down by the weight of the sea.

I want to tell her, underneath all this, deep down, there is a little sound. It is my sound, but I have to be quiet to hear it.

Then one morning I wake up and look out the window and see the sun rising behind the Mount, and the sea is pale yellow and turquoise and glows as though the sea itself is the source of light, and I lie in bed listening to the sound of the birds, and my mind is calm, pale blue and still.

4

'My God, Evie, it's been weeks! How are you? How have you been? I want to hear everything!'

'Oh, Cecile, it's so lovely to hear your voice!'

'We didn't know how to get hold of you, even Miss Pym didn't know. The number we had for you didn't work.'

'The phone was cut off, I know.'

'At your father's place?'

'Yes.'

'Where are you, then?'

'I'm at Magda's, she's got a new phone now.'

'Are you OK, Eve?'

'Magda's been amazing, Ces, I don't know what I'd have done without her. She helped with everything.'

'But are you OK, Eve?'

'Yes, well now I am. Think I went mad, Ces.'

'I'm not surprised. You've been through it, Eve. It was hard all that time he was lost, never mind the shock at the police station.'

'I know.'

'Was it OK, the funeral?'

'Yes. He's buried with my mum. It was quiet, you know.'

'How did you feel?'

'Dazed, really. But like he was there with me. It was afterwards.'

'What happened afterwards?'

'Oh Ces, d'you really want to hear all this?'

'Course I do, Eve! I'm your friend! I want to know what you've been through!'

I smile at her down the telephone.

'Well, it was after the funeral, really. I went to his cottage with Magda. Oh Cecile, it was a shambles, stuff everywhere. We took all the rubbish to the tip and loads of stuff to the charity shop, and Mr Tremethick's.'

'Who's he?'

'He's got the second-hand shop in town. He took most of the furniture.'

'D'you mean you had to clear out the house?'

'Yes, it's going back to the landlord.'

'Oh, I see.'

'Not till the end of the month.'

'Evie, listen, that in itself. Your whole childhood, everything going.'

'I know, I know, but it wasn't really that, it was when I went into the study. Oh Ces! I could just feel his despair. It went right through me. I couldn't breathe. The pain of it was horrible. I felt it somehow. Felt how he felt. All the pages of the book he'd never finish all scattered everywhere. I just couldn't think straight after that.'

'Look, Eve, it was pretty heavy what he was feeling, it's bound to leave an atmosphere, but he's free of it now.'

'I think he had lots of stories in him, Cecile.'

'I'm sure he did.'

'But I don't know, he got stuck somehow, then he just went down and down. I thought I had to find out why. Now I realize, I just have to know not to do that.'

'Well, it's good you know you don't have to follow him down there.'

'D'you know, Ces, I think that's what I've always done. Part of me got lost along with him.'

'And now?'

'And now I don't have to.'

'Well, thank goodness for that!'

'I think I'm free now, Ces.'

'Evie, I'm so glad.'

'I think he's been helping me somehow. I mean just knowing . . .'

'What?'

'I can't say it, it sounds daft.'

'Well, say it quickly.'

'There are two realities, Cecile, and one of them's invisible.'

'I know,' she says.

A silence falls between us.

'We went back down to the river, you know, Eve, and took flowers, me and Rob.'

'Oh thanks, Cecile, thanks so much.'

I look out the window and down over the fields to the bay and the Mount shrouded by mist, and the Lizard beyond, only just visible along the horizon of the sea.

'So where are you now? I want to imagine you.'

'Sitting by the window at the kitchen table, next to the stove.'

'Sounds nice and warm. What can you see out the window?'

'One looks on to the farmyard,' I say, looking out the rain-spattered window.

'Yes?'

'The barn, the big blue door to the cowshed.'

'What's the weather like?'

'Wet.'

'And the other one?'

'Down over the fields to Mount's Bay.'

'The sea? Can you see the sea?'

'Only just. There's mist today. But I can see it. Then in the far distance, there's the Lizard.'

'What colour is it?'

'Grey.'

'Have you been painting it, Evie?'

'I can't, somehow. Everything's gone blank.'

'Well, maybe it has to do that for a bit. But it'll be back, Evie.'

'How's your work going, Cecile?'

'Well, I like it. I've got into green. Everything's green. But the terrible tutors are just the same.'

'Oh no, how?'

'Honestly, I don't know. They all troop in and stand in front of the pictures and something in me just curls up and runs away. They don't even have to say anything.'

'Yes, I know the feeling.'

'But you stood up to Sergei.'

'Sort of, I was at the end of my tether, more like. It's funny, I can't really remember now. It seems like another life.'

'Well, it's like that, isn't it, when you've been through stuff. Eve, have you got friends down there?'

'Not any more. They've all moved upcountry now.'

'That's a shame.'

'What have you been doing today, Ces?'

'We were drawing with Karl.'

'Three-second poses?'

Cecile laughs. 'No, they're five minutes now.'

I feel a pang, remembering the classes, remembering charcoal and rubbers and dust and the struggle to put the model on the page.

'Will you say hello to the other two?'

'Yes.'

'And tell Miss Pym I'll be back soon.'

'Yes.'

'Otherwise they might throw me out.'

'Not with Miss Pym in charge.'

'Oh Ces, I'm so glad you're there.'

'Yes, I'm here, Evie, and I'm so glad you're there too. But I'd prefer you here.'

'I'm coming back.'

'Well, come back soon. Karl says he's going to get a shed in Regent's Park to store the materials, and do a painting project in the park now the weather's getting warmer. You have to be back for that, Eve, all the flowers will be coming out.'

'Oh Cecile, it sounds lovely.'

'Yes and we can have picnics, you know. It'll be fun. I miss you, Evie!'

'I miss you too, Ces.'

'Evie?'

'Yes?'

'I think you should burn all those papers. He doesn't need them now. It might set him free too, you know. Build a bonfire and burn them, Evie.'

'Yes, I will, Ces, I think you're right.'
'And give your sketchbook a chance.'
'OK, OK.'
Cecile laughs. 'See you soon.'

When I put the phone down, I take out my sketchbook to face the blank page, but when I look at the white, I see the white sky and the line of the horizon barely visible, and the Lizard pale blue in the far distance along the horizon of the sea. And within a few strokes the blank page has turned into the sea, the sky and the far-away land.

5

The sack of potatoes is in the shed by the back door. The potatoes are muddy, and as I pick them out, the grit gets under my nails. I put them in the colander one by one. The sack is nearly empty and the potatoes have begun to sprout. I take them into the kitchen and wash them in the big square sink under the window.

I can still smell the smoke in my hair.

I did what Cecile told me, and burned the papers. I sat by the bonfire and fed the pages into the flames one by one, and watched them licked and swallowed by the fire, and the smoke coiled and billowed round me. All except a slip of paper that was whipped out my hand by the wind. It flew into my face so I caught it against my cheek. I want to keep it to show Cecile; it's a quote from William Blake.

I peel the potatoes slowly and plop them in a pan of cold water.

It was written in dad's handwriting so I felt like he was saying it to me.

'Everything in the Universe is lit by its own inner light,' and I folded it up and put it in my pocket. I look out the window into the farmyard and see Magda coming through the blue door in the corrugated iron barn that glows in the evening sunlight against the dark grey sky.

She opens the back door, bringing a blast of cold air into the room that makes the flames flicker in the stove.

'Well now,' she, says taking off her coat, 'there's quite a wind!'

She goes to the fridge and takes out the package of fish she bought from the fish van.

'All ready for tomorrow, then?' she says.

I dry my hands and lean on the kitchen table and watch her unwrapping the fish.

'I think so, Magda.'

'Come now, you can help me,' she says, lifting down the big black pan.

I place the pieces of fish in the pan; the white flesh is bluish, the skin is striped silver.

I spread them with butter and Magda pours the milk over. She lights the gas and lifts the pan on to the stove. The butter melts into yellow puddles in the milk, and simmers gently.

'It'll be a different place without you, Eve.'

I look up at her, but she is busy weighing out the butter.

'Now get the flour down for me, love.'

I take it off the shelf and weigh out two ounces.

'So you'll be going straight to your little flat?' she says.

'Yes,' I say. 'My friend Bianca's cousin has been staying there.'

'Well now, that's good.'

Magda puts the weighed-out butter into a smaller pan to melt and hands me the wooden spoon.

'There now, love. Mix the flour in and mix it so that it's smooth.'

I pour the flour into the hot yellow liquid and stir. The mixture smoothes into a paste and begins to change texture.

Magda pours the milk off the fish into a jug and hands it to me.

'Now you can add the milk the fish cooked in,' she says, 'but slowly, so it doesn't go lumpy.'

I stir the sauce round and round, adding the milk slowly and it thickens, turning smooth and yellow.

'And she'll still be there, will she?'

'No, Bianca said she'll be gone by tomorrow.'

'So you'll be on your own.'

'Not for long. I'll see them when I go in to college.'

Magda is carefully removing the cooked white flakes of fish from their silver skins.

'She's a good friend then, Bianca.'

'Yes, she is.'

'Well, that's good. You need people to help and that's that. I don't want you to feel alone.'

'I don't. And I can talk to you now,' I say, nodding at the new phone.

She smiles. 'I'll do for some things,' she says 'but you need your friends.'

'I'll get the parsley,' I say and go outside into the wind and pick it out of the stone basin at the back door where it grows along with the chives.

Back in the warmth, Magda is mashing the potatoes. Mashing and smashing and whipping them round. I wash the parsley and chop it small.

'Oh, wait now,' says Magda looking up. 'While I remember, I dug it out for you.'

'What?'

'Open the drawer, Evie, it's in there.'

I open the drawer and see a little black and white photo with a white rim all the way round.

'This?' I say, lifting it out.

'Yes.'

My dad is in the middle, squinting at the camera, holding my mother's hand. My mother has her hair up, with a far-away look in her eyes.

'She looks so young,' I say, looking closely.

On the other side of dad, a young Magda is holding me in her arms. The wind is blowing her hair across her face.

'Can I keep it?'

'Course you can,' says Magda.

I can feel something in me, something deep down, but I don't know what it is until it comes out of my mouth in a question.

'Magda?' I say, taking a deep breath.

'Yes,' she says.

'D'you think she didn't like me?'

She stops mashing and looks at me, and for a few seconds she is perfectly still.

Then she continues stirring the potatoes but more slowly.

'Your mother, you mean?'

I nod.

'She was just too young, love. She didn't know what to do with a little thing like you. That's all. But she loved you in her own way.'

I mix the parsley and the fish into the sauce and pour it into the square brown dish.

'That's all,' she says again, as she spreads the potatoes over the top and forks them into a pattern.

'There now,' she says as she puts the fish pie into the oven and closes the door. 'All we need now are the peas.'

I look out the window at the bay. The Mount is obscured. There is a dark cloud over the sea and the sun turns out like a light.

Magda looks up. 'Oh, my washing!'

'D'you want me to bring it in, Magda?'

'That rain'll be here any second, would you, love,' she says looking out the window at the Bay.

I take the basket from outside the back door, grey wicker from being left out in the rain, and walk to the washing line with the wind blowing against me. I pull the big stick down that keeps the line propped up, and take the washing off the pegs as quickly as I can. The wind is pulling the sheets out horizontally and billowing them so they're hard to get hold of, and I grapple with them.

Magda comes out the kitchen door.

'I'm going to give you a hand with this!' she shouts, because the wind is so loud. 'Didn't realize it was so bad.'

We pull the washing off the line and bundle up the linen, there's no time to fold it, and the sky breaks just as we've pulled the last one off the line. We run, crouching, into the house, being beaten by the rain and the wind.

'Thank goodness for that!' says Magda, wiping away a wet curl from her forehead. 'That washing would have been all down the valley if we hadn't got it in!'

She builds a fire in the big stove in the kitchen and we fold up the sheets between us.

6

We stand under the televisions waiting for the yellow writing to say Paddington. It is cold inside the station and I am jumping up and down to keep warm. When it says One, we walk through the gates, along the platform, into the wind. The train slides in and we look for my carriage and stand together at the open door.

'Oh, Magda, what would I have done without you?'

'I don't know at all,' she says and smiles. 'Now don't be a stranger!'

'No,' I say, 'I'll ring you.'

'Well, if you feel like it. I just want you to know there's always a place for you here.'

'Thanks, Magda.'

I climb into the carriage and open the window and lean out.

'Magda? You know with dad?'

'Yes, love?'

'What was the argument about?'

'What?'

'With dad. Why did you argue?'

'It was over the drink.'

'Really?'

'I told him he couldn't set foot in the house if he was drunk, and I meant it.'

She looks away and sighs, then looks up at me.

'But I never meant you,' she says, and pats my hand.

'Oh, Magda, I didn't know.'

'Ah, I thought you maybe thought I was interfering.'

'No. I was a stupid teenager. I took dad's side. But really all that time, my God, I wish I'd known.'

'Ah well, what's done is done.'

She nods and pats my hand again, and the train begins to judder and make moving noises.

'Now you take good care of yourself!' she says, and takes a few steps with the train, and I lean out the window and wave and watch her get smaller, and the train curves away from the platform, until I am sitting next to the Bay and I watch as the sea turns grey under the clouds, and the Mount slips behind the marshes at Marazion. I roll up my jersey and lay my head against the window and close my eyes and see Magda standing on the platform, waving, and imagine her getting in her car and driving back up the hill to the kitchen and the warm stove and the cowshed full of cows. And I imagine dad's empty house that I know I'll never go back to.

When I'd finished burning all the pieces of paper I'd walked back down the corridor to the study. There was only the green sofa and the desk left in the empty room, and I'd lain down on the sofa like I used to. The room had felt quiet then, and peaceful, and I'd remembered the trellis of stories dad had woven across the room when I was small. In and out of the dark alleys, along the river, and under the arches of the mysterious city, while I snuggled up beside him and listened, and the wind blew outside and the rain hit the window. We'd travelled backwards and forwards in time through golden coronations and music that echoed off the water, yellow fog and griffins with red eyes, and I'd seen the riots and the blue cockades. I'd seen the cherubs on the ceiling before the crowd fell silent, and the pigeons dropping out of the sky when the city caught alight.

And as I move through the evening towards London I sink into sleep to the rhythm of the train, remembering the stories that once flowed through him.

Part Four

1

It was strange coming up the stairs to the same hole in the carpet, the same chips in the paint, and letting myself into the flat.

Bianca's cousin had left a vase of red tulips on the kitchen table, and milk in the fridge. I had to turn the lights out and sit in the dark for a while and watch the car-lights from the street whizz round the walls. I didn't want to close the curtains and sit in the dark. I just wanted to feel what it was like being back in the city.

Feels like I feel everything, and I don't know what to do about that.

But when I got under the covers and lay in bed with the curtains still open, I felt glad about being back; glad of the honking sounds and the twinkling lights and the constant hum, glad of something else too; the feeling of hope, of possibilities that London exudes.

I didn't feel it when I got up, though. I felt that naked feeling again, and I biked along the side streets to avoid the vehicles with big wheels.

When I've chained up my bike, I walk across the quadrangle into the building. I smile at Stan, who raises his black eyebrows and nods at me. I walk straight into Cecile's studio, past a boy halfway up a ladder, painting an orange stripe on to his canvas with a wallpaper brush.

The music is blaring as usual and Cecile is sitting in the corner under a big green painting of tendrils and spiral patterns

She is drawing a green labyrinth, and looks up.

'Evie! Oh, Evie, welcome back!' she says, getting up and giving me a hug. 'Sit down,' she says, pulling a stool out from behind the partition. 'How are you? How do you feel?'

'Like I've been all the way to the middle and fallen apart,' I say, looking at the green labyrinth.

'Well, now you can come back out again,' she says, 'and you'll be brand new!'

'I hope so, Cecile. Anyway, how are you doing? I like this green painting,' I say, standing up to look at the picture. 'Green is brave!'

'I'm discovering just how!' says Cecile, standing up and looking at it with me.

'On a good day I think, leaves, chlorophyll, on a not-so-good day I think pea soup, but on a bad day I think, well, mould!'

I laugh. 'That's the danger of green!'

'Yes, and everyone knew that except me!' she says, and laughs too.

'Oh, Cecile, it's lovely to see you.'

'You too! So what about the painting?'

'I'm in a muddle, Ces, I don't even know if I want to paint any more.'

'Well, I wonder that most days!' she says, and smiles. 'You'll be all right. You've fallen apart, and now you're a little shoot growing out of the rubble. Just take one step at a time.'

'I'm scared to go upstairs and even look at the half-finished pictures.'

'They'll be in the storeroom. I'll come with you,' she says.

So we take the lift up to the storeroom and collect my canvases and a bag of materials and I don't even look at the old paintings, or the half-finished paintings tied up with string.

'Thanks, Cecile,' I say when I walk out of the lift. She waves at me through the sliding doors. 'See you at coffee time,' she says as the doors close.

When I walk into the studio that I share with Rob there is a blanket over the window and one has been pinned over the skylight so the studio is dark but for candles, which flicker in jam jars on the floor. They light up the huge mud women that have been taped to every wall.

Their presence fills the studio with stillness and the smell of baked earth. I close my eyes in the flickering darkness, and wonder how Rob opened a doorway into another time.

I hear Rob walk in behind me. I open my eyes and turn round.

'Evie, you're back!' she says and hugs me. Her belly has grown big.

'How are you?'

'I'm OK,' I say.

'I'll take the blankets down I just wanted to see how they looked.'

'They're wonderful, Rob.'

We look at the figures in silence for a minute.

'Have you shown them to anyone?'

'Oh, I tried to get Tom to see the point of them but he just talked about the fire hazard. I want them to be like a cave wall, you know. Like you're deep down in the earth.'

We take the blanket off the window and fold it up, and

215

I stand on a stool and pull the pins out of the skylight so the other blanket falls down on me. I pull it off and light pours down into the space.

Rob looks up at me.

'You OK, Eve?'

'I feel a bit strange, Rob.'

'You're bound to.'

She untapes the paper so it rolls upwards.

'So the mud didn't crack?' I say.

'No, it's a good medium. It's holding it together, anyway. I'm glad you're back,' she says.

'Me too,' I say, and jump off the stool.

'Oh, I nearly forgot,' she says. I've got something to give you. Zeb left it for you when he went to Barcelona. It's in my locker. We didn't know where to send it.'

My heart beats. 'Have you heard from him? Is he coming back soon?'

'Yes, Mick knows when he's back, it's not long.'

'Really? Has he got friends out there, d'you think?'

Rob shrugs. 'Don't know.'

I follow Rob out on to the landing. She opens the locker and hands me the packet, and goes back in the studio. It has 'Evie, love Zeb' written on it in black marker, and I say his name Zeb, Zeb, Zeb, under my breath. I open it and pull out a box.

It is a big matchbox with a miniature battery attached to the base. I push it open and inside is a small tree made of gold wire, and on every branch is a tiny coloured bird, that lights up when the box slides open, and each one glows a different colour and I look at it under my jersey to see it glow in the dark.

* * *

When I walk into Bianca's studio at coffee time she gives a shrill cry and runs towards me with her arms out and kisses me twice on both cheeks.

'Evie, you look too thin! Almost as thin as me! You must come to Brixton and eat something!'

London spreads out under the white sky. There is a faint green mist over the trees. The new leaves are beginning to unfurl.

'I eat, Bianca. I do eat!'

I sit on the windowsill above the radiator and look around the room.

The work has grown larger. And sometimes a glinting person, just the shape, no features, shines from a corner, or a turquoise figure glows in the foreground on a background of gold.

Bianca sits on the chaise longue and crosses her legs. She is wearing floppy orange trousers. She hands me small boxes. 'These are just ideas for bigger ones,' she says, and I open their lids. Inside are strips of metallic paper and squares of ultramarine, green or rose, each like a doorway opening into a shrine.

'They're beautiful,' I say. 'I like them small.'

Bianca shrugs. 'Yes, maybe.'

I show her what Zeb left for me, and she slides it open and looks at it with her mouth open at the same time as smiling, because it is enchanting her.

'Ah!' she says and covers her head with a sheet so she can see it in the darkness like I did.

She is sitting with her head under the paint-spattered sheet saying, 'Bastard! Ingenious!' when Rob and Cecile walk in.

They laugh and want to know what she's looking at. So

we all get under the sheet and the coloured birds light up our faces in the semi-darkness.

'How is it, then, Evie, are you glad to be back?' says Bianca, pulling the sheet off us, her long hair gone electric and sticking to the sheet.

'I am feeling a bit weird.'

'Don't worry, we'll look after you,' says Cecile.

'Yes, we don't mind if you're weird.'

'Rob's always weird anyway.'

'Thanks,' says Rob.

'I'm glad to be back with you lot, that's for sure.'

'Me too!' says Cecile. 'Now I'm not the only one being referee!' and she points at the others with her eyes, and looks up at the ceiling.

'You know what we should do after coffee!' says Rob.

'What?'

'Stephanie's going to show a few of the first-year print-makers how to make pinhole cameras. She told me I could come if I want. There'd be space. We could always make one between us.'

'Yes, let's.'

So after coffee we walk down the stairs to the print room and sit at the high table looking over St Stephen's, and measure cardboard to the right measurement, paint it black inside when we've constructed the box, and pierce it in exactly the right place so when the light penetrates, it hits the photographic paper at the right angle to make an upside-down imprint. We make two cameras between us.

Stephanie hands out the photographic paper and sends us out to the sculpture yard to take photographs, and we pose for each other, trying to stay still for eight minutes, to take a clear picture, or move slowly, so an image is captured moving across the paper like a ghost.

We sit on the wall of the sculpture yard in the full light, in the shed in the dim light, and half-in and half-out, so the light is bright and the shadows are dark; then go upstairs and squash together in the tiny dark room to expose the pictures.

'Ces said you need a job, Evie,' says Bianca. Her lips are the same colour as her face in the red light.

'Yes, I do,' I say.

We stand in the corner, while the other two lean over the chemical baths and watch the photographic paper reveal its images. We are taking it in turns to drop the white glossy paper into the liquid. The chemical smell gets up our nostrils and stings them. Then we lift it out by the corner and hang it on the line to dry in a row.

'I've got some grant money left,' I say.

'Won't last long,' says Rob, looking up from the baths.

'I know,' I say, but I don't want to talk about it any more in this squashed space filled with chemical smells that make it hard to breathe.

'I'll ask Susie,' says Bianca. 'They often need people to waitress.'

'Thanks, Bianca.'

'Oh wow! Look at this one!' says Cecile, turning round. Even in this light you can see Cecile's lips are red.

'It's all four of us,' she says, picking it out of the bath with the tongs and hanging it on the line.

'It's nice!' and we look at ourselves in a row, staring out of the sculpture shed between sacks of plaster and a heap of wrought iron.

*   *   *

I lie awake. The curtains are open and the street light shines in. I listen to the cars passing and the sound of people walking along the street. The girl upstairs begins playing the violin and the music is gentle and sad.

'Dad?' I say, 'are you there? Are you there, dad?'

But I can't feel his presence, only his absence, and I look out the window at the night and feel a hollow feeling with no tears in it.

2

The window is open and I can hear the pigeons roo-cooing from the plane tree. Safi touches her fingers together and places them in front of her lips. They are long brown fingers and they make a pattern in front of her mouth. She is wearing a turquoise and gold sari. The gold is stitched into brown.

'It all seems too hard, that's all.'

'You've had a lot to deal with, Eve.'

'It's like the world is too much; it all seems too harsh, too noisy.'

'You are feeling vulnerable. It's only natural. You are grieving, Eve.'

'But there are so many other things to think about, I have to get a job for a start.'

'I'm sure you will find something.'

'Well, Bianca says she might know of one.'

'That's good, Eve.'

'But it's not even that, Safi.'

'What is it then, Eve?'

'Nothing makes sense. It just seems pointless.'

'What does?'

'Everything.'

'That's because you are tired. You will heal. Give it time.'

'I don't even know if I want to paint.'

'It won't be like this for ever.'

'Safi, I wish you'd tell me something.'

'What do you wish I would tell you, Eve?'

'I wish you'd tell me something beautiful, that would make it all make sense. It's just everything's gone blank.'

'That feeling is part of the grieving process, Eve.'

'What am I supposed to do? Just wait?'

'Trust in the process. Give it time. Don't expect too much of yourself, Eve. You will find your way.'

I look at the gold patterns on Safi's sari.

Then I look out the window at the plane tree and watch the breeze blowing through the newly unfurled leaves.

But I can't see the pictures when you speak, Safi, and the colours don't sing any more.

3

I sit in the studio in front of the white canvas. I feel afraid. The empty space blows a wind through me. It feels impossible to begin when my imprint is so faint I might disappear into the colours.

After the photos had dried, Cecile brought them upstairs and I was shocked when I looked at myself because it was a picture of how I was feeling; as though I had lost my edges; become insubstantial and see-through.

In one I could see the wood pile through me.

'What is that? It's spooky,' I said to Rob.

'It's because you moved,' Rob said. 'It's a very slow exposure.'

'But look, Bianca moved all the time and she comes out really distinct.'

'Well, don't move.'

'I told you I didn't move.'

'You must have,' she said.

'But I didn't.'

Behind the muslin curtain dotted with blue paint, I can hear Rob swearing under her breath. I look round and see her using her back and her splayed arms to unroll the big drawings on to the wall, but the corners keep rolling up. I stand up and go through the curtain.

'You daft idiot! Let me help you.'

'I can do it!' she says, staple-gunning the corner behind her head.

'Well, it's easier with two.'

We unroll the paper and staple the bottom corners and I look up at the new drawings. The figures are drawn in blue and their bodies are covered in pictures.

'Rob, they're great.'

'I think they're the Picts,' she says, wiping her hair away from her damp forehead, and a little out of breath. 'They were covered in blue tattoos.'

She unrolls the other two and staples them to the wall and the studio dances with the new figures.

'How's it going through there?' She inclines her head to my space.

I sigh. 'Don't know. I think I've lost my imagination.'

'Nonsense!' she says. 'Just have some fun!'

I shrug.

'Hey, I know what you need,' she says, squatting down on the floor. 'I got them in the market as an experiment.'

She empties everything out of her string bag and gives up squatting and sits down against the wall with her legs out.

'You're going to have to help me up, you know!'

'What are you looking for?'

'These!' she says, holding up a handful of triangular packets.

'What are they?'

'It's henna. You know, for drawing on your skin.'

'Where did you get it?'

'Southwark. Shall we try them? Look, you just tear the top off, it's like icing a cake.'

She hands one to me with the top torn off.

'What? Now, Rob? You mean ... oh look, it's coming out, I can't stop it!'

The henna is oozing out of the hole at a tremendous rate, and already making wiggles on the floor.

Rob sits down, lifts her skirt over her knees, and kicks her shoes off.

'Well, I didn't really mean now, but I didn't realize it was going to do that.'

You have to draw quickly at the speed it comes out the packet. I draw a climbing plant with tendrils, which wind round her calf and blossom at her knee, with leaves that turn into eyes, and faces that smile from the leaves.

'See! You haven't lost it!'

When the packet is finished I roll up my trousers and Roberta paints landscapes on my legs, the moon on my knee, and plants sprouting from my pores. She gets so carried away I let her do my hands and then my arms, which sprout wings, and birds singing, and animals, and people with the bodies of birds, and birds with the bodies of lions. We go to the bathroom to stick our limbs in the sink, and Rob has to stand still while I do her legs, and we wash off the earthy-smelling worms of henna, and the drawings are left behind in sepia, glowing from our skin.

'Let's go and show Bianca!' And we walk upstairs to the abstract floor.

Bianca wants to be decorated too, so she lies down on the floor of her studio, with her legs and arms stretched like a star and we kneel down on either side of her, an arm and leg each and continue our pictorial flow, while Bianca moans and sighs, 'Oh, this is ecstatic! Let's do this every week, I feel as if I am being transported,' and we laugh and tell her to be quiet, we're concentrating. Don't make us laugh, it makes the line wiggle.

We have become proficient and Bianca's decoration is a masterpiece of twirls and furls and laughing faces.

'My God, I am a walking mythology!' says Bianca, delighted, as she prances about after washing off the henna, with her trousers rolled up to her thighs, and in only her vest, stretching out her arms in elegant mudras to show us our skill, and pointing her feet this way and that so she looks like a painted Pierrot.

4

'Hey,' Bianca said, her painted fingers in an elegant posture. 'Susie needs someone to cover for a missing waitress on Sunday, says you'll be next in line for a job if you're any good. It's only £6 an hour, but the tips are good.'

'Thanks, Bianca,' I said, 'I'll do it,' but I've been dreading Sunday ever since.

As I walk along the street I take out the matchbox and push it open.

I need a new battery because the birds don't light up.

I look at the gold branches and imagine Zeb shaping them with his long fingers.

I asked Rob for his address. She said Mick would know it, or I could send it to the art school in Spain, and Miss Pym would have the address, but I said I'd prefer to wait and get it from Mick.

Bianca said, 'Zeb'll know you didn't get the packet straight away, don't worry, but send a postcard and tell him you've got it now.'

'He'll think I didn't care about it, it was weeks ago he left it, all that time ago.'

But Bianca said, 'Your father died, Eve! And it only seems that long to you because of what happened.'

I said, 'How many weeks is it, then?' and she counted them on her painted fingers and said, 'Seven.'

It seems unbelievable. Time doesn't always pass at the same rate, that's all, because I feel as if the whole of reality has been reconstructed, and isn't it amazing it can happen in seven weeks.

So I sat down at her table while she heated wax and resin, and filled her studio with interesting fragrance, and drew a picture on a piece of card of coloured birds flying across the blue sea to Spain. Seven weeks ago. He must have a girlfriend by now, and I said it out loud without realizing. Bianca shrugged. 'Maybe he does, but I think he loves you.' And I posted the card in the post box when I'd waited for Mick to come back.

I arrive at the corner of the road and wonder which way to turn. Bianca gave me a note with the address. I look at the numbers and follow them backwards.

There are plants growing up the walls around the door. You have to ring a doorbell.

'Hello,' I say to a tall man with blond hair. 'I'm here for the waitress shift. I'm standing in for someone.'

He nods at me, without smiling, and shows me along a corridor.

I am introduced to Susie, who shakes my hand. She has a beauty spot on her cheek.

'Come this way,' she says in a deep grainy voice. I follow her down a mustard-yellow corridor into the dining room panelled in dark wood. There is a long table in the first room, and tables of different shapes in the second room, and a conservatory that leads into the garden where there are benches among the flowers, and places to sit that are hidden behind trees.

'This is lovely,' I say.

She shrugs.

'For them!'

Susie has longer hair at the front than the back, so it hangs down either side of her cheeks like two telephones. When she leans forward she could speak into the receivers.

We go through the double doors into a large brown room with a billiard table and a fireplace and sofas and a bar, and Susie tells me she sings in nightclubs, and what she really wants to be is a singer. I say, 'You've got the voice for it' and she smiles and shouts across at the bar, 'This is the waitress today.'

'What's her name?' shouts the barmaid.

'Eve,' I say.

'Upstairs there are bedrooms where the members can stay,' she says, pointing up the staircase. 'I'll introduce you to the kitchen,' and we walk back down the yellow corridor into the dining room and through a studded green baize door into the kitchen.

The under-chef has grey hair although he is young, and a rough-looking red face. He looks up from his preparation and nods without looking at me.

There are some other boys working in the kitchen dressed in white, with dirty aprons.

'Where's Carlo?'

'Not here yet.'

'He's the head chef.'

We go through to the back.

'This is where you bring the dirty plates. This is Patrice.'

Patrice is African, with a closed face that opens into a smile.

He flicks his towel over his shoulder so it snaps.

'How do you do,' I say and smile at him.

Susie ushers me back through the kitchen where a tall bulky man is standing in a white coat and blue checked trousers. He has slicked-back hair.

Susie says, 'This is Eve, she's the waitress today.'

He nods upwards and looks me up and down.

We walk back through the swing door.

'Don't worry about Carlo,' says Susie. 'He's got the worst temper. He's a real pain in the arse.'

He bangs through the doorway, so the swing door slams against the wall.

'Susie, I want to see you!' he says. His black eyes have a closed-off look.

Susie looks at the ceiling. 'See, he's just showing off to you that he's the big boss. Honestly, he's such a child, don't get taken in.'

She winks at me and goes through into the kitchen. I am left in the corner looking at the empty tables and wishing I could go home.

A blonde girl slides in, undoing her coat.

'Oh thank God, I thought I was late. Haven't even eaten yet. Look, this is where the cutlery is, I'm Edna.'

Susie and I put white cloths on the tables between us and lay the tables in all three rooms, after we have eaten our roast beef and yorkshire pudding cooked by the under-chef. The light slants in through the windows and Susie tells me she's in love with someone who comes here with his wife. They are having an affair and each time she sees him it's agony.

'He'll come today,' she says.' He always comes on Sunday.'

Carlo opens the door and blares, 'Susie, come here!'

'See, he's doing it again,' she says, smiling. 'He just loves being in charge and manly!'

People begin to come in and sit down at the tables. Susie comes back through with a biro behind her ear.

'You can take these tables here, all right?'

I must look alarmed because she says, 'Don't worry, we're not open yet, I still have to tell you what to do!'

She shows me how to take an order, how to put it on the nail through the hatch in the kitchen, and where to collect the plates.

'Carlo or someone will put it through and call it out. Then you take it to the table, all right?'

'OK,' I say.

'He's here!' she says, suddenly blushing and pointing him out with her eyes.

The man she is in love with has a reddish face and black curly hair and eyes that are in a smile, that isn't really a smile. He slides a glance at Susie while he pulls the chair out for his wife.

'Oh, he makes my heart race!' says Susie.

'But he's revolting, Susie.'

'Oh no, you don't know him,' she says. 'He's just wonderful.'

'I don't want to know him.'

Susie takes me by the arm.

'See that woman with dyed black hair, see over there in the blue?'

I look over to the corner and see a woman dressed in bangles and jewellery and feathers, with bright red lipstick and long false eyelashes.

'She's about seventy! Well, she's going out with the under-chef.'

'Is there any service?' a woman calls out.

'We've only just opened!' says Susie.

Suddenly it seems all the people arrive at once, the dining room is filled with the noise of people talking. They are pulling the chairs out and sitting down and shouting across at each other.

I take my pad and take the order for the first table, and put my order on the nail inside the hatch.

'Hey, come back!' says the under-chef. 'What's that?'

'Two roast beef.'

'Well, you have to write it, 2, number two, *times*, understand, or I don't know what the fuck you mean, geddit?'

'OK,' I say.

I go back and forth with orders and starters.

People are sitting down at all my tables.

I take the dirty plates from the first table's starters through the swing door and through the kitchen, where there is a frenzy of cooking and Carlo growls 'Get out the way!' as though I am a dog. I go into the back kitchen where we put our dirty plates, and smile at Patrice.

He receives them with a towel over one shoulder.

'Do you want to sleep with me?' he says.

'I . . . er.'

'Do you want to sleep with me, yes or no?'

'I don't even know you.'

He takes the dishes and clatters them in the sink. He whips his towel off his shoulder.

'You English girls, you're all the same. Yes or no! I say Yes or NO! I am just asking.'

'I, er, well, no,' I say.

'Thaaankyou,' he says. 'A straight answer, that's all I am asking. A strrraight answer.'

He has an African accent.

'Did he ask you if you would sleep with him?' says Susie, when I come back into the dining room.

'Yes.'

'He asks all the girls.'

'He didn't ask me!' says Edna.

'You haven't got the tits!' says Susie.

'Maybe someone should tell him it isn't exactly the best approach.'

'Oh, you'd be surprised,' says Susie.

My two other tables are full. I approach with my note-pad and pen. I still have the faded henna on my fingers.

'Oh, very exotic!' says the young man. 'Are you exotic?'

'No,' I say. 'What would you like?'

'You look rather exotic to me,' he says.

He speaks sideways so I can see up one of his nostrils. Someone should tell him not to do that.

'Are you,' and his eyebrows flick up, 'painted all over?'

'No,' I say. 'Can I take your order?'

'And how long have you been a waitress?' he says.

'This is my first day. What would you like?' I say.

'Oh, first day! I see, how splendid! I say, Mummy what d'you want?'

Mummy proceeds to order in French. The menu is written in English with a translation in French but she has to order the whole thing in bloody French.

I hesitate. 'Is that the calves' liver?'

She says it again in French and looks at me with a blank look.

'Thank you,' I say, trying to memorize what she just said so I can look it up. I collect the menus.

'Oh, I haven't finished yet,' says the young man, his nostril pointing at me, and pulling the menu towards

233

him. 'Does the *marmite dieppoise* come in a white wine velouté?'

I have no idea, and I'm still trying to memorize what Mummy said.

'I'll ask in the kitchen,' I say.

'Well, it says it does here,' he says. 'And I'd like to change mine for a *confit de canard*.'

'Yes. OK.'

'You might need to do a bit better than that,' he says, 'if you're going to stay longer than the first day.'

When I walk through into the other dining room Carlo opens the kitchen door.

'Look, you idiot, your beef has been waiting here five minutes! It'll be COLD!'

'Sorry,' I say, and take the beef and hurry away.

'WAIT!' shouts Carlo through the hatch. 'You have to serve it at the same time as the sea bass. Are you an imbecile?'

Susie comes up behind me.

'No, she's not. Leave her alone, she's doing fine.'

'Don't you worry,' she says. 'It's OK.'

'I've got two more for that table.'

'Don't worry,' she says, winking at me. 'I'll bring them through.'

I manage to get all my orders in, but then I collect some main courses that belong to someone else and serve them, so Carlo goes spare and starts banging on the hatch table.

How does he know they're for another table?

How do I know?

The rest of the afternoon seems to be a blur of coming and going and shouting and Susie running about picking up all the orders that I can't manage. When there is a lull I say to her, 'Oh Susie, you're a gem!'

'S'alright darling, oh, if only someone else would say that to me!'

Mummy wants brandy and the nostril wants a whisky and soda so I go through to the bar with a tray.

'Do they want them on the tab in here, or are they going to be put on the bill?' says the barmaid.

'I don't know.'

'Well, you'd better find out. We can't be short at the end of the day.'

A man sitting at the bar whispers something incoherent into my neck.

'Get off me!' I say, pushing him away.

'Oh,' he groans, 'be friendly, can't you?'

She finishes putting the drinks on the tray. I lift it up and the man gets a hold of my buttock and squeezes it. I slam down the tray with the shock.

'What the hell are you doing?' says the barmaid. 'You want to break my glasses?'

'Don't you dare do that to me!' I snarl.

The man slams down his hand on the bar. 'Can't anyone get a drink round here?'

'Well, tell me what you want?' says the barmaid.

I pick up the tray and walk down the yellow corridor.

Outside the dining-room door, Susie's lover has his leg in between hers and his hand up under her white shirt.

Susie is looking blissful.

I squeeze past them into the clattering chattering dining room.

At last everyone is ordering coffee and some tables are getting their bills. Susie is doing the adding up and the dining room begins to empty. When we've cleared away the cutlery and plates and glasses and wiped down the tables, Susie brings out the cash box and opens a bottle of white wine and all the waitresses sit down at the end of the long table and have a drink.

'Oh, I don't think I've got the hang of it,' I say, putting the glass to my forehead. 'I really don't think I'm cut out for this job.'

'You did fine,' says Edna.

Susie shares out the tips. 'You got good tips, though, Eve.'

I walk out into the cool air and take out the matchbox and for a few seconds the birds light up, then flicker and go out. I close the box and put it in my pocket and walk along the street with ringing in my ears.

5

'He should have told us we were meeting there, I could have got the 159 from Brixton all the way.'

'Yes, instead of leaving a stupid note on the board.'

'He must have left it on Friday.'

'I thought we were going to Regent's Park.'

'That's the painting project, and it's not till next week.'

'Better than the bloody National Gallery, all those boring old paintings.'

'They're not boring.'

'No, they're all Italian, I know.'

'That's got nothing to do with it.'

'And there'll be loads of people.'

We are walking towards the bus stop, with our bags of sketchbooks and charcoal. Karl is meeting us at the National Gallery for the drawing class.

We wait under the tree.

The 22 comes along the road and Rob and Bianca decide we'll get it to Piccadilly and walk down the Haymarket. Cecile is busy looking in her bag, wondering if she's left her purse behind. We climb up the stairs and sit in the seats at the front.

Bianca sits down beside me.

'Hey, what was it like?' she says. 'Sunday lunch?'

'Pretty horrible,' I say.

'I spoke to Susie, she said she liked you.'

'Yes, I like Susie, but everyone else is so bad-tempered.'

'Oh, it's always like that in restaurants.'

'And everyone's having an affair with everyone else.'

'Sounds fascinating!'

I shake my head.

'Oh, tell me the gossip, what's Susie's boyfriend like?'

'Revolting.'

Bianca laughs. 'She says he's really handsome.'

'He's having an affair right in front of his wife.'

Bianca shrugs. 'Well, people do, you know.'

'I didn't like him.'

'You are a bit of a prude.'

'Maybe I am. I don't know.'

I look out the window and watch the shops flashing past in clashing colours.

I close my eyes for a moment, so only the light and shadow flicker on my eyelids. When I woke up I just wanted to stay under the covers; lie in bed and be very still listening to the quiet, because it seemed like there was too much noise, and too much to feel.

'Well, maybe you are an idealist,' she says, thinking better of it.

'Maybe that too,' I say.

'You have to live in the real world,' she says.

'I know I do.'

We clamber down the stairs and out into Piccadilly. People are gathered at the traffic lights and move along in a body. Cecile holds on to my coat through the crowds and we follow Bianca and Rob along the road, past restaurants and banks and cinemas and stairs going underground.

'You're a bit far away, Eve,' says Cecile.

We walk along the grey street in silence for a while.

'So you didn't like the waitress job much?'

'It was horrible, Ces.'

'Why?'

'Because everyone is so mean and I'm useless at it.'

We pass the *Evening Standard* news-stand and photographs of women crying over men killed in the war.

'Don't you think it's all too much sometimes, Ces?'

A car door slams and two men begin shouting at each other in an alley.

'Sometimes it's all too much, don't you think?'

Cecile nods. 'Look, I know what you mean. I feel like that sometimes too.'

'Everyone is so mean, I can't stand it! And the thing is, Ces, you just have to feel it all.'

We pass a woman huddled in a doorway, holding on to a dog.

'That's why people paint, Eve, why they write music or sing or make films. Because they can't stand it either.'

'Is it?' I say, feeling helpless.

I look up at the roofs of the buildings where the pigeons are flying and Cecile puts her hand in my arm and guides me along the street.

'Don't forget the good things,' she says as we cross Trafalgar Square between the huge lions.

We walk up the stone steps and into the building. He said he'd meet us inside but Karl is nowhere to be seen.

'Are we late?' says Bianca.

'It doesn't matter, you know he's just going to tell us how composition leads the eye round the painting and

all that stuff. Come on, let's find some paintings to draw,'
says Rob.

The floor squeaks as we walk through the galleries. The
huge rooms are almost empty of people.

We walk past Titian and Goya, Velazquez and
Rembrandt.

Cecile says Titian could make ugly people beautiful, he
paints them with such tenderness, and Bianca tells us that
the flesh colours are painted over green to make them
glow like real skin.

We look at how Titian paints velvet and Goya paints
brocade and Rembrandt's portraits glow out of the darkness.

And Rob groans, 'Old *masters*' and Bianca says, 'Idiota'
in an exasperated voice.

We look at the Duke of Wellington in his medals and
pink sash, and Bianca starts calling Rob 'Dona Isabella'
after Goya's portrait, because of the resemblance.

We look at Van Gogh, and Cézanne, Monet and Pissarro.

'Oh Evie, you'll like this one!' says Rob. 'Montmartre,
it's like the one you did when the robber ran past.'

'If only,' I say, and the night glows in beautiful colours,
reflected in the wet street.

We walk through the huge rooms on the creaking floorboards, looking at the centuries pass by in moments that
are captured in layers of oil paint, depicting beautiful and
wrinkled faces, naked bodies, light on water, landscapes,
and sunflowers and holy families.

Bianca says she wants to draw *The Baptism of Christ*
by Piero della Francesca, and Rob says, 'Bianca, you are
secretly religious!' But Bianca says, no, she isn't, she likes
the man taking his clothes off behind John the Baptist.

Cecile says, 'But d'you know he worked out the composition mathematically, and that's why if you look at it, it makes you feel tranquil?'

Cecile says she's going to try Philip of Spain's brown and silver brocade, and Rob says she'll go and draw *Diana and Actaeon* because the women have real bodies, instead of the spindly things you see in magazines.

Cecile changes her mind and decides on Van Gogh's *Long Grass with Butterflies* in spite of Rob shaking her head, saying, 'How are you going to copy all those grass stalks, Ces? You must be mad!' and I walk back to *The Baptism of Christ* and draw the tranquil composition and it's true it makes me feel more peaceful.

After the stillness of the pictures we come out into the bustling noise of traffic and rushing people. Someone is handing out leaflets for an anti-war march. Bombs are dropping across the page. The date is written in a fluorescent explosion.

As we walk across the square, the pigeons are flying all over the place, and the police have arrived because some men are fighting and there is blood on the pavement.

'Eve, this is all you need!' says Cecile, but I shrug, and smile at her, and we all catch different buses to go home.

I climb off the bus before home and walk down the street to the river. I cross the road on to the bridge.

I walk out into the middle of the bridge. Even the trees in the park look dirty.

The light has gone out of the sky and the evening is grey. I lean over and look into the water. It is dark green, and feels magnetic as though it is pulling me in, and I imagine falling.

A man walks towards me from the other direction. He has a long coat on but the sleeves are too short. He stands beside me and leans out over the water.

'It's bad, isn't it?' he says.

I can smell the alcohol and I feel sorry for him.

'Life is bad,' he says. 'It's rotten.'

I look into the dark water.

'A person could be tempted to throw themselves in,' he says.

'I know,' I say.

'There's not much to live for,' he says.

'No,' I say.

'Go on!' he says. 'Jump! I'd like to see the splash!'

I turn to him and he looks at me with mad eyes.

'It's extraordinary how quickly a person can go under!' he says, 'like he's been grabbed by invisible hands.' He fingers the air in front of my face.

'No!' I say. 'No!' as I walk backwards away from him. 'No!'

I turn round and run back to the Embankment, and I can still hear him laughing even above the traffic noise. I don't stop running till I'm two streets away from the river, and when I get home I write a list of things that are good about life.

6

'He might have been an angel,' says Cecile. 'You never know.'

We are sitting on two blocks of stone in the sculpture yard, while the other two roll out the paper.

It was Cecile's idea to paint a picture together, but Bianca and Rob took over, and went to Green and Stone to buy the roll of Fabriano, and split it four ways so it cost £5.77 each.

'He seemed more like a devil to me,' I say, watching as Rob puts a tin of paint on one of the corners so it doesn't roll up.

'Are we using the whole roll, Rob?' I call out.

She looks up. 'Why not? Don't you think?'

'It's just . . . it's massive, all twenty-three feet!'

'Liberating!' she says

I shrug. 'OK.'

'Yes, but look what you were about to do!' says Cecile.

'I wasn't going to throw myself in, Ces.'

'But you were miserable enough to!'

'Imagine how horrible that would be,' I say.

Bianca is telling Rob to pull her end along a bit, so the rest of the roll isn't in the shed. The day is sunny and their shadows fall across the white sunlit paper.

'Loads of people do, you know. Maybe it's comforting to join all the other people who've done it.'

'I don't know about comforting, Ces, sometimes you have funny ideas.'

'Is that really what he said, about how quickly a person can go under?'

'Yes, like they'd been grabbed by invisible hands! And I'm telling you he'd seen it, Ces, I'm sure he had. It gives me the shivers.'

'So it should! Apparently someone was found in Wapping who'd jumped in, and they had shrimps coming out their eyes and their nose and their mouth.'

'Oh Ces! Where d'you get these facts?'

'I read it in a book.'

'You're making it up.'

'I'm not! It's in the book, I'll show you.'

'Look, it's ready,' says Rob, the paper is rolled out. 'Let's go and get our stuff!'

We take the lift up to our studios and meet back in the lift with our boxes of materials.

Roberta has brought potatoes.

'What are those for?' says Bianca, pointing.

'Printing,' says Rob. 'We do it with the kids.'

We take our baskets and boxes and bags through the sculpture department and outside into the yard to our huge piece of paper; six feet wide and twenty-three feet long.

We lay our materials out alongside the paper, on the ground. There are jars of acrylic, tubes of printing ink, rollers and brushes and squeezy bottles of poster paint. There is charcoal and oil pastels, oil sticks and chalk, and some silver aerosol car-spray that Mick had left over. Bianca has brought sheaves of gold and metallic paper, and Cecile some corrugated cardboard and the bits and pieces she picks up off the street for collage.

We have empty jars and buckets full of water, and plastic egg cartons for mixing the paint.

'And if we don't have every colour that exists,' says Cecile, 'we can make it!'

'Well, I think we've got enough,' says Rob.

It is a warm day and Bianca ties her hair up in an old piece of cloth and looks fetching, and takes her shoes off. We decide to copy her so we can walk across the paper and stand in the middle of it if we need to. The henna tattoos that have faded on our fingers are still bright on our legs, and I like watching the decorated feet walking over the white surface.

Roberta starts straight away, rolling a colour on to the white with a printing roller. Bianca crouches down and begins to smooth gold leaf on to the surface, and Cecile starts painting a big green labyrinth.

'Don't feel inhibited!' says Rob, from the other end of the paper. 'If it isn't any good we can always go over it.'

'Thanks,' I say, sitting in front of the big white space.

'I'm just saying,' she says. 'It'll be easier when we get going.'

I try painting a crow, but it looks lost on the empty paper, so it turns into a black oblong that might be a door, and I decide instead to paint nothing in particular.

The paper begins to fill up with colours and I move around the paper putting dots on to coloured shapes and tendrils in the spaces between. I forget myself as the painting begins to have its own life.

We move round and in and out of each other's pieces of work, sometimes covering them or letting little parts of them show through, in layers of paint and collage. The colours are dark and light, ugly and beautiful, drab and glinting.

We become absorbed and silent, and sink into an exhilarated painting trance. Time stops passing and stands still, and in the long moment the picture moves and pulsates with spirals and curves, and explosions of dots.

The henna paintings on our legs get splashed too, as we walk across the paper, and seem to become part of the painting.

I watch Bianca as she crouches down on the paper, getting her knees covered in paint, printing faces and eyes and hands, with potatoes cut in half, and magenta and turquoise printing ink. Cecile's huge flowers blossom in unexpected colours, and through them, and among them wind Rob's mysterious pathways. She has brought her dried earth to mix with medium, so among the sprouting flowers some earth-caked women are squatting.

Suddenly I see something. I paint an undulating line that changes colour along the length of the painting, meandering between Rob and Bianca's feet from one end to the other. It is the edge of the river, and the buildings and their reflection in the silver, sometimes copper, water.

'It's the river!' shouts Cecile.

The picture has turned into the wildest painting of London you've ever seen. London with its ancient history, with fireworks, with its wild spirit and primeval beginnings, with fields of marigolds in Pall Mall and Mesolithic ancestors, and frenzied atmospheres and flashing neon, and places of unexpected pale blue peace. I paint Tower Bridge and Lambeth Palace and a flaming angel with jewelled eyes, and Bianca adds patches of different-coloured metallic sky.

Rob starts painting the outlines of buildings. Huge flowers are sprouting from Westminster, Big Ben is splashed with fluorescence and the outline of St Paul's contains a labyrinth.

By the time we have finished, our feet and hands and knees are covered in paint. We have streaks on our faces and paint-spattered hair, as Bianca took to flicking fluorescent pink over the paper so the dots of light would glow on the dark colours.

The sun has gone behind the buildings and the air has become cool.

'We've been at it four hours!' says Bianca, picking up her watch and putting it back on. 'Can you believe that?'

We stand together and look at the painting.

'It's amazing, don't you think?'

'Yeah, don't know how we did it.'

'Let's put it under cover,' says Rob. So we drag it into the sculpture shed, and Bianca fetches traffic cones from the bike shed and we leave it to dry, and go through the sculpture department and up in the lift with our bags and baskets, suddenly so exhausted we can hardly see.

7

I lie in bed under the covers. I don't want to move.

There is traffic outside the window and the cars are honking and hooting. I get up and close the window and put Nina Simone on the player and climb back into bed. I feel like a snail outside its shell. I can't even go through to the kitchen and make a cup of tea.

I don't want to think about the studio and the mess I've left on the canvas.

I was so glad after the wild painting we made together, because it didn't feel pointless any more. I thought, 'Now I know what I want to paint,' and I'd gathered all the colours, even gold. I'd tried painting the city, the beautiful river and the ancient past, under the metallic sky, that shines dark and light at the same time, with the mad men and the sad men and invisible hope; but the picture turned into a dirty mess. And when Andrew, my new tutor, came through the curtain to introduce himself I was sitting on the stool holding my head, next to a canvas of muddy chaos.

I liked him because he knocked on the partition when he came through the curtain, and blushed when he said hello.

'Are you all right?' he said.

'I'm making such a mess!' I said.

'Maybe you're trying to do too many things at once,' he said, and I took him out on to the landing where we'd put our painting on the wall, beside the stairwell.

'See, it has them all, the beautiful and the ugly colours,' I said.

'But it's twenty-three feet long!' he said. 'There's more space for all the colours! You can't paint all the paintings at once!'

I stood there looking at it, and knew what he meant.

'It's all right,' he said. 'You'll get there!'

But it isn't because of the painting that I want the covers over my head.

I listen to Nina singing:

'My father always promised me that we would live in
   France,
We'd go boating on the Seine,
I would learn to dance, we lived in Ohio then,
He worked in the mines,'

and I think of my dad and I lie in bed and draw my knees up to my chin, and pull the covers round me because there are too many feelings to feel, and my senses are too raw for the outside world.

8

'Come on! Let's have one more go,' says Cecile.

'But it's so nice just lying here,' I say.

'I know,' says Bianca. 'I want to live here.'

I am lying with my eyes shut. When the water splashes
it echoes against the tiled walls.

'How long have we been here?'

'Three hours, I should think.'

'Bianca!' calls a voice from downstairs.

'Coming!' she says, and gets up off the bed and pads
downstairs, wrapped in a towel.

It was Bianca's idea, of course. As soon as she saw me
she said, 'You're miserable, you look ill! You need a treat!'

I smiled and said, 'What like?'

She said, 'Come on, I've got an idea!'

Cecile was nodding, but Rob said, 'We're supposed to
be drawing with Karl, we can't just not turn up!'

'Yes, we can!'

'Come on, he'll be livid.'

'Who cares!' Bianca said. 'Eve's ill!'

'I'm not ill.'

'You weren't in yesterday,' said Cecile.

'I'm OK, honestly.'

'Anyway, we can draw in there,' said Bianca.

'In where?' said Rob.

'I'll tell you when we get there.'

So we took the Tube and next thing you know, we were walking up the stairs into the huge, warm room and the sound of splashing.

A small lady with dyed black hair brought us piles of towels and said, 'Here you are, darlings,' and Bianca started talking to her in Italian. After she'd shown us into two cubicles as big as bedrooms, hung with red curtains, we undressed and wrapped ourselves in the warm towels.

Rob said, 'But we can't draw in here!'

'Yes, we can!' Bianca said, and she was right.

The oil pastels melt in the heat and slide over the paper. I drew a picture of Rob lying on her back, her hands on her big stomach, sitting in the wooden chair in the hot room, and Cecile lying on a bench with her legs stretched vertically up the tiled wall.

Cecile and I tried drawing in the steam room and two women with long dark hair said, 'Draw us, we don't mind,' but then the paper got so damp it wrinkled, and began to tear, and it was hard to see through the steam.

We have spent the afternoon sweating in the hot room, lying around in the steam, and plunging into the icy water by turns.

'Come on,' says Cecile, 'just once more.'

'OK,' I say, opening my eyes and sitting up.

We slip through the red curtain into the huge room where women wrapped in towels are lounging among the tiled pillars, having tea, and walk down the stairs by the cool air of the plunge pool and through the double doors into the tropical heat. There is a smell of soap in the wet air, and a faint scent of pine in the steam.

Bianca is lying naked on a marble slab being soaped all over with a bristly brush by the Russian masseuse.

Through the open door of the hot room we can see Rob, who is still talking pregnancy with two old ladies. Cecile and I walk into the steam. The walls are dripping. The air is wet. We lie naked on our towels and sweat trickles down our arms, behind our knees, between our breasts, and down our necks.

When we come out Cecile is pink all over.

We pass Bianca again, who is being hosed down and pummelled. She mouths 'Help me!' as the masseuse presses down on her shoulders so her cheek slides up and down on the soapy marble slab.

We laugh, and watch her make open-mouthed and shocked expressions as the muscular masseuse cricks each vertebra all the way up her spine.

The plunge pool is ice cold. Cecile stands at the side and slowly dips her toe in. I draw her quickly as she steps into the water.

I put down my sketchbook when she is fully submerged and leap in. I gasp at the sudden icy cold. When I step out of the water my whole body is warm and tingling, and we walk upstairs and lie down.

'Feel my skin!' says Bianca, coming in and climbing on the bed. 'It is scrubbed smooth.'

'There were three in the bed, and the pregnant one said, move over! move over!' sings Rob when she comes through the curtain, and we join in until a curt 'Shsh' from the next-door cubicle makes us quiet.

So we push the beds together and lie top to tail, and look at the gold ceiling, and listen to the whirring sound of the heating system that hums downstairs.

'I don't know what we're going to tell Karl,' says Rob, 'and we've got Regent's Park tomorrow.'

'You worry too much,' says Bianca.

'Well, he's still pissed off with us because we went to the National Gallery instead of the National *Portrait* Gallery,' says Rob, looking pointedly at Cecile.

'I told him it was my fault,' says Cecile. 'I read it wrong.'

Bianca laughs. 'Don't worry!' she says, languidly hitting the air.

It was obvious he didn't believe we'd even gone to the National Gallery until we showed him the drawings; though Cecile's didn't prove anything as it was a thicket of black lines.

'What's that?' he said.

'*Long Grass with Butterflies,*' she said, surprised he didn't recognize it, 'by Van Gogh!'

He just started laughing and said, 'There's no one quite like you, Cecile.'

But when he saw *Diana and Actaeon* and *The Baptism of Christ* times two, he believed us, and said, 'OK, girls, you're forgiven,' and tapped Bianca's drawing and said, 'You've got to use your pencil as a measurement, or you'll never get it in proportion!'

'You're not really worried, are you?' I ask Rob.

She shrugs. 'Oh, who cares!'

'You know, I don't want to be a mother,' says Cecile out of the blue. 'My mother frightens me,' and Bianca says, 'Let's not get on to mothers!' and Rob says, 'Ahem! I'm just about to be one!' and Bianca says, 'But I didn't mean you!'

Rob looks at me and says, 'My God, Eve, you're an orphan!' and I feel the empty place in the world they've left behind.

'But I've got Magda!' I say, and for a moment I think of her on the farm among the cows, and the blue sea and the Lizard far away in the distance.

'And you've got us,' says Ces.

Then we talk about who wants what in a boyfriend and Rob says she just wants Mick and Bianca says, 'That's lucky!'

Cecile says she likes her husband, he's kind, and Bianca says she wants someone with a sense of humour who's maybe a bit dangerous, and Rob nods to herself as though she knew it all along. And I look at my feet next to Bianca's closed eyes on one side, and Cecile's pink cheeks on the other that make her hair look more orange than usual and think, 'I want a man with dark eyes who wants to make sculptures out of light, and says that reality's 80 per cent invisible.'

'I think we should order tea and toast,' says Bianca and all of us agree it's a good idea, but our limbs feel so heavy, and the drowsiness so pleasant, none of us can bear to get up and we continue to lie there thinking how nice it would be.

'We should be drawing,' says Rob.

'We've done a few,' says Cecile.

'I'll do mine later,' says Rob languidly.

'D'you think the baby likes it?' says Bianca.

'He's gone quiet,' says Rob.

And we hear each other's voices along with the whirring and the humming and before long we have all fallen fast asleep.

9

It was while I was sleeping I decided to go. I must have dreamed the idea because when woke up I had the place in my mind. Cecile said she'd come too, when I told her on the way to the Tube. We stepped out into Queensway in time for the rush hour, and walked through the traffic feeling delicate and clean.

'I'll come if you like,' she said, but I said, 'No, thanks, Ces, I think I'll go on my own this time,' and she nodded and gave me a kiss goodbye.

I'm glad somehow that I'm all clean; as though I'm sparkling. Doesn't make any difference of course, and anyway he's under the earth in Cornwall, but it's where he left his body and that must mean something.

Ces gave me her water bottle and I bought candles from the cobbler by the station, and when I walk up the steps from the Tube on to the pavement by the river I buy a bunch of freesias from the same woman as before.

I walk along by the river, up some steps and into the alcove. Today there is sunlight and it shines right into the dark places, lighting them up. I put the bottle in the lit-up corner, and the yellow and pink freesias glow in the sunlight. The other corner is dark and I light the candles and leave them in the shadows.

Sometimes you think something is over and suddenly it takes you by surprise.

All at once I see dad. I imagine him lying here, crying. It is déjà vu, or the vague memory of a dream. I feel pierced by his sadness and I crouch down by the flowers and start sobbing so uncontrollably that an old lady stops and strokes my hair as she passes, and leaves a pound coin by my feet.

Then something peaceful happens. It comes over me, and fills me through and through, and I feel sure this happened to him too.

And when I go out of the alcove and walk along by the river, I have to stop still, and hardly breathe. The sky is so blue and the light is so clear and the sunlight is on the water; and I feel the invisible reality of dad's presence spread through me; and the promise, and the hope, and the longing, fill the whole sky from deep within me, and glitter on the water, and spread out into the clear light.

10

'Well, we were showing him pictures of us naked if you think about it!' says Bianca, and starts laughing.

We are lying on the grass in the sunlight in Regent's Park, while Bianca unwraps boiled eggs, pears and ciabatta bread folded in tea towels.

'You know, I never even thought about that!' says Cecile. 'We were stark naked!'

'Cecilina!' says Bianca. 'Well, it's the first time he hasn't criticized my proportions!'

Rob laughs.

'It's because you drew us lying down, so we were foreshortened,' says Cecile.

'Whatever you say, Ces,' says Bianca.

When we showed the drawings to Karl he shook his head and said, 'You four are something else.' But he said it was an original alternative.

'He didn't really mind,' I say.

'No, I think he thought it was quite funny,' says Rob.

When we'd arrived in the Park in Karl's van we'd walked through the green heat and cool shadows, weighed down with easels and canvases, and bags of paint and brushes. We'd walked along paths, by hedges, across sloping lawns, and down a grand avenue, past fountains and flowerbeds laid out in colourful symmetry, that scented the air with lilies.

We walked until we came to the lake, the weeping willows dipping their new leaves into the water.

Roberta sat on a bench to paint, and Bianca walked across the grass to draw the fountain, and Cecile and I had settled by the water to paint reflections. Cecile sat under a tree because of the sunlight and her pale skin. She wanted to paint the water through a curtain of green, and we've worked all morning.

'At Goldsmiths they're making a dove,' says Bianca, putting little twists of salt next to the boiled eggs, and a jar of capers, and Parma ham wrapped in greaseproof paper.

'A dove, what for?'

'The anti-war march.'

'Are you going?'

'Of course!'

'What are they making it out of?'

'Willows.'

'And what?'

'Oven-proof paper painted with PVA.'

'Why oven-proof?'

'They want to light it up inside.'

'With candles?'

'Don't know. Might be bulbs.'

'But they can't plug it in!' says Cecile, and Rob starts laughing.

'There are batteries, you know, Ces,' she says.

'Must be candles,' says Bianca.

'I'd like to see that.'

'Does the march go on till dark?'

'There's a candle-lit vigil after.'

'In Trafalgar Square?'

'Westminster. Outside the Houses of Parliament.'

'All night?'

'Don't know.'

'We should make something,' says Cecile. 'What shall we make?'

'Are you joking?' says Rob. 'Look at me! I'm hardly gonna manage the march with this!' she says, pointing to her belly, 'let alone carrying some bloody bird!'

'Keep your hair on! I was just thinking.'

'And Bianca gets tired, you know, she's not going to want . . .'

'OK, OK.'

'Hey, this is a fabulous picnic, Bianca!'

We eat our picnic and fall silent, and the bees buzz among the flowers.

'Look, Karl's coming,' says Cecile. 'We better get back to work.'

I walk back to my easel and sit by the lake, looking at the surface reflecting the trees, and the sky and the sunlight; and butterflies flit about behind my head, twirling round each other in shadows across the canvas.

Before long a mandarin duck with a bobbing quiff swims through the water I am painting. I try to paint him into the picture as quickly as I can. He has a red streak in his feathers and yellow eyes.

11

When we gather in Hyde Park behind the long trail of people that stretches up to Park Lane we are glad we have nothing to carry. Especially Bianca, who is dancing around, talking to everyone.

We are standing behind a group of men in long white shirts and white trousers with beards and skull-caps who have posters written in Arabic in green curly letters.

The men begin to sing a mournful and beautiful song, led by one who calls out the chant.

Around us are the green summer trees of Hyde Park, the birds are singing and the bees are buzzing in the long grass. It is a clear sunlit day. The march is taking time to begin.

Cecile and I wander away towards the trees.

The anti-war march looks like a colourful carnival from here.

'Oh look, I can see it!'

'The neck's a bit long for a dove.'

'Silvia said they tried to make it a dove but the willows were too long.'

'It made itself into a swan.'

It's near the head of the march and there are four people carrying it.

The bird rises up very slowly on poles, the wings begin to flap up and down, and we realize the people are beginning to move.

Though when we get back to our little crowd it's still at a standstill, and Rob is lying on the grass on a shawl that one of the bearded men has gallantly spread down for her to lie on.

As the people begin to move she stands up with a little help from Cecile and folds up the shawl. The man bows to her when she returns it to him.

We begin to move. But Bianca wants to join the dove, so we walk briskly alongside the slowly moving people towards Speakers' Corner.

We pass a crowd of travellers in rainbow jerseys drinking cans of lager and singing about a new world, and a crowd of little girls in tie-dyed frocks doing cartwheels on the grass. We pass people holding banners and placards, people laughing and people looking bored.

Silvia and Carlotta are standing under the big white bird, along with a crowd of South Americans. Bianca is greeted with warmth and laughing and they all begin to talk at the same time.

We begin to walk down Park Lane behind the Gays Against War, some of whom are twirling about on roller blades, wearing pink tutus.

The South Americans and the Gays Against War begin to mix together and the tutus begin twirling around the big white bird so that by the time we reach Hyde Park Corner and come to another standstill they have devised a choreographed piece which they perform to the delight of the tourists in a roofless tourist bus, who all stand up on the top deck and applaud.

We move slowly along beside Green Park, and a group of serious-looking people dressed in black and grey, who do not smile, push past us, carrying posters of dead soldiers.

Maimed and swollen faces, bloody limbs, bounce off the placards into my eyes. 'The unpublished pictures,' 'the real face of war,' say the placards. Then come several posters of death tolls and statistics and a truly horrifying picture of dead children, which Rob looks away from with her eyes shut and her mouth open.

Bianca doesn't see them; she is busy wobbling unsteadily on roller blades five sizes too big, holding the hand of a huge man in a pink tutu, who walks along barefoot past the Ritz. She is screeching with laughter.

There begin to be more and more policemen standing in the roads leading off Piccadilly; some are on horses.

The tall buildings of the Royal Academy and Fortnum & Mason seem to close in on us. I begin to feel claustrophobic. There is a scuffle with the police in Piccadilly Circus, when the people with dyed black hair and black eye make-up, with chains in their clothes, decide to sit down in the road.

We walk down the Haymarket. There are red and white barricades at the mouth of all the roads, and police with riot shields. The march gathers in Trafalgar Square. It is crammed. People are talking on a stage. Their voices echo off the walls of the National Gallery. Placards are being raised up and down. An unquiet feeling throngs the air. I can see people climbing up on to the lions. Rob says, 'D'you know they're made from. . . .' 'Melted down guns,' I say, nodding.

I am surprised she isn't affected by the violence in the air. Cecile looks like a frightened rabbit. We catch each other's eye.

'Let's go into the Underground!' she says. Bianca feels it too, and we push our way through the seething crowd.

A pole smashes through a window. There is a surge forward. People are throwing stones. I see a policeman hiding his head. I see a girl in a green skirt being pulled into the back of a van. The air has become strange.

I look round to see where Bianca is, and a crowd of people dressed in black are pushing past, raising their placards and shouting.

I am separated from the others. I can hear Rob shouting, 'Eve!' I see Cecile's red hair slip between the people, and the crowd surges away from the centre of the square. I am pulled along in a mass moving up St Martin's Lane. I am squashed in the press of bodies. A bang explodes behind us. The crowd begins to panic and run. I run along with them, and slip down a side street and run up an alley, away from the noise. I see a pub. I push the door open and fall in. I close the door, and stand against it, breathless, my heart pounding.

The landlord comes out from behind the bar and looks over the frosted glass window.

'What's it like out there?'

'Mayhem,' I say.

He locks the door, and we watch through the back-to-front 'Beer and Ale' etched into the window, as the people run past in both directions.

I buy a half of cider and my hands are shaking when I lift the glass. I hope the others are all right.

I look round at the dark brown pub, crimson flock velvet on the benches and stools. It is dingy and smells of smoking. An electric organ instrumental of 'Danny Boy' is playing on the jukebox.

'Were you on the march?' says a girl in a rainbow jersey.

'I got separated from my friends,' I say.

'You poor thing.'

I walk over and sit down.

'I hope they're all right, one of them is pregnant!'

She pats my shoulder reassuringly. 'Doesn't do any good to worry.'

We discuss the march, and how it had begun so peacefully. It turns out she's from Cornwall too, and we talk about missing the sea, and the stupidity of war and my hands stop shaking and outside it grows quiet.

'Are you going to the vigil?'

'We were planning to,' she says, inclining her head to the boy beside her.

'Looks like it's getting dark outside.'

He gets up and begins to feed money into the slot machine.

Suddenly she turns to me and says, 'You look WOW!' and puts her hand up to my face. 'It's like, geometric!'

'Are you on something?' I say.

'I think it's just kicked in!' she says, looking about her slowly with an open mouth. 'Sometimes he just slips it in my drink,' she says, nodding towards the boy, 'and I say to him, "No, you haven't, you *haven't*," and then I realize, "Yes he has!"' and she starts giggling. 'He most certainly has!'

This is all I need, I think to myself.

'Well, it's quietened down out there,' I say, standing up and nodding.

'Far out!' she says, stroking the air around me as though it is soft.

'Nice to meet you anyway.'

When I walk out into the evening I see the damage; shop windows are smashed and I crunch through the glass strewn over the road. I pass a scaffolding pole smashed through a windscreen of a car, surrounded by police tape. There is hardly anyone on the streets.

A neon cockerel says 'Take Courage.' Maybe the others will be at the vigil.

Flyers are being blown across the road by the wind or plastered to the tarmac by the drizzle. I walk over the bricks and cans on the paving in Trafalgar Square and the photographs on the discarded placards are covered in footsteps.

The square is deserted after the riot, the traffic lights change colour even though there are no cars. There is an eerie feeling, as though the buildings are listening to me. Watching me.

The placards have been chucked in the fountain and photographs of dead soldiers look up from under the water that reflects the orange sky.

There are strips of police tape flying about. I walk between the fountains. I turn to look at the National Gallery and to my horror it shouts at me. It shouts so loud I put my hands to my ears in case they bleed, but the sound is still overwhelming. I scream and can't hear the sound. Then I realize it's my own thoughts which are loud and the sound is echoing off the buildings.

I collapse on the rim of the fountain and put my hands in the water. The sound subsides.

'Maybe he spiked my drink, too,' but the thought does not shout back.

Then I look in the water and see dismembered soldiers calling to me through their own thin red blood. Their hacked limbs are waving and running.

'Oh God, oh God.' I put my head in my hands and the water cools my hair. I put my face up to the light of the moon that has come out from behind an orange cloud, and the light touches me.

I am blinking my eyes, seeing the ripples of reflected moon.

'Please don't let me see anything else.'

There is a terrific boom. I look up at Nelson's Column and the air throbs. The sound evaporates into the enraged sky and the lions begin to melt back into guns.

I run between the fountains of blood, and men with green faces spew water from their mouths.

The silver angel from the *Evening Standard* is flying about above the steps down into the Tube, which seems like the mouth of hell.

There is a face down there in the dark, his hair is long and matted, his eyes glint at me. I hurry past. Lion-headed, claw-fingered creatures with scary roaring mouths have jumped on to the lamp-posts. Winged children without legs look down from a pillar. I run away down Whitehall towards the river, past a cloaked man high up on a horse, but he is no help.

People have left empty clothes hanging on a plinth. They have turned to stone. Their emptiness reminds me of death and I smell the musty stone smell of a tomb that echoes when you whisper. I stop running and walk along the pavement.

The feeling of the night changes and becomes desolate. The wind makes an eerie sound along the hollow pipes of the scaffolding like many sad singing voices. The grief-stricken wind blows through me and tears pour down my cheeks. I feel burdened by the pain in the world. I walk past a huge poster of a dry river bed. Skeletons lying on the bank, with their skin still on, open their mouths. Their eyes revolve upwards and swivel in fear.

I reach Westminster and Big Ben looms up.

I cross the road to be by the water. The river is high and laps against the walls.

A brick-red shadow steps out of me and slips off into the darkness and I realize I've been looking through the eyes of despair.

There is a crowd of people standing outside the Houses of Parliament. I can see the dove but it isn't lit. I look for the others but they aren't among the crowd.

The people are humming and the sound has pictures in it; I feel them changing the atmosphere as they rise up into the night. A breeze blows from the river into my face.

Then everything stops. No noise. The water does not flow. The trees make no sound. There is no movement.

The world is passing through a still point.

The stillness is like a prayer. The air is potent.

I stop breathing and listen, and out of the silence I hear a beautiful sound. I open my hands and raise them to touch the air it passes through. It lights up every atom and makes my breathing sweet. It hums in my ears and glows behind my eyes with gold light.

All at once there is a dong. It is Big Ben.

Big Ben stops booming and little lights are being lit among the crowd. I see the dove being lit up from within and carried over and placed on Boudicca's chariot so it looks as if she's riding a bird.

I cross the road and pass through the luminous people. The sky is dark blue. An angel is looking out of my eyes, and everything is made of coloured light. A man gives me a night-light to hold. People begin humming again and the sound is soothing. I feel washed with relief.

A small girl looks with longing at my candle and I give it to her, she smiles shyly at me, and I decide to go home. I walk away from the humming people past the tall stately buildings and through the plane trees that hang over the river.

A Japanese man with black-rimmed glasses walks up to me. 'Excuse me, Downin' Street?' he says, adjusting his glasses. I can't think what he wants there at this time of night but I point him in the right direction.

Then just before I step on to Lambeth Bridge I seem to hear the leaves tinkle together in the night breeze, and look round.

There are birds here, small and lit-up. They glow with colours and emanate their coloured light. They are turquoise and rose-pink and orange. The songs they sing into the vast London night are complex and beautiful melodies. They fly up and about from branch to branch as birds do, never interrupting their song. Then they rise up in a swift synchronized motion and swoop up into the night. They leave the echoes of their harmonies and change the dark into something that is alive, that touches you and wants to open you, and I walk back along the river all the way home.

12

The birds flit about in my mind as I walk into college, and fill me with stillness although they are moving.

I walk up the stairs and meet Bianca coming down.

'Hi, Evie, were you OK? We lost you. Did you go to the vigil?'

'Yes, what happened to you lot?'

'We went down into the Tube.'

'All of you?'

'Yes. Cecile went home with Rob, she was a bit shaken.'

'I'm glad. I had visions of her being trampled or something horrible.'

'What about you?' says Bianca.

'Oh blimey,' I say, 'I was in a stampede.'

Bianca nods.

I open my mouth to tell her what I saw, but can't fit the words together to describe it, and instead I say, 'The birds are flying round my head.'

She looks at me with a frown. 'Are you all right, Evie?'

'Sort of.'

I want to tell her what happened but I can't.

'Come to the print room with me,' she says. 'I've got to finish my etchings, and I'll show you how to do monoprints, you missed that.'

All the images and feelings are in me and I can't speak about them, so maybe I will make them into pictures, and I nod, 'Yes, yes, that's a good idea. Monoprints. Show me how.'

The sun is slanting through the tall windows of the print room, cutting the room into triangles and rectangles of light and shadow. The big room is empty and all the tables are washed clean.

The window next to the etching press looks in the same direction as Bianca's studio but two floors down, so we can't see over the tops of the trees, but into the leaves and among the branches.

'Here! I'll show you,' says Bianca, pulling out a piece of plastic-coated chipboard from a box under the table and two rollers and some ink from the shelf above.

She sits down on the stool and leans over the chipboard palette and squeezes some black ink on to the shiny white surface.

'Did they light the bird?' she says, looking up at me.

'Yes, it was beautiful. Everything was so . . . surreal.'

'Did you see Silvia?'

'No.'

'She must have come home. OK, you take your roller.'
I smile because she lifts up the roller to show it to me.

'And you smooth the ink out like this.'

She makes a rectangle of ink with the roller.

'Make sure it's not too thick, and it's evenly spread out.'

'Let me try.'

She gives me the roller to roll the ink. It makes a sticky sound.

'Did you get home all right?'

'I walked along the river.'

'At that time of night?'

'I just felt like it.'

'OK, now you take a piece of card,' and she starts drawing into the oblong of ink. The lines are white.

She gives me the card and I draw into the ink.

'I like this.'

'Then all you do is put the paper on top and roll the clean roller over it.'

I lift my hands to let her do it. Then she nods at me to peel the paper back; the white lines and shapes glow out of the black ink.

'Wow.'

Bianca slips off the stool and goes to the other side of the room to cut paper, and soak it in the paper bath ready for her etching, and I sit down to work.

I make pictures of the frightened faces, the dismembered bodies and the lions melting into guns. I peel the pages off the palette and tape them to the shelves.

I draw the clock and the bridge over the water. I print the shining swan, and a figure in the dark, and people lit from within. I make the river of black ink in the background, or leave it white so it shines in the foreground, and as I work the birds begin to fly outside my head and out the window.

I lose sense of time as I draw into the ink, one after the other, the images pouring out of me like dreams. And as I print I see the paintings I will paint emerging from them, of someone in despair who remembers hope, and know that now I've found my own way of working.

'My God,' says Cecile bursting through the double doors, 'I've been looking everywhere for you two.'

'Cecile!' says Bianca.

'It's Rob!' says Cecile.

'What?' we both say together, standing up at the same time.

'The baby's coming!' says Cecile. 'It started this morning; her waters broke!'

'Oh no!' Bianca's hands cover her mouth, she doesn't like thinking about things like that.

'Where is she now?' I say.

'She's in hospital, with Mick.'

'Oh, I'm glad Mick's there.'

'So are you coming or not?'

'Where?' says Bianca.

'To the hospital! She's just about to have it!' says Cecile, holding the doors open.

'O Dio, I hope we don't have to watch!' says Bianca, covering her eyes at the thought.

I take her arm and glance back at my prints taped to the shelves; they'll be all right. 'Come on, Bianca, let's go.'

We fetch our coats and run out into the road. Standing on all three corners to make sure we get the first taxi that comes. Bianca calls out and whistles and we all clamber into the back of a cab.

'Where to?' says the cabby.

We look at Cecile, who tells him which hospital.

'Our friend is having a baby!' says Bianca through the glass.

'I'll get you there quick!' he says, doing a U-turn so we fall against each other, and putting his foot down so we zoom along the road.

'He's not joking!' says Cecile.

'Is she all right? I mean, it's not dangerous, after yesterday and everything?' says Bianca.

Cecile shrugs. 'They don't know. They were asking her all sorts of questions when I left.'

'Oh God. I hope it's all right.'

We arrive along with ambulances and climb out of the cab and through the big white doors into a turquoise hall. We run along a green corridor following signs and down a moving stairway.

'It's like a bloody airport!' says Cecile.

'I hate the smell of hospitals,' says Bianca, holding her nose. 'I hope she's had it,' she whispers to me.

Every desk we come to, and think we have arrived, we get directed somewhere else.

'Go up two floors, and turn right, and then left,' says the nurse with the telephone next to her ear.

We have to take a lift along with a man attached to a drip, and a bandage round his forehead.

'That's 'cos of the bump,' he says, pointing to his black eyes. 'I haven't been in a fight or anything,' he says.

'No,' says Cecile, shaking her head, then nodding so he knows she wouldn't have thought it.

We get out the lift and walk along a violet corridor past collages made with real flowers, and through double doors with oval windows, and ask another nurse at another desk, who tells us to wash our hands, please, and go along the corridor and turn left. No one has told us yet if Rob is all right, but when we walk along the corridor and turn left, the lilac curtains of the end cubicle are drawn back and there is Rob sitting up in bed, with Mick leaning close to her, both looking at a bundle with a furry black head.

'Oh my God, she's had it!' squeals Bianca, running along the corridor. 'Oh, we should have brought you flowers!' she says.

Rob looks up, and down again as if she can't bear to look away.

'Hello, you lot!' she murmurs, her eyes glued to her baby.

We gather round him and admire his little pink fingers and tiny ears. Rob looks down on him with a gentleness I've never seen before, and I lean over to look into his blinking mystified eyes, and smell his sweet baby fragrance. His presence has a stillness that fills the room and the corridor, so we fall into a quietness and just watch his ancient newborn face move slowly through emotions and then fall asleep. We look at each other. 'He's fallen asleep,' we whisper, while Rob and Mick continue to gaze.

'I hope you'll be well in time for my birthday,' says Bianca, breaking the spell.

'Well?' says Rob. 'I'm not ill!'

'Up and about, I mean,' says Bianca. 'We could have been twins,' she says into the baby's ear.

'Of course I will,' says Rob, looking up for a brief second.

'Good! I want to go to tea at the Ritz!'

'Trust you!' says Rob.

'You can bring Mick,' says Bianca.

'Thanks,' says Mick, smiling. 'I'll carry the baby.'

'No, you won't,' says Rob.

'Zeb'll be back then,' says Mick.

'I will invite him too,' says Bianca.

'Don't you want to be alone with a horde of women?' says Rob, looking up at Mick.

The rhythm of my heart has changed pace.

'Is he back soon?' I ask.

'He'll probably be in college next week,' says Mick, gently rubbing the fluffy head of his son.

I look at the floor, then the lilac curtain. I want to find a place to look so I can repeat the words and still breathe. Next week! Zeb will be back next week!

13

Every day I come in, and look through the window in the door of the mezzanine studio, expecting to see Zeb, but he isn't there.

Today is Friday and I rush up the stairs and look through the window in the door. But the studio is empty and dusty and I walk up the stairs, disappointed.

If Zeb isn't back by the degree show I won't see him till the autumn. By the time I've reached my floor, he might not come back at all.

The studio has become spacious without Rob and the canvases I have stretched and sized for the new pictures are lined up round the wall. I have mixed the primer from titanium pigment and rabbit-skin glue, and as I kneel down and begin to prime the surface in layers, I look into the white with Zebedee on my mind.

But when I tape the prints to the wall, and draw them out in charcoal on the canvas, and flick off the dust with a rag so only the line remains faintly visible, when I begin to imagine them in colour, and which colour, and what tone, his dark eyes begin to fade, and the white surface shows me other pictures.

At break time Cecile comes through the door.

'Oh, I like these new pictures, Evie!' she says.

'Well, they're only ideas so far.'

'I can see them as paintings. They're like London and dreams mixed together.'

'I don't know what they are, but I'm enjoying it, Ces!'

'About time!' she says.

I laugh. 'I know.'

'Shame I have to pack them up so soon, before they've even been painted,' I say as we walk up the stairs.

'You know we can paint in the annexe over the summer?'

'Can we?'

'Yes, as soon as the degree show goes up; in the studios above the ballet school.'

'Are you going to?' I say.

'Definitely. I used to go to that ballet school,' says Cecile, looking wistful, as we reach the abstract floor, and I imagine Cecile as a little girl in a tutu doing a plié, with her red hair tied in a bun.

The abstract studios are hot in the sunlight, and Bianca is sitting in the corner, wearing a hat she has made out of newspaper.

'Bianca, you can make a paper hat look elegant!' says Cecile.

The windows are open and the day is still.

Cecile takes the coffee pot out the door to fill it with water.

'Still no sign of him?' says Bianca.

'No,' I say, collapsing on to the chaise longue. 'He's probably decided to stay.'

And I think of Zeb all brown with a Spanish girlfriend.

'Oh, he'll be back,' says Bianca.

'Who you talking about, Zeb?' says Cecile, coming through the door.

277

Bianca nods.

'He's back! But they've put him in the sculpture yard because of the explosions!'

'He's back?' I say, standing up suddenly.

'What explosions?' says Bianca.

'Oh, I don't know, stuff like fireworks, coloured smoke, you know him. It's a new dimension to his work. I only spoke to him for a minute when he came through our studio with all his stuff.'

'A new dimension?'

'He'll have all eleven soon,' I say, aware of the blood rushing in my veins.

'Well, we can take him some coffee,' says Bianca.

I swallow and look out the window and suddenly don't know what to do with my hands.

'Yes, let's,' I say.

So after we have brewed our own pot we brew another for Zeb and take it down in the lift along with the sugar while I struggle with my heart rate, trying to calm myself, because he didn't write back to my postcard and he made the matchbox of birds ages ago, and anyway that was because he knew about dad. He didn't come and find me, but then I was in late. Anyway, he's bound to have found someone else by now.

Bianca keeps glancing at me, while Cecile scrapes the paint off her fingers, unawares.

Why do I feel like this? It's just stupid, I mean what good does it do? I think to myself as we walk through the big studios on the ground floor and through the sculpture studios.

On the other side of the sculpture yard, under the corrugated roof, I see his figure in the dark shed.

He is kneeling on one knee, the other leg square, his arm on his thigh, leaning over something he is lighting. His body makes a beautiful shape. The sleeves of his dark blue shirt are rolled up and his black hair falls down his back, tied in a plait like an Apache. I don't want him to look up.

There is a smell of gunpowder.

He kneels on both knees and sits back on his heels.

POW! A blue flame explodes with pink sparks, and momentarily lights up the interior of the dark shed, followed by a plume of smoke.

Bianca puts down the coffee pot and claps.

He looks up.

'Zebedee!' she cries.

'Hello, Bianca!' he says, getting to his feet and putting out his arms to greet her.

'Here! We have brought you coffee!' she says and hugs him, and I suddenly feel absurd, holding the sugar.

He looks at me. 'Evie, how are you?' He puts his arms round me and hugs and I feel the warmth of him on my skin. We pull apart quickly.

'Have you seen the baby?' says Bianca, pouring the coffee for him.

'Not yet,' he says. 'I got back yesterday.'

His face is brown. He smiles and nods at Bianca as she hands him the coffee and I see his asymmetrical dimples.

'His dad is happy, that's for sure,' he says, sipping the coffee.

'Mick is over the moon!' says Cecile.

We sit down on the dirt floor of the shed and talk about Barcelona and Miró and the Gaudí mosaics.

Bianca talks about the gold mosaics in Ravenna and I

279

look at his face and his hawk nose and his black eyebrows and for a moment he looks round and catches my eye and I look down. When I look up he is still looking at me. It makes my heart turn over.

Bianca asks him about the fireworks, and he tells us it's just an experiment, and he wants to make sculptures out of sunlight that disappear when the sun goes in.

We stand up and brush the wood chips and plaster dust off our clothes.

'See you later,' says Bianca. 'Come to my birthday tea!'

'I'm coming,' says Zeb. 'Mick already said.'

We are standing in the shed and I can't speak, I feel as if there is a force that pushes me away from him like a repelling magnet.

Then just as I turn to leave, he catches me by the arm.

'Evie,' he says.

'Yes,' I say, suddenly breathless.

'I'm so sorry about your dad.'

I shake my head then nod. 'Yes,' I say. 'Thanks, Zeb, it's OK now, and thanks, you know, for the beautiful tree,' and again I pull away too quickly.

'He likes you!' says Bianca as we leave Cecile in her studio on the ground floor and take the lift up together.

'But maybe it's because he feels sorry about dad,' I say.

'Oh, for God's sake, Evie.'

'He might just feel ... I mean, I know he's a good friend.'

'Bollocks!' says Bianca in a high-pitched voice. 'I could ask him for you!'

'Oh, don't do that, Bianca, please don't do that,' I say as the doors open to my floor and I step out.

But Bianca's expression doesn't convince me that she won't, so I step back in before they close.

'Don't! Will you, Bianca, please?'

'All right, don't panic!' she says, 'but don't be such a wimp.' The doors open and she steps out.

'Just grab him, Evie! What do you really want?' she says as the doors close, and the lifts moves down again.

I want to look into his eyes, I want to break through this awkwardness, I want to hug him and kiss him and feel his heart beating, I think to myself, and find I've missed my floor.

14

'No, it's because your baby is wrapped in a tablecloth, and they thought you were a gypsy!' says Bianca as we walk up Piccadilly.

'It's not a tablecloth! It's from Morocco,' says Rob.

'Well, it might have been because of my gym shoes,' says Cecile.

'Or the paint on your trousers! It doesn't really help that you're wearing them under a dress!' says Rob.

'They would have let the boys in,' I say. Mick and Zeb are walking on ahead.

'That's because the doorman fancied Zeb,' says Bianca.

'Well, he certainly didn't fancy us!'

'He couldn't keep his eyes off him!'

He's not the only one, I think to myself, as I look down at the pavement, or up at the tall buildings of Piccadilly, trying not to look at Zeb all the time; but I can always see where he is, like a blue light in the corner of my eye.

'We've all got paint on our clothes somewhere!' says Cecile, and Bianca looks round at herself to see if it's true.

'You could have managed it, Bianca, you look like you've stepped out of some bohemian version of *Vogue*,' says Rob.

Cecile comes up beside me and says in a low voice, 'I

do actually think it was Rob's Doc Martens with socks and a skirt.'

I start laughing. But whatever the reason they wouldn't let us in to have Bianca's birthday tea at the Ritz.

'Oh poor Bianca!' I say, walking up beside her and putting my arm in hers. 'We'll get dressed up and come back another day.'

'There would be no point,' she shrugs. 'Anyway, the cakes are better at Patisserie Valerie.'

Zeb and Mick have stopped on the pavement and are pointing at the RA.

'What?' Bianca calls out.

Mick is looking at his watch.

'D'you want tea at teatime, Bianca, or shall we treat you to Picasso on the way?'

She lifts her hands up. 'I am in the hands of the gods!'

'Good!' says Mick, lifting up his hands and Zeb's too. 'They're good hands!'

When we walk through the archway some of the RA students are outside, painting. Mick knows two of them and we talk to them in the sunlight.

'Why don't you take our passes,' says the girl with a long plait, who is painting a tree. 'If you're going to see the Picasso, you might as well.'

'But don't they know you?' says Bianca.

'They don't know us at the ticket desk. As long as you look like painting students.'

'Sometimes it helps to have paint on your clothes,' says Cecile as we walk into the exhibition for free. 'We're like the band of raggle taggle gypsies-oh,' she says, as we walk behind Rob with the baby in a bundle, Zeb and Mick, and Bianca talking to everyone in a loud voice.

In the first room Picasso looks at us through close-together eyes from a gentle boyish face, wearing a white shirt, and painting his own portrait with black and white and Indian red on his palette.

'I'd quite like to try that,' says Cecile, 'paint with those three colours.'

We walk around and stand in front of the pictures.

The picture of his studio is filled with shapes, turning the painting into a room with far-away places in it.

'He's brave, isn't he? Black and white and all the colours,' says Rob, pointing to the picture.

'Then all the shapes and stripes,' says Cecile. 'Sometimes it's all curves.'

'I think he's curvy, really,' says Rob, moving along to look at a woman whose blue profile kisses her own face with gentle violet lips. 'He's just playing with the squares.'

'He's playing with everything!' says Zeb.

A blue woman reclines with her legs stretched vertically on a red and white cloth. It looks like Cecile in the steam room.

'Wish I'd seen this before we went to the Turkish baths,' I say. 'I'd've painted you blue, Ces.'

Cecile is busy in her sketchbook, copying a figure in a red coat who has a pattern for a face and holds a blue feather in a feathery hand.

'God, everyone starts looking like a Picasso painting!' whispers Cecile, glancing at a man near us, with big eyes and long stubble and black eyebrows that meet in the middle.

'Here's someone who knows how to copy the "old masters",' says Bianca, collecting Cecile and me by the elbow, one on each side, and steering us into the next room to look at his copy of Velazquez's Infanta in her square dress. In the foreground the outline of a figure steps out of the sunlight.

'What would Karl say if we had a go at copying them like that? Bet he doesn't measure!'

Cecile laughs. 'You should try it, Bianca!'

'He's called Lump, you know,' says Bianca.

'Who?'

'Picasso's dog!' says Bianca, pointing at the long white dog in the picture, 'called Lump!'

Suddenly Bianca draws her breath in. 'Oh my God, no!'

'What?' we say together, looking round.

'Not in the gallery!' says Bianca, closing her eyes.

Rob has sat down on the black square bench, and opened her shirt and begun feeding the baby, who sucks loudly and makes little squeaking sounds.

'She could at least have chosen the room with the naked women in it!'

Cecile and I laugh. 'Come on, Bianca!' says Cecile.

'Next thing it will be puking!' says Bianca, walking away into the other room, saying, 'No! I really can't bear it!'

The guard looks confused, and pretends not to notice, and eventually moves into the other room, too.

Cecile shrugs and we follow them.

Zeb and Mick are standing together, looking at a painting.

Between them I see a skull and a black lamp, and sea urchins on a white plate in diagonals of light, but I can't help looking at the figure in blue who stands with his weight on one leg, and his hands in his pockets, with a long black plait falling between his shoulder blades.

Rob comes in, doing up her shirt. Mick turns round. 'I'll take him now, love,' and Rob hands him the bundle tied in the red and white shawl, and he holds him easily against his shoulder with one big hand.

'Come on,' says Cecile, putting her hand in mine and drawing me through the doors. 'Look! It's the picnic!'

Bianca is standing in front of the picture of a blue lake in a green forest. Clothed and naked people sit among the trees having a picnic.

'He's copied Manet!' says Cecile.

'And did you know Manet copied Raphael?' says Bianca.

'Oh well, that's the way to do it!' says Cecile, taking out her sketchbook to copy Picasso.

'Let's go on a picnic!' says Zeb, coming behind us, and looking at the picture between me and Bianca.

'Yes, with Evie and me!' says Bianca, pointing to the naked woman and the other bathing.

Zeb smiles and blushes slightly, and we look at each other for a second and the light from his eyes seems to jump into mine, and dances there when I look back at the painting.

'Come here!' says Cecile, holding my arm. 'I want to show you *The Rape of the Sabines*.'

'Do you have to?'

Bianca is laughing at the funny little man who is lying with his feet in the air.

'Isn't it wild?' Cecile says, taking out her sketchbook and frantically drawing the women and their mounted captors.

Bianca turns to the picture of a woman who falls backwards off a horse.

'Look! You can see its arsehole and its bollocks!' she says, pointing at the horse.

'You like that word!' says Rob, coming over to look and patting the baby, who is now tied diagonally over her breasts.

The man holds a carving knife next to the flaring nostrils of the horse.

'You shouldn't show him such violence at such an early age,' says Bianca, smiling and patting him too.

When Mick and Zeb saunter over we decide it's time for birthday tea.

So we go to Patisserie Valerie and have pyramids of strawberries and chocolate éclairs, and custard tarts and Bianca gets mesmerised by a couple who start kissing outside the glass door. They keep trying to part and kissing again, pulled together like two magnets, and get so carried away they put their hands under each other's clothes.

Bianca claps and the shop assistants watch them through the shelves of cakes, and even the manager goes to knock on the window and then shrugs in a French way, and says to the café, 'That's what French cakes can do for you,' and leaves them to it.

'It's my birthday,' says Bianca.

'Bon anniversaire!' he says, and brings her a cake gratuit with caramel icing, and a candle burning on top, and we sing 'Happy Birthday', and the manager sings in French, and some of the other customers join in.

15

The floor has been painted grey and all our spots of paint have disappeared.

The muslin curtain has been taken down, and the doors are open to the landing.

The technicians are putting up partitions and there are the sounds of hammering and sawing in the studios. They are transforming the college into an exhibition space.

The third-years are running about, calling questions to each other up and down the stairwell about, 'Where is this?' and 'How much?' and 'Can you get mine done at the same time?' in a frantic rush to get their work mounted, framed and hung in time for the degree show.

The first- and second-years have to pack up paintings and put them in the storeroom, and gather what we need for the summer, and transport it to the annexe.

'When do we need to be out, then?'

'Five o'clock, I think, but the van is going up to the annexe this morning.'

'D'you know who is going?' says Cecile.

'Only us lot from our year, and some second-years,' I say.

We are putting Rob's materials into boxes to load into the van.

'Is Zeb coming?' says Cecile.

And I remember yesterday, when we were hidden behind the crowd.

'Yes,' I say, 'he is.'

We'd all walked along Shaftesbury Avenue after the birthday tea to catch our buses, and waited at the bus stop among a crowd of people. I stood next to Zeb on the steps of the Casino, and heard the dringing sounds of the slot machines, the mini sirens and ding-dong of the pinball, and he'd leaned over and said, 'Are you going to the annexe?'

'Yes,' I said. 'Are you?'

He nodded and his eyes looked at me like sunlight.

'We've got the whole summer,' he said.

'I'd like to hear about Spain,' I said.

'I'd like to tell you,' he said.

And then his eyes had turned dark and deep.

'And you, I want to hear about what happened with you, all of that, Evie. I want to know.'

His eyes had reached into mine, and I had to hold on to his arm; tears were pricking the back of my eyes.

'I know,' he said. 'I'm sorry, Eve. Not now. It's not the place.'

And I dropped my hand, and he caught it and held it, and I heard him say, 'Evie,' close to my neck.

Then all the people were moving at once. Cecile was shouting through the people, 'It's our bus, Eve!' and grabbed my free hand through the crowd, and I'd looked back at him and he'd squeezed my hand before he let it go, and I felt the pressure all the way home.

'What about the fire hazard?' says Cecile.

'What?'

'Zeb. The fire hazard.'

'Oh, it's all right, he's going to work on the roof,' I say. 'Trust him!'

When we've finished the boxes we take them downstairs and pile them up with the rest. And when I've swept the studio and emptied my locker, I go up to Bianca's studio, and she is lying on the chaise longue with a hand over her forehead.

'Oh, it's unbearable!' she says. 'I can't bear to leave! I don't want to pack anything!'

'But we can unpack it again today,' I say. 'We can start painting again tomorrow.'

'Oh, it's so traumatic!' she says. 'I can't bear to leave my lovely space!'

Cecile comes upstairs and we sit down together and help dismantle Bianca's studio into boxes, and take it downstairs in the lift.

When the van arrives, everyone packs in their paintings and Karl flicks his eyes up to the sky when Bianca comes through the door of the college carrying the chaise longue upwards, with her hands round the middle as though she's dancing with it.

'Bianca, do you have to?'

'Yes,' she says. 'Yes, of course. I can't do without it!'

So when the big canvases have been tied to the roof rack and we are sitting in two rows next to a stack of materials and smaller paintings piled up behind Karl's seat, he and Bianca lift the chaise longue into the van and lie it along our knees.

I am wondering where Zeb has got to when a second-year comes out of the door with a big box and stands at the door of the van.

'Another box?' says Karl, scratching his head.

'Zeb's not coming,' he says, resting the box on the step, filled with an assortment of copper tubing, rolls of wire and plugs and metal shapes. 'But could you take this for him? He says he'll bring the rest later.'

'OK,' says Karl, pushing the box into the van so we have to lift up our feet. He closes the door and we are jammed together in the back. He starts the engine and we judder forward.

I am disappointed that Zeb isn't coming. But when I look back at the college my heart sinks and my breath quickens as I see him in the corridor, having an intense conversation with Suzanne.

We arrive at a tall red-brick building and the studios are on the top floor. We walk up flights of stairs, and the green tiles on the walls make our voices echo. We can hear the sounds of the bouncing muffled feet of little ballet dancers, and the plink-plink of the piano keys behind the closed doors, as we carry our boxes and stretchers up the stairs.

The studios have tall windows that look over the trees and houses all the way to Putney and Wandsworth.

We sweep the floor and choose our spaces and Bianca finds a good position for the chaise longue.

'Let's go back and pack up the pictures now,' says Bianca. 'I feel homesick!'

'I'm going to stay here a bit,' I say.

So everyone troops out of the double doors, and I hear their footsteps echo on the tiles of the stairwell.

I unpack my pictures in the silence and arrange them on the floor around the walls. I take out the photograph Magda gave me and put it on the windowsill next to the palette.

I look at the faces of my mum and dad, looking so young and unsure, and decide that somewhere I will put them in the paintings, maybe surrounded by blue.

I unpack my paints and put them on a table and unwrap my brushes so everything is ready. I look at the pictures again and imagine the colours. I am ready to go back.

Before I reach the door, I turn around and look at the big studio, with the boxes of materials stacked in the corner; tubes of paint, rolls of paper and canvas, tins of media, primer and glue, and in the quiet I can feel something is waiting; an invisible reality more vast than this one. That's why Bianca wants the glinting colours, and why Zeb wants the exploding light, and Rob the presence of her ancestors caked in mud; because part of us is from there, and longs for there, and we want to touch that place, and let it through somehow.

I close the door and walk down the stairs, and try not to think too much about Suzanne.

When I get back to college the ground floor is already a gallery with pristine white walls and work on display. Upstairs, our studio space has been divided by white partitions.

I walk up to the top-floor storeroom and find Bianca wrapping her work in bubble wrap.

'I'm scared it will get nicked, actually,' she says, 'but it needs protecting anyway. Here's a good space for yours, Evie. Let's put them together, safety in numbers!'

She looks up. 'Did you start painting?'

'No, I was just unpacking.'

'Oh, Zeb was looking for you,' she says, moving her eyebrows up and down quickly.

'Was he?' I say.

'Yes, he said to tell you he'll see you at the degree show.'

I look at her for a minute.

'Why didn't he come?'

'Oh, the third-years finally decided it wouldn't steal the show but enhance it to have his fireworks, as long as he didn't attach them to his sculptures, so he had to sort them out. Suzanne was making a song and dance about it, though.'

'I saw them talking in the corridor,' I say.

She looks at me for a moment. 'Did you think he was getting back with her?' She smiles. 'You idiot, Evie!'

And I look into the dark corner at the back of the store-room and shake my head at myself.

16

'Come and get ready in Brixton with us,' Bianca said. 'Silvia is coming too, it'll be fun!'

So I went back with her on the 137, clutching my dress for the degree show in a plastic bag, and watched the sun slip over the water from the top deck while Bianca took the dress out the bag and told me not to wear 'that old thing'.

After we'd climbed the stairs through the glass-stained sunlight, Bianca made fennel tea and we went and sat in the scented bathroom where Silvia was in the bath, washing her hair. I tried on the dresses from the rail, and Bianca gave her opinion from the armchair, and every now and then Silvia turned round to look. By the time Silvia had rinsed her hair, and was stepping out of the bath with the towel wrapped round her, I'd decided on the dress with roses on, that I'm wearing now.

We took it in turns to sit in the armchair and after another pot of fennel tea, everyone had decided what to wear.

We caught the bus and teetered down the road to college, Silvia in a deep red dress with a blue-black boa around her naked shoulders, and Bianca with feathers in her hair, in a Chinese dress of gold silk.

We turned the corner, and people were spilling out of the glass doors and standing around the Henry Moore sculpture with wine glasses in their hands. 'Fine Art Degree Show' was written in red letters on the glass wall, and the quadrangle was bedecked in bunting made of white-fringed flags, printed with red and black drawings.

The tutors looked strange in their smart clothes. Paul was gleaming in a silver suit with a yellow tie and long shiny shoes, which looked like crocodile skin.

Bianca said, 'Oh my God,' and made a face behind her hand.

We walked through the doors and into the noise of people talking and I noticed Miss Pym resplendent in turquoise, and Terry wearing a tie.

Bianca wanted to go upstairs to her space, but Silvia said, 'I'm going this way,' pointing to the sign that said 'Sculpture Department'.

'I'm looking for a strong sculptor!' she said, flicking the feather boa around her neck, 'not a wimpy painter!' and she kissed the air with her eyes closed.

I didn't think about it then, when I watched her cross the hall. I don't know why. It's only now as I look over the banisters, through the crowds of people, that I think of Zeb.

We watched Terry catching sight of her and following her with a wine bottle and an empty glass. I even said, 'Will she be all right with the terrible Terry on her trail?' and Bianca flicked the air with her hand. 'Silvia? She's from Sicily!'

It was when they both disappeared down the corridor to sculpture that I began to think about how everyone loves Silvia.

'Come on,' says Bianca. 'Let's go upstairs to the abstract floor.'

'D'you think Silvia's got anyone in mind?'

'No, she just likes flirting!'

We pass Geoff, wearing a Hawaiian shirt, and Bianca whispers, 'I am a born-again Christian looking funky!'

I smile at her, and decide to put the whole thing out my mind.

I look through the crowds of people at the paintings we have watched emerge, and the spaces without their grime suddenly make the paintings stand out, cut clean of their beginnings.

Maria Ines and Anna are on the landing and they greet Bianca in a shower of Italian.

'Come through!' she says. 'I will show you where I have been working. Ah, my beautiful space!'

Bianca's old space is filled with people and hung with blue paintings that belong to Mona, the third-year student. Bianca takes no notice of the paintings or the people and points out the window, showing Anna and Maria Ines the view of London. Mona is hovering round her space with a wine bottle, introducing her friends to each other, and looks a little ill at ease.

I walk upstairs and find the colour harmonies I once saw in a sketchbook, turned into paintings as long as the wall.

They fill the room with clear colour sounds and I stand and look, and listen to them sing.

I wander through the unfamiliar spaces, partitioned into corridors and alcoves, looking at the paintings in between the crowds. The third-year students, with wine bottles in their hands, talk very fast, smile a lot and hand out their cards.

I look over the banisters and see the top of Cecile's head and walk downstairs to the next floor with relief.

'Oh I'm glad to see you!' I say. 'All these people!'

Cecile looks elegant in a green dress.

She puts her arm through mine. 'Me too. Let's wander about! Where's Bianca?'

'Upstairs in her space.'

'Her space!' Cecile laughs. 'Poor Mona.'

I shrug. 'You know what she says about the paintings?'

'I know,' says Cecile. 'Dishcloths. Isn't she awful!'

We walk downstairs to the figurative floor and the sounds of people talking echo up the stairwell. On the landing are paintings of a man with a cow, and chickens in a farmyard. The paintings are colourful and splashy.

I see Sergei wearing his same old jacket, walking round the pictures, eyeing them up close, with his hands behind his back and the strange quivering sneer on his lips.

But as I pass by I notice his hair is all fluffy on the back of his head, like he's been sleeping on it, and hasn't brushed it out. It reminds me of a little bird.

'Cecile, I feel sorry for Sergei!'

'Quick, let's get away, that sounds dangerous,' she says.

We walk around the figurative floor, past the model painted from many angles lying on a blue curtain, through landscapes and cityscapes and portraits, discussing the pictures we like, and every now and then I take a look out the window to see if I can catch a glimpse of Zeb in the sculpture yard.

'You like him, don't you,' says Cecile.

'Yes,' I say, smiling at the floor.

'Let's go down,' I say, looking up.

'Come on then,' she says. 'I want to see the sculptures, and they're doing a piece of performance art in a minute.'

We meet Rob on the stairs with Mick and the little bundle, who is now called George. She smiles a tired smile.

'It's mayhem here!' she says, and Mick puts his arm round her shoulders. 'I'm beginning to feel claustrophobic!'

'Come outside with us,' I say.

So we all walk downstairs, and I meet Safi coming up, dressed in a brown and silver sari.

'Eve, how glad I am to see you!' she says, folding her hands over mine.

Around her the air feels less crowded and more peaceful.

'You look very beautiful today, my dear,' she says. I love the melody in her words.

'Thank you, Safi,' I say, and I walk down the stairs to join the others, feeling very beautiful today.

A crowd of dishevelled students pass us as we cross the hall, talking about 'Our sculpture department is better equipped! And aren't the studios dark', and Rob and Cecile look at each other and say, 'Royal College'.

We meet Bianca in the doorway. She is talking to Giacomo and Cesar, and everyone is getting a bit drunk.

'There's going to be music outside!' says Bianca, looking excited and flushed. 'I want to dance with you!' she says, putting her arms round Giacomo, who lifts her off her feet.

We walk through the studios; past sculptures made of glass and mirrors, carved wood and plaster figures, and metal geometry in three dimensions, through Suzanne's space, past the wobbly sculpture on a plinth, and Suzanne in a rubber dress talking to two men in sunglasses, and out into the sculpture yard.

In the back of the shed I see Zeb in a red shirt, busy with some boxes. Cecile looks at me, smiling, and I wish that she wouldn't.

We watch a piece of performance art involving a large rusty metal wheel, and two people make gestures that are sometimes in synchrony and sometimes not, but none of us can work out what it signifies. Everyone claps, except Rob, who says, 'Performance Fart!' in a loud voice.

Then someone tinkles a glass and Paul gives a speech about the third-years and Zeb punctuates it with fireworks with pink tails and unexpected colourful explosions in the dark shed, which make everyone laugh with surprise.

Afterwards I watch him as he moves around the shed with a bucket, kneeling down to collect the spent fireworks. He must feel my eyes on him, because he looks up and smiles.

People begin to disperse or linger and someone turns on the twinkling lights that are threaded round the yard, and music starts playing through the speakers that are hidden in the piles of wood and bags of plaster.

Cecile says, 'There's my husband!' and goes to join a man with grey hair who greets her with kind blue eyes.

People begin to dance where they are standing, and I don't know if it's the dimming light, but the air feels charged and vibrant, as though something secret is happening under the music; and the sculpture yard slowly changes its atmosphere and becomes intimate.

I look above me and the sky has turned violet.

When I look down I see Silvia leaning against the wall, talking to Zeb.

Her feather boa is flung around her naked shoulders and her hand slowly strokes her other arm. She blinks slowly at him and smiles with her mouth open.

I look down. I look away. Everyone around me is talking and the music confuses me. I walk through the people into a dark corner. What if he likes her more than me? I stand there, breathing. They're just talking, I say to myself. For heaven's sake, Evie! and just as I turn round I feel the warmth of him, and he is holding both my hands.

'Hello,' he says, drawing me towards him and away from the dark corner. 'I've been wanting to talk to you all evening,' he says.

'Hello,' I say, looking up at him.

His face is in shadow but I can see the light in his eyes.

'Shall we dance, d'you think?' he says.

'Yes,' I say, 'I feel like dancing.'

'So do I.'

I put my arms round him and it's like holding a tree that sways in the wind.

Stevie Wonder is singing sadly about an empty well.

'Come on now, Stevie, cheer up!' says Zeb, smiling down at me.

But Stevie goes on to shattered dreams and we start laughing at how miserable the words are. I feel his body trembling with laughing next to mine, and he holds me just a bit closer.

'Now it's worthless years!' I say, looking up at him. He shrugs and looks down at me and that's when it happens. Something slides down between us and collapses; a wall that has kept us apart. It crumbles, and suddenly we are in the same world. It is glowing. It must be one of Zeb's dimensions that you slip into, and he looks at me with naked eyes, that say, 'Here I am, this is me,' and the look is so beautiful I cannot look away. Then my cheek is touching his cheek and my arms are circling his neck and I feel his breath by my ear. He holds me close to him so we are almost one person, and a river of light slips through us. Then his lips are on mine and we are kissing, and Stevie is singing, 'it will be for ever,' and circles of coloured light are exploding behind my eyes, because the world is being born.

ACKNOWLEDGEMENTS

With special thanks to Marigold Farmer, for helping me to finish this book, and to Richard Farmer, both for their kind hospitality.

Many thanks to Alexandra Pringle, as always, for her amazing ability to see the final book in the first chaotic draft.

Thanks also to my agent Victoria Hobbs, and my editor Victoria Millar, to Barbara Turner, Katy Noura Butler, Oonagh Harpur, Angel Green, Erica Jarnes, Audrey Cotterell, and everyone at Bloomsbury.

Many thanks to Buz de Villiers for helping me through the book's darkness.

Thank you to the Hawthornden Foundation, the Royal Literary Fund, the Author's Foundation, DW Gibson and Ledig House USA, and Arts Council England.

And thank you to Peter Ackroyd for his two wonderful books, *London – A Biography* and *Thames – Sacred River*, both of which feature in this book.

A NOTE ON THE TYPE

The text of this book is set in Berling roman, a modern face designed by K. E. Forsberg between 1951 and 1958. In spite of its youth it does carry the characteristics of an old face. The serifs are inclined and blunt, and the g has a straight ear.

GHOST GIRL

It's the 1970s, and whilst London is taken over by punk rock, thirteen-year-old Cath is sent to a Catholic convent. She is afraid of the nuns, unused to the restriction and terrified of God. However, her elder sister Very is at art school in London and when Cath escapes the convent for a visit, she enters Very's wild, chaotic world filled with bedraggled artists, outrageous homosexuals and shadowy nightclub owners. The two sisters whirl through the city, along Chelsea Embankment, through the alleys of late-night Soho. Cath persuades Very to call the convent and say that she is sick, giving her fears another few days respite. But London, too, holds its dangers, and Cath must find her own way through.

'This exciting, highly-visual writer chooses the first burst of sexual love and lust as her subject . . . Unforgettable'
Sunday Express

'Compellingly written, this is a sensitive depiction of the trials and tribulations of growing up'
Time Out

'Frequently moving and as haunting as its title suggests'
Mail on Sunday

BLOOMSBURY